The Mayo Clinic
Cardiac Catheterization Laboratory

David R. Holmes Jr. • Robert L. Frye
Paul A. Friedman • Donald J. Hagler
Thomas M. Munger • Erik L. Ritman
Editors

The Mayo Clinic Cardiac Catheterization Laboratory

History, Research, and Innovations

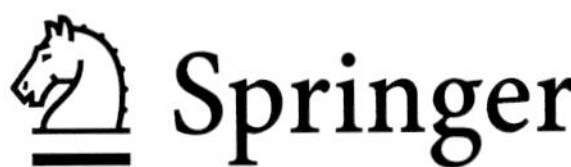

Springer

Editors
David R. Holmes Jr. (ID)
Department of Cardiovascular Diseases
Mayo Clinic
Rochester, MN
USA

Robert L. Frye
Department of Cardiovascular Diseases
Mayo Clinic
Rochester, MN
USA

Paul A. Friedman
Department of Cardiovascular Diseases
Mayo Clinic
Rochester, MN
USA

Donald J. Hagler
Department of Cardiovascular Diseases
Mayo Clinic
Rochester, MN
USA

Thomas M. Munger
Department of Cardiovascular Diseases
Mayo Clinic
Rochester, MN
USA

Erik L. Ritman
Department of Cardiovascular Diseases
Mayo Clinic
Rochester, MN
USA

ISBN 978-3-030-79331-9   ISBN 978-3-030-79329-6   (eBook)
https://doi.org/10.1007/978-3-030-79329-6

This Springer imprint is published by the registered company Springer Nature Switzerland AG
The registered company address is: Gewerbestrasse 11, 6330 Cham, Switzerland

Authored Books

By Author

Robert L. Frye, MD

- **Cardiovascular Disease**
- *Clinical Medicine Volume 6, Hagerstown: Harper & Row, 1981*

W. Bruce Fye, MD

- **Caring for the Heart**
- *Oxford University Press, 2015*

Donald J. Hagler, MD

- **Two-dimensional Echocardiographic Atlas. Volume 1 Congenital Heart Disease**
  - James B. Seward, MD
  - A. Jamil Tajik, MD
  - William D. Edwards, MD
  - Donald J. Hagler, MD
- *New York: Springer-Verlag, 1987*

- **Visual Guide to Neonatal Cardiology**
  - Ernerio T. Alboliras, MD
  - Cecilio Lopez, MD
  - Donald J. Hagler, MD
  - Ziyad Hijazi, MD
- *New York: John Wiley & Sons, 2018*

Stephen C. Hammill, MD

- **ECG Board Review and Study Guide**
  - James H. O'Keefe Jr, MD
  - Stephen C. Hammill, MD
  - Mark Z. Zolnick, MD
  - David M. Steinhaus, MD
  - Pierce J. Vatterott, MD
- *Amonk NY: Future Publishing Inc, 1994*

- **The Complete Guide to ECGs**
  - James H. O'Keefe Jr, MD
  - Stephen C. Hammill, MD
  - Mark S. Freed, MD
- *Birmingham: Physician's Press, 1997*

- **The ECG Criteria and ACLS Handbook**
  - James H. O'Keefe Jr, MD
  - Stephen C. Hammill, MD
  - Mark S. Freed, MD
  - Steven M. Pogwizd, MD
- *Birmingham: Physician's Press, 1998*

- **CPT Coding Guide for Electrophysiology and Pacing Procedures 1999-2000**
  - Stephen C. Hammill, MD
- *North American Society of Pacing and Electrophysiology, Washington DC, 1999*

- **CPT Coding Guide for Electrophysiology and Pacing Procedures 2000-2001**
  - Stephen C. Hammill, MD
- *North American Society of Pacing and Electrophysiology, Washington DC, 2000*

- **The Complete Guide to ECGs, Second Edition**
  - James H. O'Keefe Jr, MD
  - Stephen C. Hammill, MD
  - Mark S. Freed, MD
  - Steven M. Pogwizd, MD
- *Royal Oak: Physicians' Press, 2002*

- **The ECG Criteria Book**
  - James H. O'Keefe Jr, MD
  - Stephen C. Hammill, MD
  - Mark S. Freed, MD
  - Steven M. Pogwizd, MD
- *Royal Oak: Physicians' Press, 2002*

- **Cardiac Repolarization: Bridging Basic and Clinical Science**
  - Ihor Gussak, MD
  - Charles Antzelevitch, MD
  - Stephen C. Hammill, MD
  - Win K. Shen, MD
  - Preben Bjerregaard
- *Totowa: Humana Press, 2003*

- **The Complete Guide to ECGs, Third Edition**
  - James H. O'Keefe Jr, MD
  - Stephen C. Hammill, MD
  - Mark S. Freed, MD
  - Steven M. Pogwizd, MD
- *Sudbury: Physicians' Press, 2010*

- **The ECG Criteria Book, Second Edition**
  - James H. O'Keefe Jr, MD
  - Stephen C. Hammill, MD
  - Mark S. Freed, MD
  - Steven M. Pogwizd, MD
- *Sudbury: Physicians' Press, 2010*

- **The Complete Guide to ECGs, Fourth Edition**
  - James H. O'Keefe Jr, MD
  - Stephen C. Hammill, MD
  - Mark S. Freed, MD
- *Jones & Bartlett (Burlington MA), 2016*

- **The Complete Guide to ECGs, Fifth Edition**
  - James H. O'Keefe Jr, MD
  - Stephen C. Hammill, MD
  - Mark S. Freed, MD
- *Jones & Bartlett (Burlington MA), 2021*

David R. Holmes Jr., MD

- **A Practice of Cardiac Pacing**
  - Seymour Furman, MD
  - David L. Hayes, MD
  - David R. Holmes Jr., MD
- *Mount Kisco, New York: 1986*

- **PTCA: Percutaneous Transluminal Coronary Angioplasty**
  - Ronald E. Vlietstra, MD
  - David R. Holmes Jr., MD
- *F.A. Davis Co. Philadelphia, 1987 Mayo Foundation*

- **A Practice of Cardiac Pacing**
  - Seymour Furman, MD
  - David L. Hayes, MD
  - David R. Holmes Jr., MD
- *Mount Kisco, New York: 1989*

- **Interventional Cardiology**
  - David R. Holmes Jr., MD
  - Ronald E. Vlietstra, MD
- *Philadelphia: F.A. Davis Co, 1989*

- **Atherectomy**
  - David R. Holmes Jr., MD
  - Kirk N. Garratt, MD
- *Blackwell Scientific Publications, 1992*

- **A Practice of Cardiac Pacing, Third Edition**
  - Seymour Furman, MD
  - David L. Hayes, MD
  - David R. Holmes Jr., MD
- *New York: Futura Publishing Co Inc., 1993*

- **Coronary Balloon Angioplasty**
  - Ronald E. Vlietstra, MD
  - David R. Holmes Jr., MD
- *Boston: Blackwell Scientific Publications, 1994*

- **Strategic Approaches in Coronary Intervention**
  - Stephen G. Ellis, MD
  - David R. Holmes Jr., MD
- *Baltimore: Williams & Wilkins, 1996*

- **Current Review of International Cardiology, Third Edition**
  - David R. Holmes Jr., MD
  - Patrick W. Serruys, MD
- *Philadelphia: Churchill Livingstone, 1997*

- **Saphenous Vein Bypass Graft Disease**
  – Eric R. Bates, MD
  – David R. Holmes Jr., MD
- *New York: Marcel Dekker Inc, 1998*

- **Strategic Approaches in Coronary Intervention, Second Edition**
  – Stephen G. Ellis, MD
  – David R. Holmes Jr., MD
- *Philadelphia: Lippincott Williams & Wilkins, 2000*

- **Cardiogenic Shock: Diagnosis and Treatment**
  – David Hasdai, MD
  – Peter B. Berger, MD
  – Alexander Battler, MD
  – David R. Holmes Jr., MD
- *Humana Press, 2002*

- **Atlas of Interventional Cardiology, Second Edition**
  – David R. Holmes Jr., MD
  – Verghese Mathew, MD
- *Philadelphia: Current Medicine, 2003*

- **Strategic Approaches in Coronary Intervention, Third Edition**
  – Stephen G. Ellis, MD
  – David R. Holmes Jr., MD
- *Philadelphia: Lippincott Williams & Wilkins, 2006*

- **Coronary Artery Disease: New Approaches Without Traditional Revascularization**
  – Gregory W. Barsness, MD
  – David R. Holmes Jr., MD
- *London: Springer-Verlag, 2012*

Erik L. Ritman, MD

- **Imaging Physiological Functions: Experience With the Dynamic Spatial Reconstructor**
  – Erik L. Ritman, MD
  – R. A. Robb, MD
- New York: Praeger, 1985

Hartzell V. Schaff, MD

- **Vasoactive Factors Produced by the Endothelium: Physiology and Surgical Implications**
  - Hartzell V. Schaff, MD
  - John F. Seccombe, MD
- *Austin: R G Landes Co, 1994*

- **Mayo Clinic Practice of Cardiology**
  - Bernard J. Gersh, MD
  - Michael D. McGoon, MD
  - David L. Hayes, MD
  - Hartzell V. Schaff, MD
  - Emilio R. Giuliani, MD
- *St. Louis: Mosby Inc, 1996*

- **Redo Cardiac Surgery in Adults**
  - Venkat R. Machiraju, MD
  - Hartzel V. Schaff, MD
  - Lars G. Svennson, MD
- *New York: Springer, 2012*

Ronald E. Vlietstra, MD

- **PTCA: Percutaneous Transluminal Coronary Angioplasty**
  - Ronald E. Vlietstra, MD
  - David R. Holmes Jr., MD
- *Philadelphia: F.A. Davis Co, 1987*

- **Interventional Cardiology**
  - David R. Holmes Jr., MD
  - Ronald E. Vlietstra, MD
- *Philadelphia: F.A. Davis Co, 1989*

- **Concise Cardiology**
  - Martin Kaltenbach, MD
  - Ronald E. Vlietstra, MD
- *Steinkopff Verlag Darmstadt, 1991*

- **Coronary Balloon Angioplasty**
  - Ronald E. Vlietstra, MD
  - David R. Holmes Jr., MD
- *Boston: Blackwell Scientific Publications, 1994*

Earl H. Wood, MD

- **An Atlas of Congenital Anomalies of the Heart and Great Vessels**
  - J. E. Edwards, MD
  - T. J. Dry, MD
  - R. L. Parker, MD
  - H. B. Burchell, MD
  - E. H. Wood, MD
  - A. H. Bulbulian
- *Springfield IL, Thomas, 1954*

- **Evolution of Anti-G Suits: Their Limitations, and Alternative Methods for Avoidance of C-Induced Loss of Consciousness**
  - EH Wood, MD
- *Mayo Foundation, 1990*

Preface

We decided to write a history of the Mayo Clinic Cardiac Catheterization Laboratory because it is a fascinating topic and many younger colleagues have asked about its origins. To tell the story, we chose to first focus on origins of the lab and explore the fascinating contributions of Dr. Earl Wood, who set the stage in developing technology to monitor human circulation while studying G forces to protect dive bomber pilots during World War II.

We then approached past and current participants in the cardiac cath lab to share their perspective on how the laboratory developed in specific areas of interest such as congenital heart disease, the introduction of coronary angiography with videometry and videodensitometry, hemodynamics, physiologic studies of coronary reactivity, valvular heart disease, coronary and valvular intervention, and heart failure. Electrophysiology, which also has been a part of the cardiac cath lab from the earliest days, is also a topic of great interest and represents a large component of the current activity in the lab. We also devote several chapters to specific time periods to give a perspective of how the practice evolved. Thus, this is not a single narrative in strict chronological order.

This has been a humbling endeavor as one reflects on how it all began and the extraordinary advances in knowledge and interventions to enhance care of patients with cardiovascular disease. The historic record given in the following chapters provides confirmation of one of Dr. William J. Mayo's famous quotes: "The glory of medicine is that it is constantly moving forward, that there is always more to learn." We have focused on contributions and events at Mayo Clinic but wish to acknowledge the contributions of many institutions and individuals to the progress we all share as a profession in providing care for our patients with cardiovascular disease.

One might question how all of these activities were supported, which is also a part of the historic record. Until the late 1950s, Mayo Clinic did not accept outside funds but relied on funds from the practice to support education and research. But the world changes. Donations and competing for funds are both now essential to support research and education responsibilities. We thus wish to recognize the donor who provided funds to endow the Mayo Clinic Cardiac Catheterization Laboratory as the Dr. Earl Wood Cardiac Catheterization Laboratory.

We have been supported and learned much from the people who helped put this all together. Many thanks to all the contributors, and we also wish to recognize Linda Lee Stelley and the staff of Scientific Publications, without whom this would not have actually happened.

Rochester, MN, USA   David R. Holmes Jr.
Rochester, MN, USA   Robert L. Frye

Acknowledgments

Histories are always built on a foundation of multiple layers beginning from the ground floor, and the concepts and the ideals which constitute that ground floor, and, as importantly, the people who put into place the things that become the underpinnings of the history, the foundation for the future. The ground floors of this Mayo Clinic Cardiac Catherization Laboratory History are based on the ideals of Mayo Clinic wherein projects are developed, then designed to address the clinical needs and questions of the people who we are privileged to serve.

In addition to the patient components who formed the basis for all of this, the "people components" were Mayo Clinic employees, as a rule, from all walks of life, many from this area of the country, some of who had been born and raised here, and they, in aggregate, formed the base upon which this history was fashioned. Most importantly, the people who came to be treated, the technical people, the infrastructure people, the technicians, the patient care advocates, the nursing staff, the research associates (often from around the world), the fellows, all of the other professional staff, the administrators, the inventors, all of whom are too numerous to name individually. To all of these individuals and groups, we owe a debt of gratitude because without them and from where they had come, this history, would never have been made, would never have been fashioned and grown now to be celebrated in this book of our collaborative history. To all of these unstoried but essential people, we owe our incredible debt of gratitude to them as we tell their and, now, our story.

Contents

Contributors

Mohamad Alkhouli Department of Cardiovascular Diseases, Mayo Clinic, Rochester, MN, USA

Samuel J. Asirvatham Department of Cardiovascular Diseases, Mayo Clinic, Rochester, MN, USA

Malcolm Bell Department of Cardiovascular Diseases, Mayo Clinic, Rochester, MN, USA

Barry A. Borlaug The Department of Cardiovascular Medicine, Mayo Clinic, Rochester, MN, USA

Yong-Mei Cha Department of Cardiovascular Diseases, Mayo Clinic, Rochester, MN, USA

Michel T. Corban Department of Cardiovascular Diseases, Mayo Clinic, Rochester, MN, USA

Paul A. Friedman Department of Cardiovascular Diseases, Mayo Clinic, Rochester, MN, USA

Robert L. Frye Department of Cardiovascular Diseases, Mayo Clinic, Rochester, MN, USA

Donald J. Hagler Professor Emeritus, Department of Cardiovascular Diseases, Mayo Clinic, Rochester, MN, USA

Stephen C. Hammill Department of Cardiovascular Diseases (retired), Mayo Clinic, Rochester, MN, USA

David R. Holmes Jr. Department of Cardiovascular Diseases, Mayo Clinic, Rochester, MN, USA

Paul R. Julsrud Department of Radiology, Mayo Clinic, Rochester, MN, USA

Suraj Kapa Department of Cardiovascular Diseases, Mayo Clinic, Rochester, MN, USA

Hon-Chi Lee Department of Cardiovascular Diseases, Mayo Clinic, Rochester, MN, USA

Amir Lerman Department of Cardiovascular Diseases, Mayo Clinic, Rochester, MN, USA

William R. Miranda Department of Cardiovascular Disease, Mayo Clinic, Rochester, MN, USA

Thomas M. Munger Department of Cardiovascular Diseases, Mayo Clinic, Rochester, MN, USA

Rick A. Nishimura Department of Cardiovascular Disease, Mayo Clinic, Rochester, MN, USA

Peter A. Noseworthy Department of Cardiovascular Diseases, Mayo Clinic, Rochester, MN, USA

Douglas L. Packer Department of Cardiovascular Diseases, Mayo Clinic, Rochester, MN, USA

Guy S. Reeder Department of Cardiovascular Disease, Mayo Clinic, Rochester, MN, USA

Charanjit S. Rihal Department of Cardiovascular Diseases, Mayo Clinic, Rochester, MN, USA

Erik L. Ritman Department of Cardiovascular Diseases, Mayo Clinic (retired), Rochester, MN, USA

Gurpreet S. Sandhu Department of Cardiovascular Diseases, Mayo Clinic, Rochester, MN, USA

Hartzell V. Schaff, MD Department of Cardiovascular Surgery, Mayo Clinic, Rochester, MN, USA

Win-Kuang Shen Department of Cardiovascular Diseases, Mayo Clinic, Phoenix, AZ, USA

Trevor J. Simard Mayo Clinic Scholar, Rochester, MN, USA

Hugh C. Smith Emeritus member, Department of Cardiovascular Diseases, Mayo Clinic, Rochester, MN, USA

Umberto Squarcia University of Parma, Parma, Italy

Ronald E. Vlietstra Former Member, Department of Cardiovascular Diseases, Mayo Clinic, Rochester, MN, USA

Watson Clinic (retired), Lakeland, FL, USA

Chapter 1
1950–1970s: Where We Came From

Erik L. Ritman, David R. Holmes Jr., and Robert L. Frye

The precursor Mayo Clinic Cardiac Catheterization Laboratory opened in 1951 on the first floor of the Medical Sciences building (Fig. 1.1). The initial conference room (Medical Sciences 2-154) was of particular importance, as it was surrounded by the offices of a unique collection of multidisciplinary physiology talent, which included the early pioneers Drs. Earl Wood, Charles Code, Ed Lambert, John Shepherd, David Donald, James Bassingthwaighte, Reg Bickford, and Ward Fowler as well as clinicians and engineers (Section of Engineering located in the same building) among others. It was this close geographic association on an everyday basis that contributed importantly to the success of the early cardiac cath lab. Beyond this rectangular arrangement of offices around the conference room 2-154, on the rest of the Medical Sciences floor was the office of Dr. Jesse Edwards, the world's iconic and most experienced cardiac pathologist, with an extensive collection of anatomic material that formed the basis of formulating strategies of care both for diagnostic imaging in the cath lab and for surgical planning. These multiple disciplines were available for formal and informal discussions and speculations from which came a steady stream of new approaches, new technology, and new scientific insights. This unique environment was the think tank of the future.

The initial grounding for the development of the tools needed for a modern-day cath lab resulted from Earl Wood's work after he was hired in 1942 to use the Mayo Clinic human centrifuge to investigate and establish the cause of acceleration-induced loss of consciousness (G-LOC) and then develop a strategy to mitigate it (Fig. 1.2). This resulted in the G-suit (Fig. 1.3a, b), which had a dramatic safety

E. L. Ritman (✉)
Department of Cardiovascular Diseases, Mayo Clinic (retired), Rochester, MN, USA
e-mail: Erikritman2@charter.net

D. R. Holmes Jr. · R. L. Frye
Department of Cardiovascular Diseases, Mayo Clinic, Rochester, MN, USA
e-mail: Holmes.david@mayo.edu; rfrye@mayo.edu

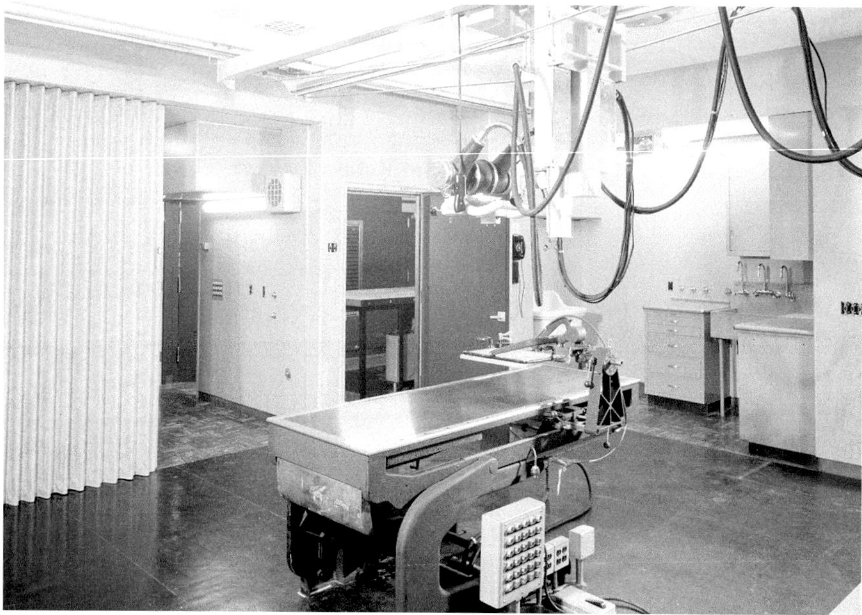

Fig. 1.1 The catheterization laboratory included a single plane angiographic system, with multiple input and output circuits seen under the base of the table used for recording and analysis and data accumulated during extensive physiologic studies. (Used with permission of Mayo Foundation)

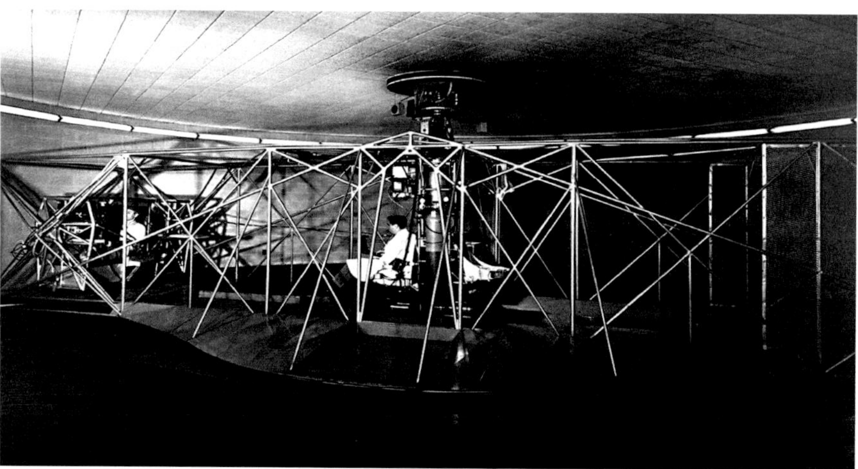

Fig. 1.2 An early focus of Wood's career involved the construction and implementation of a human centrifuge designed to investigate the cause of acceleration-induced loss of consciousness and resulted in the development of the G-suit. In this picture, Wood serves as the monitor for the experiment and the "volunteer" is seen on the left. (Used with permission of Mayo Foundation)

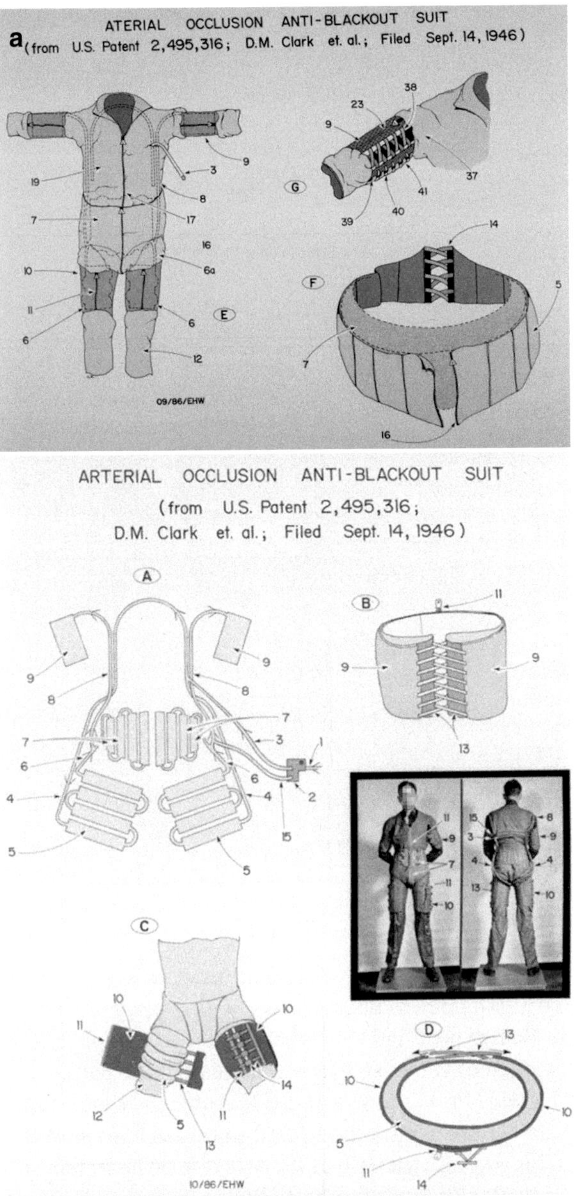

Fig. 1.3 (**a**) Patent application (2,495,316) filed on September 14, 1946, which resulted in the development of the G-suit with inflatable bladders on the calves, thighs, and abdomen. As the g-forces increased, bladder inflation resulted in peripheral arterial compression so that blood pressure increased sufficiently to maintain blood flow to the brain. (**b**) Physiology staff Ralph Sturm in G-suit. (Used with permission of Mayo Foundation)

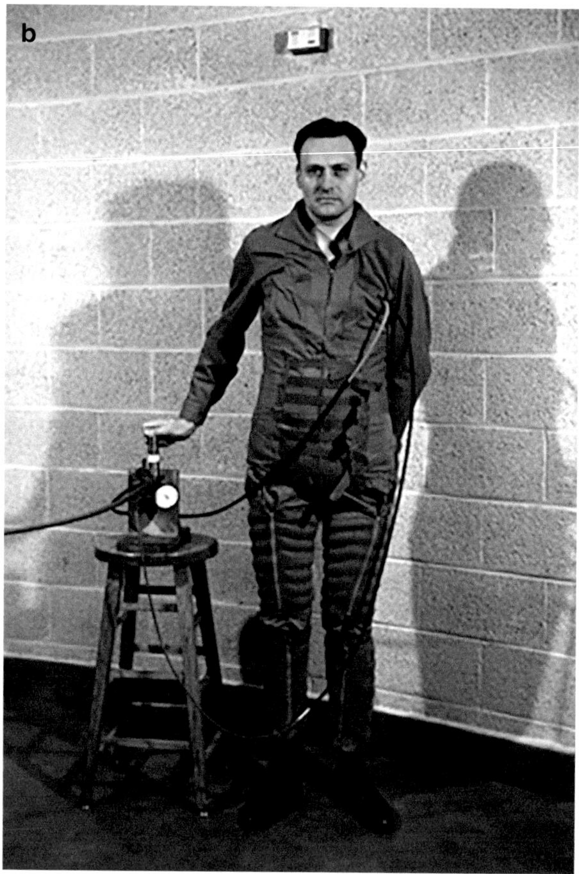

Fig. 1.3 (continued)

benefit for pilots. The basis of this work and his incredible scientific and intellectual heritage has been highlighted in the most recent biography of Earl Wood by Ritman [1]. Elements in that project had immediate and direct implications for the entire field of cardiac catheterization. Two novel instruments of particularly early importance were developed. Pressure-measuring transducers were fabricated (Fig. 1.4) and made suitable for use with a fluid-filled intravascular catheter [2]. They were used to measure blood pressure (BP) at the level of the heart and simultaneously at head level by holding one catheterized radial artery in the wrist at heart level and the other wrist held at head level, respectively [3]. The other instrument that was developed was an earpiece device that measured the blood content of tissue by using infrared transmission (Fig. 1.5) [4]. Both were incorporated rapidly for investigational studies and then applied widely in clinical practice.

Other elements in the field facilitated the application of open-heart surgery, which was made possible by the development of the heart-lung bypass machine, as well as antibiotics. Unfortunately, the early success rate was very poor, in large

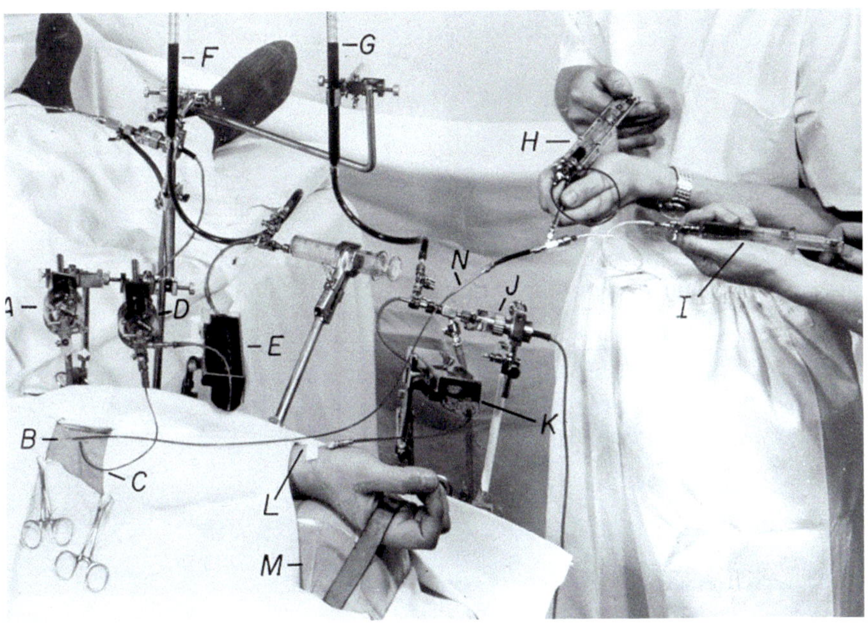

Fig. 1.4 Pressure transducers, blood oxygen content, and indocyanine dilution measurements were an integral part of physiologic experiments and procedures. They allowed measurement in a variety of clinical settings such as supine bicycling and measuring simultaneous pressures in different vascular beds. (Used with permission of Mayo Foundation)

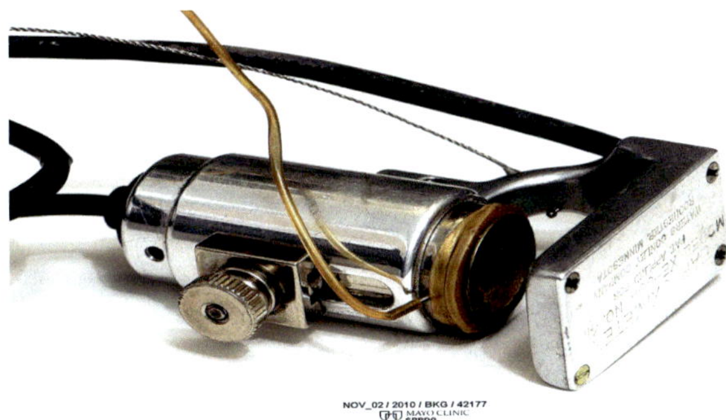

Fig. 1.5 The development of an earpiece oximeter in Dr. Earl Wood's laboratory at Mayo Clinic used light source and plunger in fully retracted position, with air tube to support inflation of rubber membrane against the pinna. This allowed rapid measurement of the blood content of tissue. The sensor could also provide a signal proportional to the oxygen saturation. (Used with permission of Mayo Foundation)

measure, because of inaccurate diagnosis of the anatomic problem [5]. Subsequent to the initial experiences and addressing lessons learned from Dr. John Gibbon working in Philadelphia, work continued at Mayo Clinic's Department of Physiology

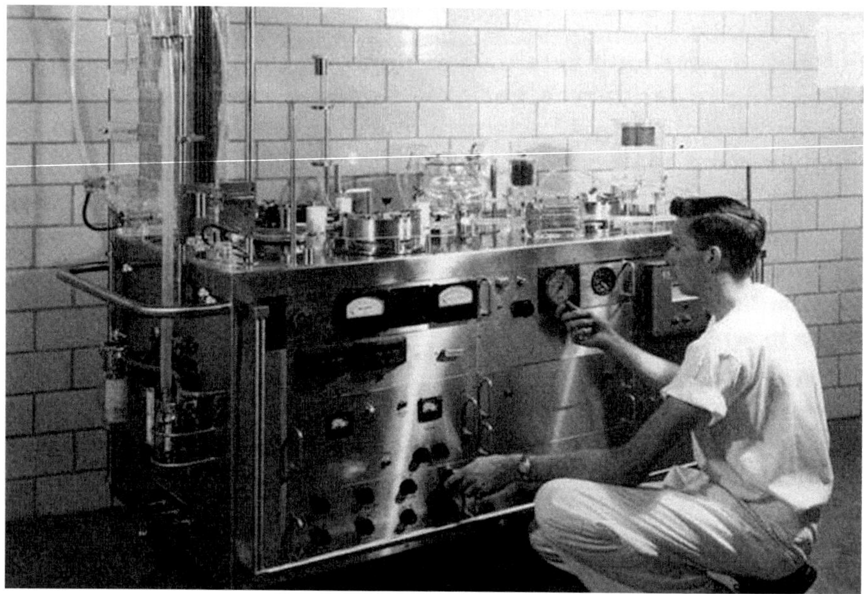

Fig. 1.6 The initial Mayo-Gibbon heart-lung machine developed by Mayo Clinic in combination with Dr. John Gibbon was used in experimental procedures and then, in 1955, was used in an operation to close a large ventricular septal defect. (Used with permission of Mayo Foundation)

and the Section of Engineering and resulted in the Mayo-Gibbon heart-lung machine (Fig. 1.6), which was first used on March 22, 1955, by Kirklin in a 5-year-old girl with a large ventricular septal defect. In other patients with congenital heart disease and right-to-left shunts, there was mixing of non-oxygenated blood with oxygenated blood; the oxygen content of blood was therefore decreased, resulting in the clinical condition of "blue" babies [6].

Optimizing patient selection criteria and outcome was, in large part, dependent on the instruments Wood and his team developed for monitoring cardiovascular parameters for use during physiologic studies with the centrifuge and then applied in the clinical arena to increase diagnostic accuracy. Of special note is the incidental observation that the earpiece device (Fig. 1.5) for monitoring tissue blood content showed a change in signal due to the passage of a bolus of intravascular saline injected to flush the needle in the radial artery. This formed the basis for utilizing the shape and time distribution of indicator dilution curves to demonstrate the presence of intracardiac anatomic short circuit shunts.

Indicator dilution curve studies played a central role. However, a saline injection resulted in a small signal, so a dye was used to enhance the signal. For this, the indicator dye is injected into the arterial vascular bed or chamber under study. After rapidly injecting a known quality of the dye, there is mixing with flowing blood. After injection, the blood is then withdrawn at a constant speed downstream from the injection site through a device calibrated to detect the dye concentration. Flow can be calculated by the formula of the amount of dye injected, the mean

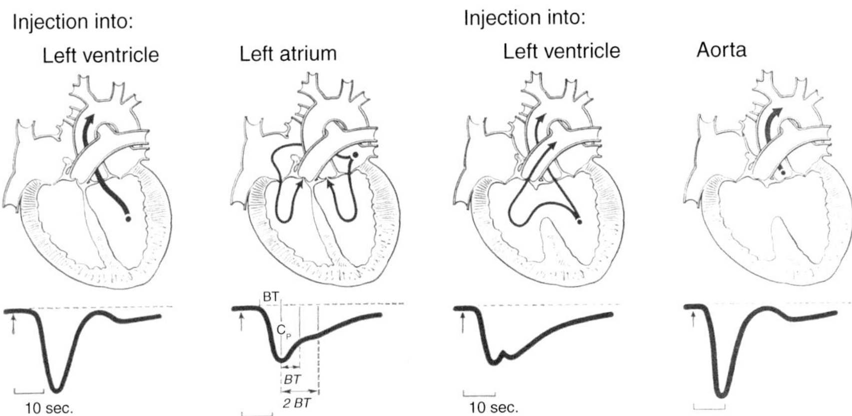

Fig. 1.7 Application of indicator dilution techniques in congenital heart disease. With injection into the left ventricle and sampling downstream, cardiac flow can be measured. An important component is complete mixing of the indicator, in this case in the left ventricle. The shape of the indicator dilution curve could provide information about intracardiac anatomic defects, as illustrated in this cartoon. (From Wood [7]; used with permission)

concentration of the dye, and the time of the concentration curve to the downstream detector, so as to provide the quantitative data needed to solve the Henriques-Hamilton principle [6] and determine flow. This method can be used for calculations of cardiac output as well as detection of intracardiac shunts in which there is recirculation of the dye (Fig. 1.7).

At that time, Evans blue dye was commonly used as the indicator for generating the dye curve rather than saline, as it generated a much more obvious dilution curve than did saline. The problem though was that in congenital heart disease, the blood is often poorly oxygenated (blue babies), and hence even the Evans blue curve would have reduced specificity and accuracy.

The focus of early studies evaluated the physiology of cardiac flow and function initially in experimental models and then in volunteers (Fig. 1.8) who were typically "recruited" Mayo Clinic fellows and graduate students interested in the field. Many of these fellows and students subsequently became leading Mayo Clinic staff physicians in cardiology, cardiac surgery, pulmonology, and physiology, while others moved to prestigious medical institutions throughout the world. Given their recruitment for multiple studies during training, it has been said that early cardiologists trained by Earl Wood often had absent radial pulses related to the frequent use of this artery for monitoring blood pressure during studies (a precursor of the now dominant use of percutaneous radial approaches for cardiac catheterization). As previously mentioned, studies involved the validation of an indicator dilution technique to evaluate flow patterns using Evans blue as the indicator for the measurement of flow and to evaluate recirculation patterns for detection of intracardiac shunts [8–10]. This indicator was subsequently discontinued, as it resulted in

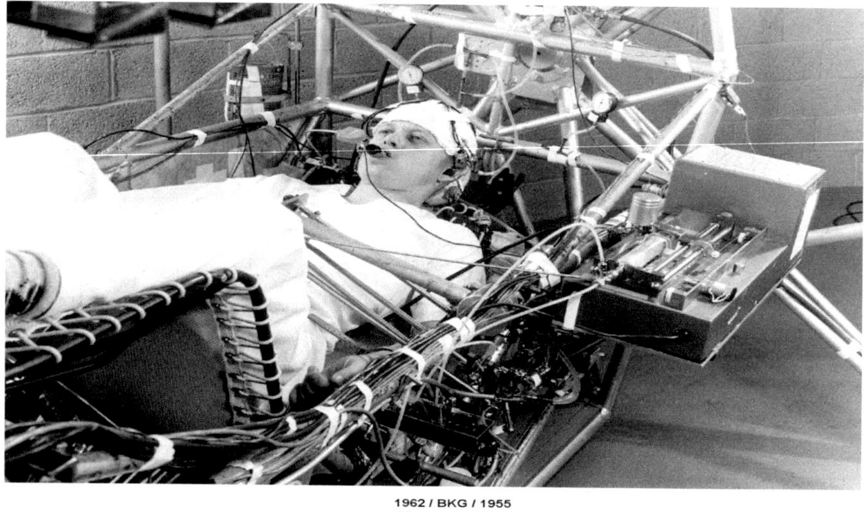

Fig. 1.8 Cockpit of Mayo Clinic centrifuge, depicting "Project Mercury" experimental astronaut "couch," human volunteer wearing earpiece oximeter on the right ear, and powered injection syringe for indicator dilution studies of cardiac function. (Used with permission of Mayo Foundation)

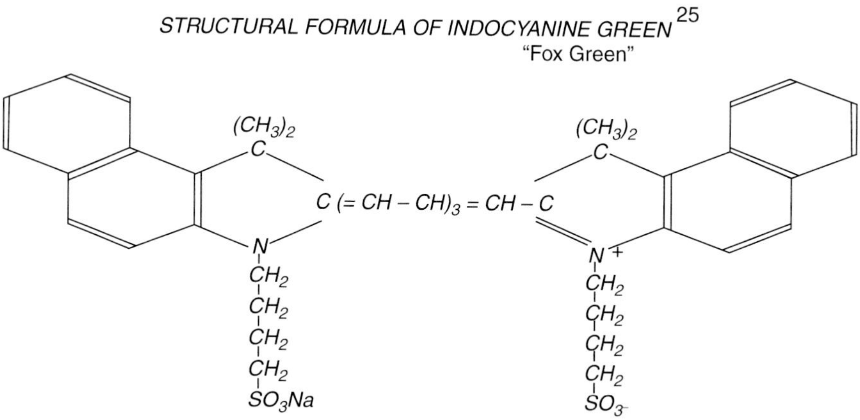

STRUCTURAL FORMULA OF INDOCYANINE GREEN [25]

"Fox Green"

$$C\,(=CH-CH)_3=CH-C$$

$(CH_3)_2$ $(CH_3)_2$

Fig. 1.9 Chemical structure of indocyanine green which became standard for catheterization indicator dilution studies. Its advantage was that its signal was not affected by the oxygen content of the blood

transient bluish coloration of the lips of the volunteers who were then easily identifiable by others as fellows in training.

Subsequent to the use of Evans blue, in 1957, indocyanine green dye (Fig. 1.9) developed by I.J. Fox, then a fellow, working in Earl Wood's laboratory [11, 12], became the standard. This dye subsequently became the worldwide standard for indicator dilution studies and forms the basis for indicator dilution approaches for assessment of cardiac function. Subsequent indicators have been incorporated in pulmonary arterial catheters (aka Swan-Ganz catheters [10]) using temperature as the indicator or use of microbubbles in ultrasound imaging [11].

During this early time, clinical efforts were focused mainly on two groups of patients – those with congenital heart disease, both children and adolescents who were often cyanotic and patients with rheumatic heart disease, typically rheumatic mitral stenosis. Dramatic advances were being made in the surgical arena focusing, in part, on a Mayo Clinic program for performing open-heart surgery. John Kirklin (cardiovascular surgery) and Earl Wood met with the Mayo Clinic Sciences Committee to discuss the "production and experimental use of a mechanical heart in certain types of cardiac surgery" (p. 208) [13]. The team assembled at this time consisted of a research associate in physiology (Dr. H.J.C. (Jeremy) Swan), the Section of Engineering (Richard Jones), and a veterinary surgeon and physiologist (David Donald). This initiative plus other major collaborating work from pioneers throughout the country led to the field of open cardiac surgery and the initial experience with the Mayo-Gibbon heart-lung machine (Fig. 1.6).

Simultaneously, through this time period, there was the development and introduction of open surgical techniques for the treatment of structural heart disease, including both stenosis and regurgitant lesions of both the aortic and mitral valves, typically the result of rheumatic heart disease.

These advances, taken together, required continued development of techniques to evaluate and diagnose both congenital and valvular heart diseases. Accordingly, the new catheterization laboratory became increasingly busy, focusing predominantly on the application of indicator dilution techniques to accurately diagnose congenital heart disease aimed at evaluating patients for open-heart surgical procedures.

Initial catheterization procedures [2, 4, 14] included direct measurements of intravascular pressure, obtaining blood samples for oxygen content, which were used for assessing cardiac and extra-cardiac shunts and flow and for confirmation using indicator dilution studies. The same catheters used for sampling of blood could also be used to deliver radiographic contrast for the new and evolving field of angiocardiography. Earl Wood helped to co-author a 1953 AHA report [15] on the field, which advised that the use of angiocardiography be limited to established laboratories and institutions to obtain the maximum benefit from the clinical studies. An important impediment to the application and wider use of angiocardiography was image quality. Early studies required that the operators use red-tinted goggles (dark adaptor goggles) prior to the procedure to accommodate their eyes to the dim images generated by the X-ray passing through a flat, fluorescent screen (Fig. 1.10). (One of the authors actually used red-tinted glasses for fluoroscopic studies at a remote rural laboratory in Iowa during his moonlighting days in training.) Subsequent to these early dim experiences, in conjunction with biophysicist Ralph Sturm, the laboratory worked to identify X-ray image intensifiers that not only improved image quality but also decreased radiation [14]. Those development efforts, however, were less fruitful at that time (largely because of the inability to record the fluoroscopic image sequences). This resulted in the effect that emphasis remained focused on indicator dilution approaches for evaluating congenital heart disease patients.

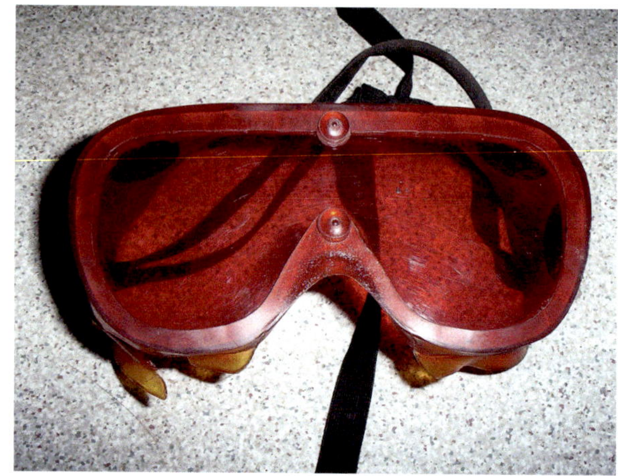

Fig. 1.10 Dark adaptor goggles used to allow operators' eyes to adapt to the low-light features of fluoroscopic procedures. These googles implied that the user was close to the fluorescent screen and therefore exposed to the X-ray passing through the fluorescent screen

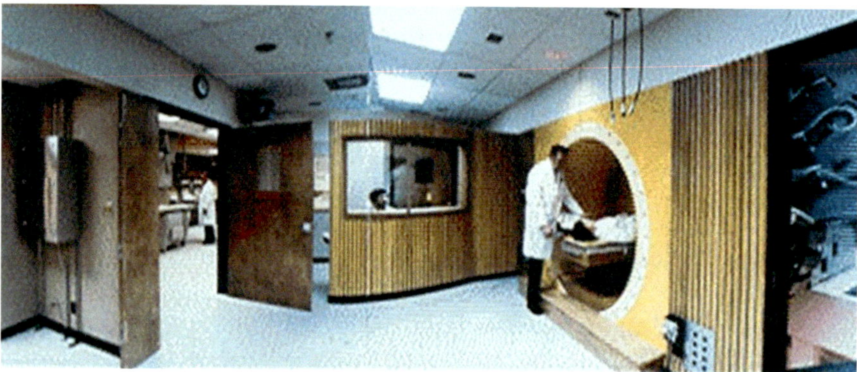

Fig. 1.11 A panoramic view of the DSR facility in the Medical Sciences building, close to the early cath lab. On the *left* (through the open door), the cath lab preparing the subject prior to the scan. To the *right* of the door is the control desk. Further to the *right* is the entry to the DSR scanner. The patient table advances into the scanner. On the far *right*, through an open door, is a partial view of the multi-X-ray source scanner. (From Ritman et al. [16] used with permission)

While the Mayo Clinic cath lab was located at the Medical Sciences building, the large majority of patients were hospitalized almost 1 mile away at St. Mary's Hospital. Concern arose because of the need for transfer back and forth by ambulance with medical assistance, usually physically, by a cardiology fellow in training with oversight by a staff cardiologist involved in the patient care. This same rather inefficient process was to be repeated some 20 years later, when adult and pediatric patients were transferred by ambulance from St. Mary's Hospital for clinical studies performed in the first fully 3D, cardiac CT scanner – the dynamic spatial reconstructor (DSR) (Fig. 1.11) [16]. One of the first clinical patients evaluated in this way is remembered by Dr. Hugh C. Smith, who had worked in Earl Wood's program and then became focused in clinical cardiology and the catheterization laboratory.

The patient had suffered a large anterior myocardial infarction with a resultant left ventricular aneurysm. Clinical considerations revolved on the ability of cardiovascular (CV) surgery with Dr. Hartzell Schaff to resect the aneurysm and whether that operation would be able to be targeted such that enough viable myocardium remained for patient survival. The DSR images obtained facilitated that discussion and the patient care decision that followed.

During the latter 1950s, those concerns about transfer of patients from St. Mary's Hospital to the "downtown" Medical Sciences building became increasingly more relevant because some of the children were very ill and the catheterization studies with multiple indicator dilution injections were very lengthy. After a very long study, moving into an ambulance for transportation back to the hospital and then returning the patient to their hospital room was fatiguing and a source of concern. These issues formed the basis of robust discussions involving multiple stakeholders – physiologists, cardiologists, cardiovascular surgeons, the Mayo Clinic Sciences Committee, and the Board of Governors. Two main topics were identified relating to somewhat different, although closely related, goals of the cath lab.

1. On the one hand, there were clinical catheterization procedures focused on making or substantiating a clinical diagnosis or used in making decisions as to the therapy or prognosis for the disease or for planning a therapeutic procedure for the specific patient under evaluation.
2. On the other hand, there were catheterization studies more focused for investigative (research) and educational purposes along with diagnostic evaluation as part of graduate school training in cardiovascular physiology [17].

In the summer of 1958, after considerable debate, the Mayo Clinic Board of Governors agreed that a new cath lab would be constructed on the grounds of St. Mary's Hospital, focusing more specifically on clinical diagnosis and establishing treatment strategies. However, as part of these considerations, there was an agreement that the facilities at St. Mary's Hospital would be closely associated and aligned with an angiographic (radiology) center, which would include all routine clinical catheterizations. This close association was specifically meant to encourage collaboration between radiologists and cardiologists; however, it had important and long-lasting implications in that radiologists were required to dictate all formal catheterization reports on clinical adult cardiology and pediatric cardiology patients despite the fact that all the procedures were performed by the cardiologists. That "collaborative arrangement" between cardiology and radiology lasted for approximately 15 years, during which time there were often very "frank and open" opinions ventured by cardiology concerning the need for radiology, including George Davis, Owings Kincaid, and Franz Hallerman, among others, to oversee coronary angiographic procedure reports. There were other important issues in the Board of Governors decision that related specifically to catheterization personnel, which also had major implications. A specific recommendation identified that "the best interests of the clinic would not be served in asking members of the Section of Physiology to devote valuable time and effort in the management of diagnostic procedures."

The result of this decision was that the new facility was independent and was formed under the direction and leadership of Swan (p.249) [13], who had been initially a research associate in physiology working under the supervision of Earl Wood. The direction given was that Swan was to confine his research activities to such investigations as "are derived from the clinical work of the laboratory" (p. 249) [13], relinquishing his research interests in other fields of physiology. This former research associate in physiology subsequently became a doyen of clinical cardiology and the President of the American College of Cardiology (1973), among other duties and honors, making fundamental strides and progress in the evaluation and care of patients for the rest of his brilliant career. Throughout that time, Swan influenced generations of physicians and scientists to come. He also continued to blend principles learned in the physiology laboratory under Earl Wood's tutelage, such as indicator dilution techniques with clinical unmet needs, resulting in the development of the ubiquitous "Swan-Ganz" catheter for pulmonary arterial catheterization for measurement of pulmonary flow and pressure in concert with Dr. William (Willie) Ganz in 1970 at the Cedars-Sinai Medical Center of UCLA in Los Angeles [10]. In parallel with that of Swan, Wood's multidisciplinary career as a physiologist continued to flourish and had profound influence on generations of physicians and scientists to come and who became prominent scientists and leaders in their own right. These individuals often maintained close relationships with Earl Wood. Of interest, one prominent biomedical engineer, Peter Osypka, who had trained in a post-doctoral position from 1963–1965 under Earl Wood, became a leading innovator and scientist in Germany. He started his company in the 1970s in Rheinfelden, Germany, after returning home from working in Earl Wood's lab. While in the lab, he developed the first split screen video display of the two biplane, angiographic images, which made Ralph Sturm's videometry feasible [18]. Osypka developed an extensive technological and biomedical engineering facility and large charitable foundation dealing with medical care. His initiatives resulted in a very successful German company, somewhat the equivalent of Medtronics in the United States. In 2002, to honor Earl Wood, Osypka renamed and dedicated the "Earl H Wood Strasse" in Rheinfelden, where the Osypka facility is located (Fig. 1.12). The road was named for Earl Wood as a token of appreciation of Wood giving Osypka his first opportunity to show his capabilities. This is another example of the indirect but significant influence of the cath lab beyond the direct cath lab needs. A notable achievement for Earl Wood was his selection as the tenth scientist who was identified as a "career investigator" of the American Heart Association; he also received the Presidential Certificate of Merit from President Harry Truman in 1947 for his contribution to Operation Paperclip. He would continue and expand his focus on scientific research that would be applied by both clinicians and physiologists in the clinical arena to improve imaging, solve complex physiologic problems, and continue to lead the way for addressing unmet clinical needs in both pediatric and adult patient populations. Both Earl Wood and Swan were the stuff of legends.

- Initially, the cardiac cath lab at St. Mary's Hospital under Swan's leadership remained administratively in the Department of Physiology. Dr. Don Ritter, a

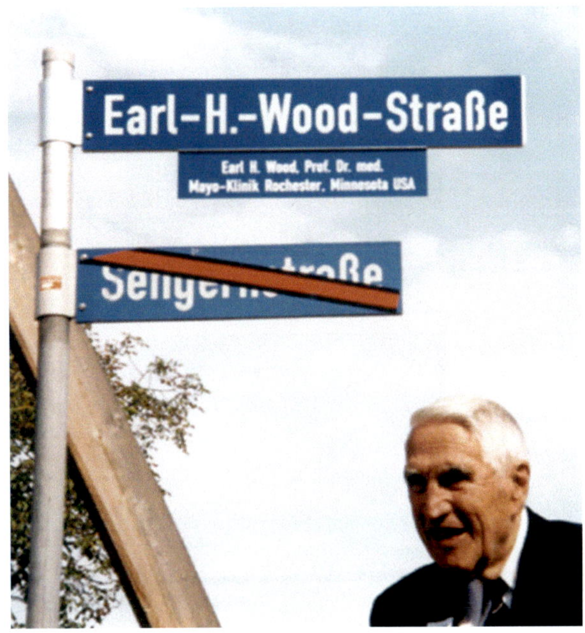

Fig. 1.12 In 2002, the Osypka facility in Rheinfelden, Germany, dedicated a street as "Earl H. Wood Strasse." (Photo courtesy of Dr. Erik L. Ritman)

pediatric cardiologist, was the first clinician to participate at the staff level in the cardiac lab. Many fellows from all over the world came to work with Swan. Gradually it became apparent there should be more involvement of clinical staff in the lab, and Dr. Robert "Bob" Frye was given the opportunity to work in the cardiac lab. That decision had major implications, which have lasted throughout the entire field, as he later trained generations of cardiologists. At that time, responsibility was not divided between pediatric and adult outpatients as well as hospitalized at St. Mary's, but Ritter and Frye would perform all cases regardless of patient age every other day. This all changed with Dr. F. Mason Sones introduction of coronary angiography [18] and led to an exponential increased demand for coronary angiography in adults. This resulted in adult cardiology commitments totally focused on meeting the demands of the adult patients. Pediatric cardiology activities also continued to expand with the subsequent involvement of Drs. Doug Mair, Bob Feldt, and then Don Hagler, working closely with cardiac radiology and Dr. Paul Julsrud in the study of increasingly complex patients with pediatric and adult congenital heart disease.

Because of the checkered history and results of surgery for coronary artery disease with Beck's talc in the pericardium and even the Vineberg internal mammary direct intramyocardial implantation procedure, which was quite popular even before the development of coronary angiography, there was considerable skepticism as to the benefits of any surgical procedure for coronary artery disease. The first coronary angiographic procedure at Mayo Clinic was performed on March 29, 1966, by Frye Dr. Ben McCallister, using a right brachial artery cutdown, with injections of 6–8 cc

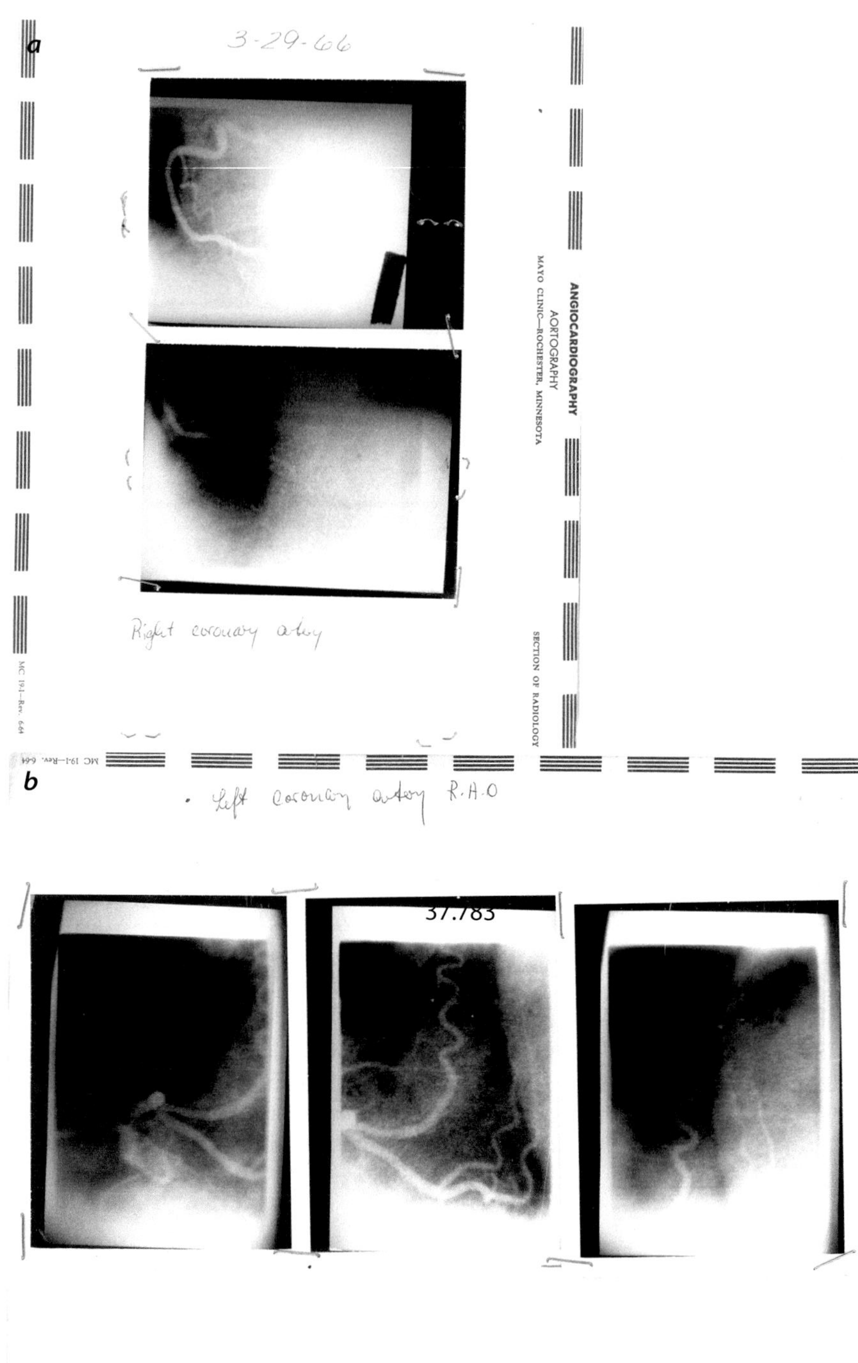

Fig. 1.13 Right and left coronary artery injections during the first angiographic study performed at Mayo, March 29, 1966, by Frye and McCallister. Two angiographic views of the right coronary artery proximal and distal (**a**). Frames from the left coronary artery taken in a right anterior oblique view (**b**)

of 76% Renografin using a #7½ 100 cm Sones catheter. Films were taken at 60 frames per second (Fig. 1.13a, b). The patient was a 51-year-old man referred by an endocrinologist for a "tension anxiety state and ischemic heart disease with angina." As can be seen, although the study was performed by a cardiologist, the report was generated and signed by a radiologist, Dr. F.J. Hallermann. That arrangement had been put in place when the decision to move the catheterization laboratory to St. Mary's Hospital had been implemented and have it focused on joint cardiology and radiology clinical decision-making. Of interest, the coronary artery study was then sent to Dr. Mason Sones at the Cleveland Clinic, and the final report was the integrated version after Dr. Sones' observations (Fig. 1.14). The patient subsequently underwent coronary surgery with a Vineberg operation. He returned on April 20, 1967, for a follow-up angiogram which documented that "the internal mammary transplant was patent including the intra-myocardial section. Faint small vessels are seen to originate from the implant and diffuse into the myocardium." As previously stated, the study was again performed by cardiology and then overread by the same radiologist (Hallermann). These studies were performed with the end-hole Sones catheter, which was also used for contrast left ventriculography. During angiography using this end-hole catheter, there were frequent VPCs or runs of NSVT, making the analysis of LV function problematic.

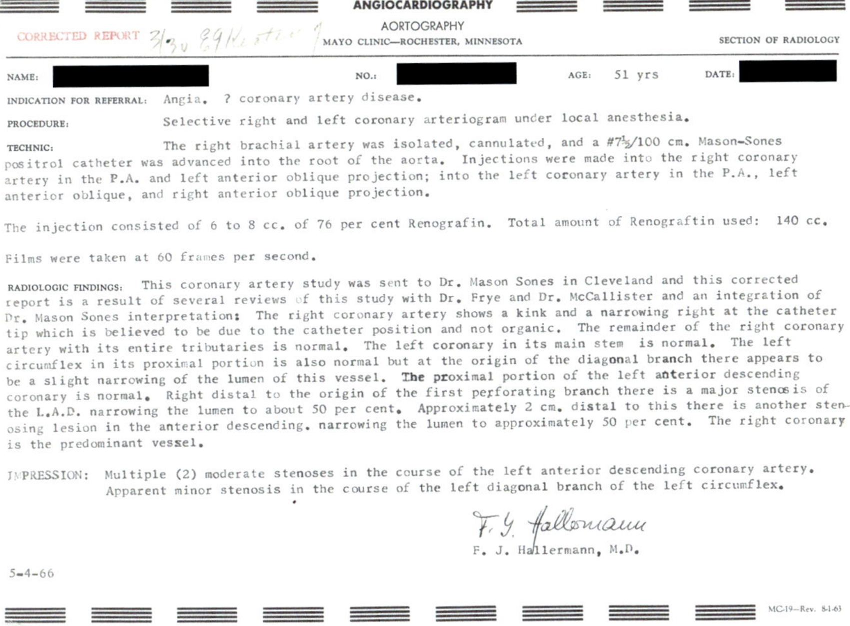

ANGIOCARDIOGRAPHY
AORTOGRAPHY
MAYO CLINIC—ROCHESTER, MINNESOTA

CORRECTED REPORT

SECTION OF RADIOLOGY

NAME: NO.:   AGE: 51 yrs   DATE:

INDICATION FOR REFERRAL: Angia. ? coronary artery disease.

PROCEDURE: Selective right and left coronary arteriogram under local anesthesia.

TECHNIC: The right brachial artery was isolated, cannulated, and a #7½/100 cm. Mason–Sones positrol catheter was advanced into the root of the aorta. Injections were made into the right coronary artery in the P.A. and left anterior oblique projection; into the left coronary artery in the P.A., left anterior oblique, and right anterior oblique projection.

The injection consisted of 6 to 8 cc. of 76 per cent Renografin. Total amount of Renograftin used: 140 cc.

Films were taken at 60 frames per second.

RADIOLOGIC FINDINGS: This coronary artery study was sent to Dr. Mason Sones in Cleveland and this corrected report is a result of several reviews of this study with Dr. Frye and Dr. McCallister and an integration of Dr. Mason Sones interpretation: The right coronary artery shows a kink and a narrowing right at the catheter tip which is believed to be due to the catheter position and not organic. The remainder of the right coronary artery with its entire tributaries is normal. The left coronary in its main stem is normal. The left circumflex in its proximal portion is also normal but at the origin of the diagonal branch there appears to be a slight narrowing of the lumen of this vessel. The proximal portion of the left anterior descending coronary is normal. Right distal to the origin of the first perforating branch there is a major stenosis of the L.A.D. narrowing the lumen to about 50 per cent. Approximately 2 cm. distal to this there is another stenosing lesion in the anterior descending. narrowing the lumen to approximately 50 per cent. The right coronary is the predominant vessel.

IMPRESSION: Multiple (2) moderate stenoses in the course of the left anterior descending coronary artery.
             Apparent minor stenosis in the course of the left diagonal branch of the left circumflex.

F. J. Hallermann, M.D.

5-4-66

MC-19—Rev. 8-1-63

Fig. 1.14 As per the "agreement" reached in the development of the cardiac catheterization laboratory, Hallermann, a radiologist, overread the film and made the final report. Of great interest is the fact that this first study was sent to Dr. F. Mason Sones in Cleveland for his interpretation and the corrected report was the integration of the interpretation of all four individuals – Frye, McCallister, Sones, and Hallermann

Surgery for coronary artery disease was viewed with considerable skepticism at the time, but many Vineberg procedures were being done. Our coronary angiography program started with the initial surgical procedure being the Vineberg and later coronary artery bypass with vein grafts as described by Favoloro. We sought an objective physiologic measurement at the time of coronary angiography which might provide insight on efficacy of the surgery performed. We thus decided to study LV hemodynamics with a 3-minute period of exercise with a catheter in the left ventricle prior to routine coronary studies. Since the angiographic studies used a brachial cutdown approach for Sones technique catheterization, the exercise was based on supine exercise with a bicycle ergometer. This facilitated the observation made on the measurement of the LVEDP at rest and then with feet elevated. As can be seen (Fig. 1.15), in some patients with leg elevation, the end-diastolic pressure increased markedly. This finding would later become one of the hallmarks of diastolic dysfunction and form the basis of a diagnosis of HFpEF and is now used as an objective indicator for this condition. The coronary practice grew rapidly after the introduction of coronary bypass with a saphenous vein bypass graft. With the emphasis on obtaining objective data on LV function and coronary flow in the setting of coronary revascularization, a data link led by Dr. Erik Ritman connected data from the clinical catheterization laboratory to the experimental laboratory at Medical Sciences. The introduction of television fluoroscopy was important because X-ray angiography became more clinically valuable related to the introduction of the videotape recorder and subsequently the videodisc recorder (Fig. 1.16). This led

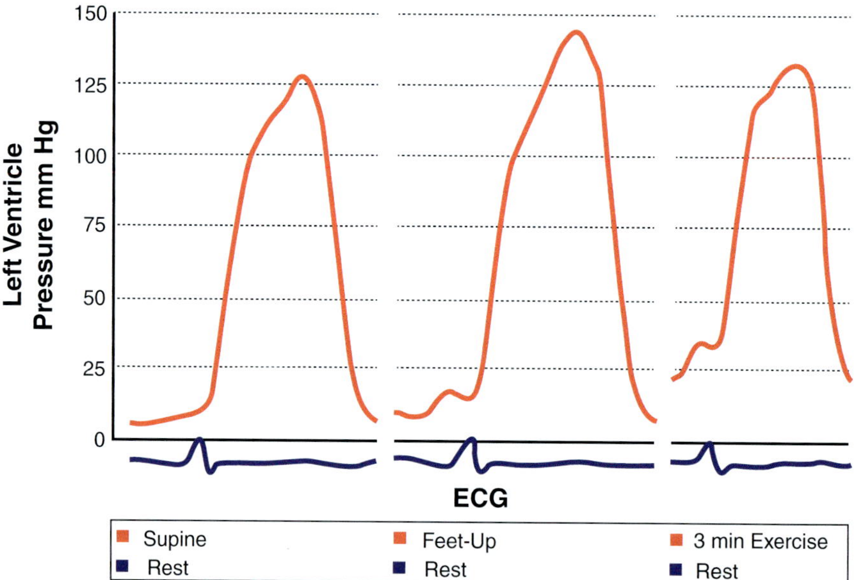

Fig. 1.15 The effect of changes in leg position on LVEDP. With 3 minutes of exercise, there is a marked increase in LVEDP, which had been normal at baseline. This was an initial documentation of the finding that symptoms with exercise were often related to increase in LVEDP. This has become part of the framework of invasive exercise studies in which the effect of exercise is to result in excessive elevation of pulmonary arterial pressure and is now part of the syndrome diagnosed as heart failure with preserved ejection fraction

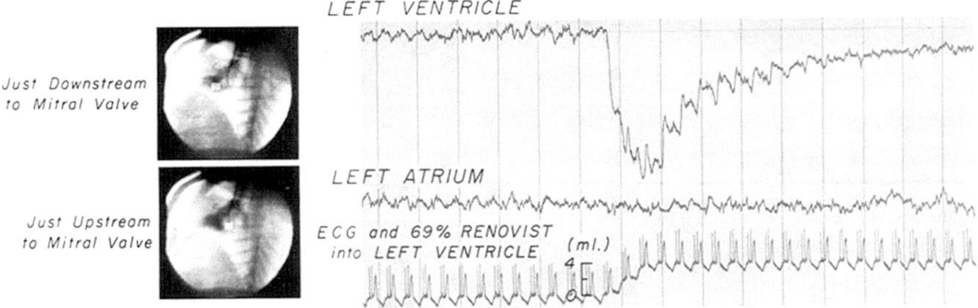

Fig. 1.16 Video fluoroscopic recordings obtained during a left ventricular angiogram shown on the panels on the right, the *upper panel* with video-densitometric sampling over the left ventricular chamber, the *lower panel* showing the measuring window over the left atrium. The angiographic dilution curves over the left ventricle (*upper*) and left atrium (*lower*) show no regurgitation into the left atrium. (From Ritman EL, Sturm RE, Wood EH. Roentgen-video-techniques for dynamic studies… 1978;23–44; used with permission)

to the ability to perform instant playback. In addition, the "density" of contrast in these video images was shown to generate accurate measures for application of techniques used for indicator dilution curve timing and concentration. The videotape recorder also allowed repeated, immediate playback of the image during the clinical catheterization procedure so that different areas within the imaged heart could be separately analyzed, yet effectively at the same time, within the one angiographic sequence. This was important in that it opened the possibility for research of cardiovascular structure and function, utilizing both animal models and patients' fluoroscopic data by eliminating the need for placing multiple intravascular sampling catheters within or downstream to the heart. Ralph Sturm developed the video-densitometer [19], a device that allowed obtaining indicator dilution curves generated by the passage of a bolus of injected intravascular contrast agent.

In the late 1960s, the development of the videodensitometry allowed quantifying arrival times and anatomic location of a contrast bolus as it passed along an artery or through the cardiac chambers.

These studies were used to assess a variety of clinical conditions. In the evaluation of mitral valve function, video-densitometric analysis of a videofluoroscopic image sequence with a sampling window position upstream and downstream to the mitral valve can be performed (Fig. 1.17) [1]. It documents simultaneous dye dilution curves in the LV and left atrial (LA) chambers. The area under the LA curve shows a marked increase due to the development of mitral valve incompetence resulting from dilation of the LV chamber, consequent to increased aortic BP.

These techniques were also applied to saphenous vein bypass graft flow (Fig. 1.18). Evaluation of this involves a sampling window at the proximal and one at the distal end of the graft [20]. This generated two curves with different mean transit times; the difference in those timing values was the transit time of the bolus of contrast through the graft. The image was also used to calculate the vein's lumen volume between these two sampling sites as its volume divided by the transit time equals flow in the vein. This information could not be obtained with catheter sampling without advancing a catheter though the vein to that distal end, thereby compromising the vein's lumen volume and flow.

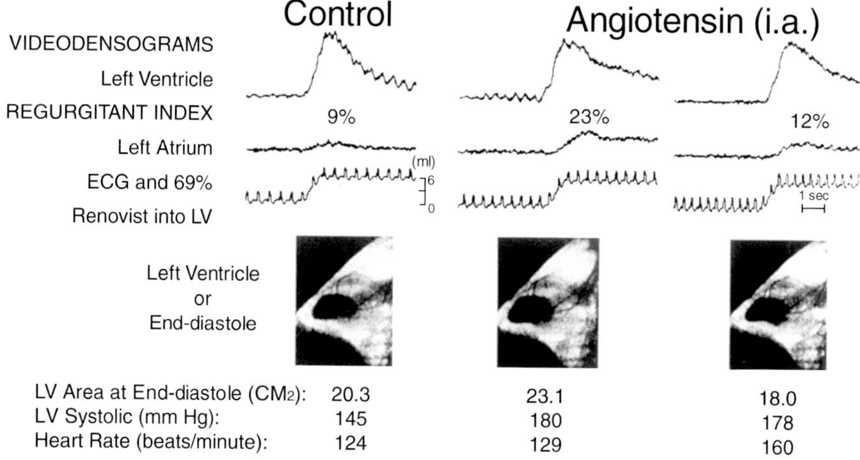

Fig. 1.17 These studies were used to assess a variety of clinical conditions. In the evaluation of mitral valve function, video-densitometric analysis of a videofluoroscopic image sequence with a sampling window position upstream and downstream to the mitral valve can be performed. (Adapted from Ritman [1] used under open access license)

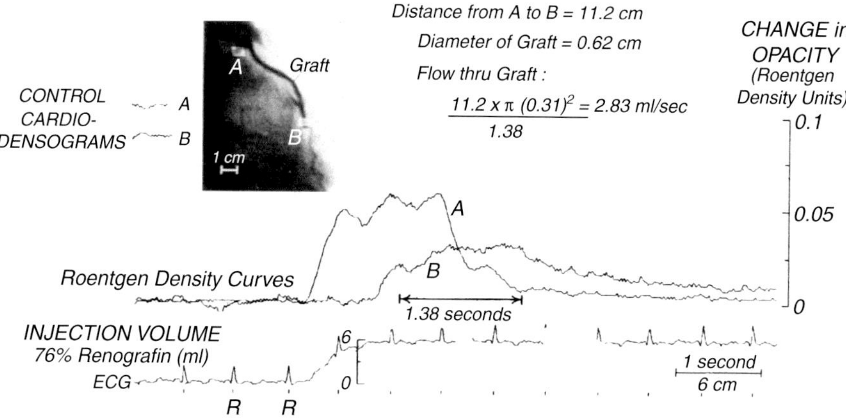

$$\frac{11.2 \times \pi \ (0.31)^2}{1.38} = 2.83 \ ml/sec$$

Fig. 1.18 Left upper panel is a single frame of a video-angiogram of a saphenous vein bypass graft. The video-densitometric curves, shown in the lower half, are measured at location A (proximal) and location B (distal). The distance along the graft between A and B and the average diameter of the graft can be measured from the angiogram and used to compute blood flow in the graft. (From Smith et al. [20], Used with permission of Mayo Foundation)

This technique could also be applied to the coronary arteries. However, there was a problem in that type of analysis; if the vein or artery lumen was not necessarily circular in cross-section, then the calculated volume depended on the angle of view relative to the vein's different diameters. This problem's resolution had to wait for fast 3D computed tomography imaging such as now routinely provided by commercial multi-slice high-speed CT scanners. Moreover, the volume of and work performed by the myocardium perfused by the graft or coronary artery was not known so that the match (or mismatch) between blood supply and myocardial and cardiac function could not be answered. Nonetheless, this methodology was used successfully in research studies in the human cath lab.

Video-fluoroscopic ventriculograms were also transmitted to the Wood lab at Medical Sciences for evaluation under the direction of Ritman. The introduction of the videometer by Ralph Sturm allowed real-time outlining of the contrast within the left ventricle and of its free epicardial surface (Fig. 1.19) [21]. Using such data, Drs. Jean Dumesnil and James Chesebro performed original work defining quantitative wall thickening as an index of regional and global and regional LV wall

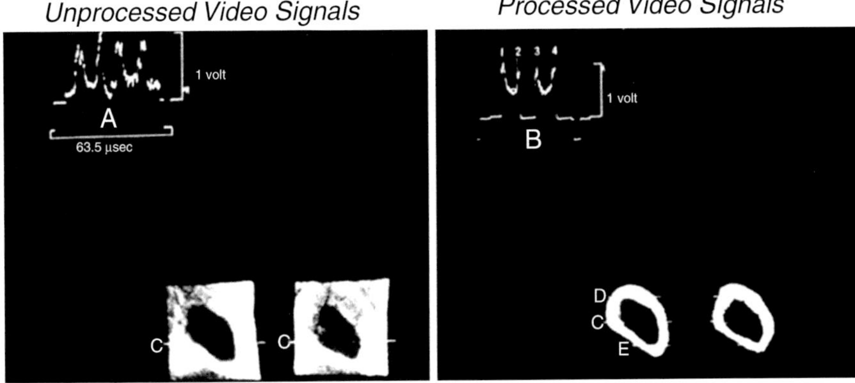

Fig. 1.19 Video-fluoroscopic ventriculograms were also transmitted to the Wood lab at Medical Sciences for evaluation under the direction of Ritman. The introduction of the videometer by Ralph Sturm allowed real-time outlining of the contrast within the left ventricle and of its free epicardial surface. (From Ritman et al. [21]; used with permission)

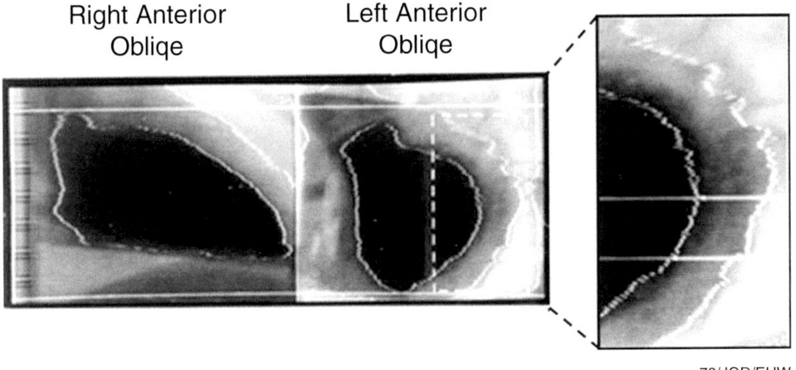

3609

Fig. 1.20 Left panel biplane views during a left ventriculogram in a 55-year-old patient. Note the automated highlighting of the endocardial and epicardial surfaces. The inset on the right shows a region of the ventricular wall used to measure wall thickness throughout the cardiac cycle. (From Dumesnil et al. [23]; used with permission)

function (Fig. 1.20) [22, 23]. With NIH funding under Dr. Bruce Kottke's NIH SCOR grant (HL14196), a comprehensive study of revascularization with coronary artery bypass grafting combining regional wall function with graft flows all measured with the videometry and videodensitometry systems in the Wood lab was performed. For these analyses, multiple components were required, working in either parallel or sequential sequences.

The stage was set on this background of science, physiology, clinical observation and study, patient needs, new technology, and new strategies to move the field on to the next decade.

References

1. Ritman EL. Earl Wood – a research career noted for development of novel instruments driven by the power of the indicator dilution concept. J Appl Physiol (1985). 2014;117:945–56.
2. Wood EH, Sutterer W. Improved resistance wire strain-gauge manometers adaptable for biologic measurements. J Lab Clin Med. 1955;45:153–8.
3. Brown GE Jr, Pollack AA. Intraarterial blood pressure in patients with coarctation of the aorta. Proc Staff Meet Mayo Clin. 1948;23:129–34.
4. Montgomery GE Jr, Geraci JE, et al. The arterial oxygen saturation in cyanotic types of congenital heart disease. Proc Staff Meet Mayo Clin. 1948;23:169–76.
5. Wood EH. Special instrumentation problems encountered in physiological research considering the heart and circulation in man. Science. 1950;112:705–15.
6. Hamilton W, Walker Moore J, Kinsman J, Spurling R. Simultaneous determination of the pulmonary and systemic circulation times in man and of a figure related to the cardiac output. Am J Cardiol. 1928;84:338–44.
7. Wood EH. Diagnostic applications of indicator-dilution technics in congenital heart disease. Circ Res. 1962;10:531–68.
8. Nicholson JW 3rd, Wood EH. Estimation of cardiac output and Evans blue space in man, using an oximeter. J Lab Clin Med. 1951;38:588–603.
9. Nicholson JW 3rd, Burchell HB, Wood EH. A method for the continuous recording of Evans blue dye curves in arterial blood, and its application to the diagnosis of cardiovascular abnormalities. J Lab Clin Med. 1951;37:353–64.
10. Mook GA, Osypka P, Sturm RE, Wood EH. Light reflection measurements on blood by fiber-optic catheter. Acta Physiol Phamacol Neerl. 1966;14:67–9.
11. Fox IJ, Brooker LG, Heseltine DW, Essex HE, Wood EH. A tricarbocyanine dye for continuous recording of dilution curves in whole blood independent of variations in blood oxygen saturation. Proc Staff Meet Mayo Clin. 1957;32:478–84.
12. Fox IJ, Swan HJ, Wood EH. Intra vascular catheterization 1959:609–636.
13. Fye W. Caring for the heart, vol. 672. New York: Oxford University Press; 2015.
14. Fox IJ, Sutterer WF, Wood EH. Dynamic response characteristics of systems for continuous recording of concentration changes in a flowing liquid (for example, indicator-dilution curves). J Appl Physiol. 1957;11:390–404.
15. Cournand A, Bing RJ, Dexter L, et al. Report of committee on cardiac catheterization and angiocardiography of the American Heart Association. Circulation. 1953;7:769–73.
16. Ritman EL, Robb R, Harris L. Imaging physiological functions: experience with the dynamic spatial reconstructor, vol. 302. Westport: Praeger; 1985.
17. Wood EH. Graduate training in cardiovascular physiology at a clinical center: an analysis of 15 years' experience. Proc Staff Meet Mayo Clin. 1961;36:567–78.

18. Proudfit WL, Shirey EK, Sones FM Jr. Selective cine coronary arteriography. Correlation with clinical findings in 1,000 patients. Circulation. 1966;33:901–10.

19. Sturm RE, Wood EH. The video quantizer: an electronic photometer to measure contrast in roentgen fluoroscopic images. Mayo Clin Proc. 1968;43:803–6.

20. Smith HC, Frye RL, Donald DE, et al. Roentgen videodensitometric measure of coronary blood flow. Determination from simultaneous indicator-dilution curves at selected sites in the coronary circulation and in coronary artery-saphenous vein grafts. Mayo Clin Proc. 1971;46:800–6.

21. Ritman EL, Sturm RE, Wood EH. Biplane roentgen videometric system for dynamic (60-sec) studies of the shape and size of circulatory structures, particularly the left ventricle. Am J Cardiol. 1973;32:180–7.

22. Chesebro JH, Ritman EL, Frye RL, et al. Videometric analysis of regional left ventricular function before and after aortocoronary artery bypass surgery: correlation of peak rate of myocardial wall thickening with late postoperative graft flows. J Clin Invest. 1976;58:1339–47.

23. Dumesnil JG, Ritman EL, Frye RL, Gau GT, Rutherford BD, Davis GD. Quantitative determination of regional left ventricular wall dynamics by roentgen videometry. Circulation. 1974;50:700–8.

Chapter 2
1970s: Growth and Innovation

Hugh C. Smith, David R. Holmes Jr., and Ronald E. Vlietstra

The year 1970 ushered in a decade of remarkable growth in the number and complexity of procedures and in clinical, angiographic, computer applications, and interventional innovations in the Mayo Clinic Cardiac Catheterization Laboratory (cath lab).

The stage for this growth was set in the final years of the previous decade. Most angina medications achieved benefit by reducing myocardial oxygen demand, while surgical efforts in the 1960s focused on enhancing blood flow supply; in patients with coronary disease, both approaches had somewhat mixed results. The merits of the most widely performed surgical procedure, the Vineberg internal mammary artery myocardial implantation, were hotly debated. Some studies showed clinical benefit and angiographically patent implantations, but in many cases, blood flow seemed suboptimal, and the subjective benefits were not matched by objective evidence of improved myocardial perfusion. Two small but important studies, by Cobb et al. [1] and Dimond et al. [2], demonstrated that a sham operation had similar symptomatic benefit to a Vineberg procedure, underscoring the power of the placebo effect. The absence of a prospective evaluation of an adequate series of patients with defined objective endpoints impaired its broad acceptance.

H. C. Smith (✉)
Mayo Clinic (retired), Rochester, MN, USA

D. R. Holmes Jr.
Department of Cardiovascular Diseases, Mayo Clinic, Rochester, MN, USA
e-mail: Holmes.david@mayo.edu

R. E. Vlietstra
Mayo Clinic (retired), Rochester, MN, USA

Watson Clinic (retired), Lakeland, FL, USA

This debate was rendered moot when, in 1967, Rene Favaloro performed the first direct interposition of a saphenous vein graft (SVG) between the ascending aorta and the coronary artery distal to a major obstruction in a 51-year-old woman. In 1970, he reported a subsequent series involving the placement of 1086 SVGs in 951 patients, with an operative mortality of 4.2% [3]. This groundbreaking surgical achievement was made possible by his close association with F. Mason Sones at the Cleveland Clinic. In 1958, during an injection of contrast media into the aortic root of a 26-year-old male with rheumatic heart disease during an angiographic study under Sones' direction, the force of the injection caused the catheter to inadvertently "fire hose," so that the tip lay nearly in the orifice of the right coronary artery, and the world's first selective coronary angiogram was obtained. Sones recognized the potential benefit of selective coronary angiography, and, in 1962, he and E.K. Shirey published a description of this technique and findings [3]. Favaloro regularly studied these angiograms with Sones prior to 1967 (a forerunner to the Heart Team of today). The benefits of SVG bypass surgery were objectively documented by other academic medical centers in 1968 and 1969. By 1970, the indications for cardiac catheterization and coronary angiography had markedly changed, as these diagnostic techniques could now, for the first time, guide an effective surgical therapy for sustained improvement in coronary blood flow.

This was the clinical environment for the cath lab staff in the 1970s, and their annual catheterization and angiographic numbers clearly reflected this paradigm shift. Coronary angiographic case numbers in the 1970s tripled those of the 1960s. Periods of change and challenge required that teams step up individually and collectively. The best teams are made up of individuals who complement each other's skills, fit well within the organizational structure, communicate well with each other, and respect each other's contributions. New ideas are welcomed. Such had been the case for every decade of the evolution of the cath lab, and throughout all of Mayo Clinic.

Robert "Bob" Frye was a prime example. He had trained at Johns Hopkins and was Dr. Eugene Braunwald's first cardiology fellow at the National Institutes of Health (NIH). He brought the lessons he had learned at these two illustrious institutions to Mayo Clinic when he was recruited by Howard Burchell in 1962. During the late 1960s and the first half of the 1970s, he was the director of the adult section of the cath lab, and cultivated an atmosphere of hard work, leavened by wisdom and humor. His technical skills were exemplary, and he was tireless in conveying them to his colleagues and fellows in training. He was always available. In 1970, Gerry Gau and Barry Rutherford staffed the cath lab on a rotational basis under Bob Frye's direction.

Gerry Gau had trained at Mayo Clinic under Bob Frye and Shahbudin "Sabu" Rahimtoola. He had completed medical school and internal medical training in Alberta, Canada, and had a fondness for things English. When the opportunity arose, he took additional training in John Goodwin's department at Hammersmith Hospital, London. His exercise physiology training added another diagnostic tool to the cardiac laboratory's evaluation of valvular heart disease and to the educational content of the fellow's program in the cath lab.

Barry Rutherford joined the cath lab staff in 1970 after training under Bob Frye in the late 1960s. He had come to Mayo Clinic from New Zealand, following in the footsteps of Brian (later, Sir Brian) Barratt-Boyes and Pat Ongley, both of whom had distinguished Mayo Clinic careers, the former in cardiac surgery and the latter in pediatric cardiology. In addition to his abilities in invasive cardiology, Barry had a deep interest and expertise in managing patients with acute myocardial infarction and was a key figure in developing automated continuous monitoring and enhanced care in the coronary care unit.

These invasive cardiologists had gained experience in selective coronary angiography, following Ben McCallister's visits with Sones in 1968. Don Ritter directed the pediatric section of the cath lab, but this age boundary was flexible, as adult cardiology fellows would scrub in and learn the diagnostic techniques necessary to define the anatomic sites, direction and magnitude of intracardiac and major vessel shunts, and other abnormalities in adults with complex congenital heart disease.

The learning experience for a cardiology fellow in the laboratory at this time was intense and incredible due to the evolving technologies and the experience, technical skills, and teaching abilities of the staff, particularly the co-directors, Don Ritter and Bob Frye.

There is an innate conflict in any medical procedural teaching. On the one hand, the mentor wants the fellow to gain experience, skill, and confidence, which, at Mayo Clinic, comes from an extended "see many, do many, teach" hands-on experience. How many is adequate depends upon the mentor, the trainee, and the complexities or technical skills required in each individual case. But the safety of the patient is paramount, and the need to obtain the necessary unambiguous data from this invasive diagnostic procedure in the most expedient and safe manner prevails. Thus, the mentors can experience tension, as they seek, in each case, to find the optimum compromise between these conflicting goals. When the fellow has evidenced significant technical skills and clinical judgment, the patient is clinically stable, and the procedure is straightforward, the fellow learns by doing, with the mentor assisting and advising by his or her side. In less stable clinical situations, and those cases with the greatest demands on technical skills and experience, the fellow learns best by assisting and closely observing the mentor. This learning experience was enhanced by in-depth, one-on-one and small group postprocedure teaching sessions where the conduct of the case, procedural options, and outcomes were reviewed. Nowhere else during the fellowship program was there such an extensive knowledge gain in cardiovascular anatomy and function in health and disease.

These learning experiences differed markedly between procedure room 73, where patients with congenital cardiac disease were studied under Don Ritter's direction, and rooms 74 and 75, where patients with valvular, myocardial, and coronary artery disease were studied under Bob Frye's direction. These experiences were complementary. Because the other cath lab staff were in the laboratory on a rotational basis, Drs. Frye and Ritter were the chief educators of the invasive component of the cardiovascular fellows' program.

Don Ritter had an encyclopedic knowledge of congenital heart disease and a quick sense of humor that he employed effectively to reduce tension – his own and

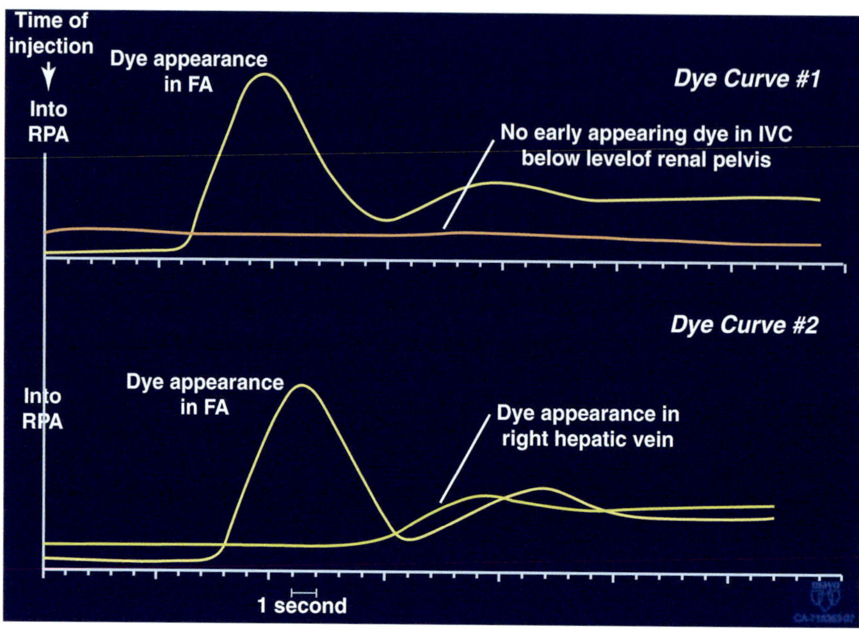

Fig. 2.1 Indicator dilution curves had been the focus of interest from the earliest days of the Mayo Clinic Cath Lab. They were indispensable for assessing outputs early on during their development and even more indispensable in congenital heart disease for shunts. Both single and double sampling studies were performed along with the assessment of O_2 saturations. For correct diagnosis to facilitate surgical repair, they were part of every preoperative assessment. In this particular case, indocyanine green dye is injected into the right pulmonary artery (RPA). Sampling is performed in the femoral artery and the inferior vena cava (IVC) below the level of the renal pelvis. There is no early appearance of the dye in the IVC (dye curve #1). For dye curve #2 the early appearance of dye in the right hepatic vein helps to document the presence and location of a shunt

the fellow's – during difficult situations. Due to the pioneering work and national reputations of skilled Mayo Clinic cardiac surgical colleagues, particularly Drs. John Kirklin and Dwight McGoon, there was a large Mayo Clinic referral practice of patients with complex congenital heart disease. Ultrasound imaging was in its infancy and not clinically available, so invasive studies were the only means for providing the accurate preoperative determination of the anatomic sites and hemodynamic severity of their often-multiple defects. These studies generally began with a right heart catheterization, with the extensive use of indocyanine green dye curves and oxygen saturations obtained progressively from different cardiac and vascular structures to assess flow and shunts (Fig. 2.1). These studies were data directed, and it was necessary to "think on one's feet" as initial results guided subsequent diagnostic steps necessary to fully define the congenital defects with the least number of catheter moves and the most efficient procedure duration.

Only after several weeks of observation, experience, and demonstrated competence would the fellow begin a procedure, with Don Ritter not scrubbed in, but standing closely behind, asking questions about what had been learned so far and providing guidance. The fellows quickly learned that there were "auditory clues" as to how well they were doing. If only a quiet discussion of findings or gentle suggestions ensued, they knew they were doing well and should continue. Don Ritter's laboratory shoes squeaked when walking, and upon hearing the squeaking, the fellows knew that Don was pacing behind them and that they had only a few minutes to get the catheter to the correct anatomic site and make progress. The sound of water running at the scrub sink was a sure sign that he was scrubbing in and would soon assume direction. It was amazing how these nonverbal cues inspired critical thinking and manual dexterity.

Bob Frye had a calm demeanor and an aura of quiet capability and confidence, reenforced by a soft Oklahoma drawl. Unlike the predominantly right heart congenital heart studies, most adult catheterization and all selective coronary angiographies involved the left heart and required two persons scrubbed in side by side. One, the operator, directed the procedure and manipulated the catheter, while the assistant helped with catheter exchanges, saline flushes, injections of contrast media for coronary angiography, or indocyanine green dye curve studies for cardiac output determinations. Consequently, early on, the fellow was the designated assistant and Bob Frye was the operator; these roles gradually shifted as the fellow became more experienced, and Bob's confidence in them grew.

There was a long learning curve to performing selective coronary angiography with a Sones catheter (Fig. 2.2). A small surgical incision and exposure of the brachial artery in the right antecubital fossa was required for catheter entry. The Sones catheter had a tapered distal 4 inches and an end hole for contrast media injection. The catheter was generally advanced into the aortic root, where, ideally, with a forward and twisting motion, the catheter would bend at its region of narrowing and "seats" in an aortic valve cusp with the distal portion curved cephalad toward the coronary ostia. Minor catheter rotations with close observation of the motion of its tip and small puffs of contrast media were employed to confirm correct position at the coronary ostium, and contrast media was then injected for selective coronary angiography. Moving the catheter tip through three dimensions, guided only by two-dimensional fluoroscopic images, required excellent hand-eye coordination and spatial orientation, a mental image of where the coronary ostia should be, and close attention to the subtle fluoroscopic image cues of catheter position in the aortic root. Not all cardiology fellows, no matter how bright or diligent, were able to master these skills.

During attempts to engage the right or left coronary ostia, an unstable Sones catheter position could result in the catheter "slipping" into the proximal or even mid-coronary artery (most commonly the RCA). In the early 1970s, the prevailing thinking, globally, and in the cath lab, was that the coronary arteries were sacrosanct and that only bad things such as dissection could happen when a catheter went into them. It was only during these events that Bob Frye's voice betrayed his outward calm, and his fellows can all recall his quick words "pull back, pull back" when this occurred. Thus, the report by Andreas Gruentzig [4] of successful coronary

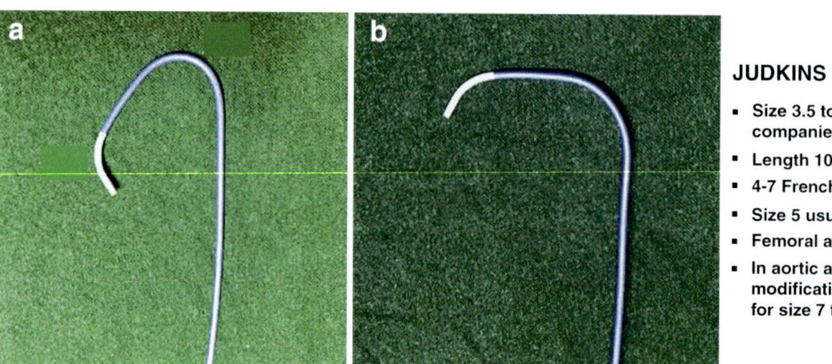

Fig. 2.2 (**a**) The Sones catheter was inserted using a brachial artery cutdown. It had a tapered distal tip and an end hole for contrast injection and could be used to intubate both right and left coronary arteries. It was also sometimes used to perform left ventriculography although that specific procedure was typically associated with frequent ventricular ectopy related to the end hole injection. (**b**) Judkins catheters were designed to be placed from a percutaneous transfemoral approach. There were separate catheters for intubating the left and the right coronary arteries. There was also a pigtail shape and design for left ventriculography

angioplasty only a few years later [5] truly represented a radical departure from prevailing thought and practice.

Given the need for an antecubital incision, brachial artery cut down and repair, and the challenges in positioning the Sones catheter in the coronary ostia, there was great interest in the published report by Melvin Judkins of percutaneous selective coronary angiography [6]. Barry Rutherford visited Judkins's laboratory to learn this technique firsthand and initiated this procedure in the cath lab in 1970. Judkins catheters were inserted percutaneously in the femoral artery in contrast to Sones catheters which required brachial artery cut down. They were single-use heat-treated preformed catheters advanced to the aortic root over a guide wire, with unique shapes for each specific purpose – a pigtail multi-holed catheter to retrogradely cross the aortic valve for pressure measurement and contrast media dispersion for left ventricular angiography, a right coronary catheter, and a uniquely shaped left coronary catheter. These three one-time use catheters came in sterile packs in several sizes, to match patient size and anatomy (Fig. 2.2b). Occasionally, patients with a severely dilated ascending aorta were encountered, where commercially available Judkins catheters were too small. We were aided in these circumstances by George Davis, a very experienced vascular radiologist who would steam shape catheters with a teakettle to match the patient's aortic dimensions. George had a twinkle in his eye and hands that showed extensive radiation skin changes, giving testimony to many years spent in close proximity to X-ray systems. He had a cheerful collaborative disposition and enjoyed teaching fellows about radiologic systems, image intensification, and optimizing angiographic images. He was vital in directing the maintenance and enhancements of the cath lab radiologic systems and in providing key selection criteria and vendor assessment for the next generation of radiologic equipment the lab would require.

Over the next several years, fellows were trained in both Judkins and Sones techniques, providing opportunity to examine the relative merits and shortcomings of each technique. Smith described their chief difference as follows: "It takes considerable skill and work to properly engage the Sones catheter in the coronary ostia. It takes modest skill and work to keep the Judkins catheter out of the coronary ostia." The percutaneous access, shorter learning curve, and more stable catheter position in the coronary ostia resulted in quicker procedures and better quality angiograms and became the dominant coronary angiographic procedure. It was important for staff members to be skilled in both techniques, as occasionally, extensive aorto-femoral atherosclerosis, aortic aneurysm, or chronic dissection made cardiac access via the femoral artery problematic.

Cardiac catheterization and selective coronary artery angiography, as invasive procedures in patients with coronary artery disease, were not without risk. The major complication rates of these procedures were reported from the Society of Coronary Angiography registry in 1984 in 53,581 patients [7]. Death occurred in 0.14%, myocardial infarction in 0.07%, and stroke in 0.07%, for a total major complication rate of 0.28%. There was an assumption that all major cardiovascular events during and 24 hours following a procedure were complications of the procedure. However, the general instability of patients referred for coronary angiography was underscored by an informal Mayo study into the reasons why patients scheduled for coronary angiography were cancelled in the 24 hours before their scheduled procedure. Stroke, infarction, and death accounted for most cancellations and were seen in 0.13% of all scheduled patients. Accordingly, a "rule of thumb" was that 1/2 of major cardiac events in the 24 hours before, during, and 24 hours after coronary angiography are procedure related and 1/2 are disease related. This informal study reinforced clinical impressions about the general instability of patients hospitalized with coronary artery disease. It engendered a sense of urgency in our cardiology colleagues to schedule these hospitalized patients as quickly as possible for coronary angiography now that there was an available surgical therapy that had the potential to dramatically alter and improve outcomes. Consistent with this urgency, the cath lab developed a standing policy to always accept unstable patients immediately and schedule all elective patients for later in the day or for the next day at the latest.

In 1970, Mayo Clinic and IBM, both located in Rochester, Minnesota, began a collaboration to develop computer monitoring and analytic techniques for the coronary care unit (CCU), the cardiac surgical ICU (CSICU), and cardiac cath lab (CCL). Mayo knew these areas could benefit greatly from automated systems, and IBM was eager to employ their new System 7 mid-range computer designed for process control. Ralph Smith, an early pioneer of computer analysis in the electro-cardiographic laboratory, provided overall direction and developed what he called his "British Empire" team with Barry Rutherford (New Zealand) directing the CCU portion, Erik Ritman (Australia) directing the CCL portion, and Hugh Smith (Canada) directing the CSICU portion. Barry Rutherford had completed a year with Homer Warner in a Computers in Medicine program in Salt Lake City, with particular emphasis on continuous monitoring technology in intensive care units. The experience was extraordinary; Dr. Warner was far ahead of the time and had already computerized his institution such that when patients were seen, the ECGs, blood work, and X-ray images had already been entered into an electronic health record by computer programs and were available. Dr. Rutherford was trained in Fortran programming for intensive care units, an expertise that he brought back to Mayo and then transferred his experience with it to IBM. Not all the time spent in Salt Lake City was work. During the winter Dr. Warner's fellows would arrive at work at approximately 7:00 AM. After working for a few hours, if there had been new powder snowfall in the mountains, the work team would drive up to the slopes and enhance their already considerable skills. They would then return to the lab mid- to late afternoon to continue programming. It is important to note that that strategy did not become part of the workflow at Mayo Clinic on Dr. Rutherford's return.

Erik Ritman and Hugh Smith were research fellows in Dr. Earl "EH" Wood's state-of-the-art computerized cardiopulmonary research lab, where becoming proficient in software development was at least a hope, if not an expectation. These three were responsible for the clinical priorities, algorithms, logic, instrumentation, and human-computer interfacing, while IBM was responsible for the computer software and hardware development to support these functions. These IBM-Mayo Clinic collaborative efforts resulted in enhanced performance in all three cardiovascular areas and provided important patient-computer-physician interaction experience at an early stage in all three careers.

The cath lab benefited significantly from its close association with the advanced cardiopulmonary research laboratory of EH Wood. Many technical advances developed in this laboratory – pulse oximetry, indicator dilution indocyanine green dye curve technology, integrated multi-channel video image, hemodynamic and electro-cardiographic recording, computer analysis of videoangiograms (video densitometry and videometry), and the dynamic spatial reconstructor (the forerunner of all dynamic CT scans), all of which came into subsequent clinical use worldwide.

In 1970, Earl Wood's laboratory had NASA funding for advanced cardiopulmonary animal research into protective measures against the anticipated G-forces upon the hearts and lungs of astronauts. This was a large extremely sophisticated research effort with G-forces created by a 40-foot diameter centrifuge and required Dr. Wood, 4–5 research fellows, and 10–12 technicians to conduct a single series of G-force experiments, which took 10–16 hours to perform (Fig. 2.3). State-of-the-art recorders captured 12–20 channels of physiologic and technical data simultaneously, which then took 2–4 weeks to analyze. Each Wood research fellow worked upon some aspect of this G-force research but was encouraged to develop research projects of their own interest. All fellows received software training in both Fortran and Compass, the assembly language for the CDC computers then in support of Dr. Wood's research. The fellows were expected to write the software for their own projects, but several skilled programmers on EH Wood's team helped the fellows over the rough spots. This training was helpful to future cath lab computerized analysis and recording developments.

The scientific and technical exchanges between EH Wood's research lab and the cath lab were enhanced by both fellows and technical staff who worked in both areas. Two Wood research fellows, Ritman and Smith, explored the application of video analysis techniques developed in the Wood lab to clinical studies in the cath lab. Jim Fellows, who subsequently became the supervisor of the cath lab, Don Cravath, and Merrill Wondrow brought significant video and computer software and hardware expertise from the Wood lab to the cath lab.

Erik Ritman was Earl Wood's most experienced and capable research fellow, and the key intermediary between the Wood lab and the cath lab for the next two decades. His youthful appearance belied extensive experience and knowledge in physiology, physics, instrumentation, and the scientific approach to problems. He was particularly interested in automated improved measurements of ventricular function. There was growing clinical evidence that a key determinant of survival in patients with coronary heart disease was the left ventricular (LV) function, measured as left ventricular ejection fraction (LVEF), or percent of diastolic volume ejected during each systole. The prevailing method of manually tracing two-dimensional systolic and diastolic frames of LV cineangiograms, and applying simplified geometric assumptions to calculate three-dimensional systolic and diastolic volumes and LVEF was time consuming and inexact. Erik developed latex cast models of the left ventricles in systole and diastole and developed and confirmed the three-dimensional geometric formulas and software to calculate LVEF from line-by-line video/computer

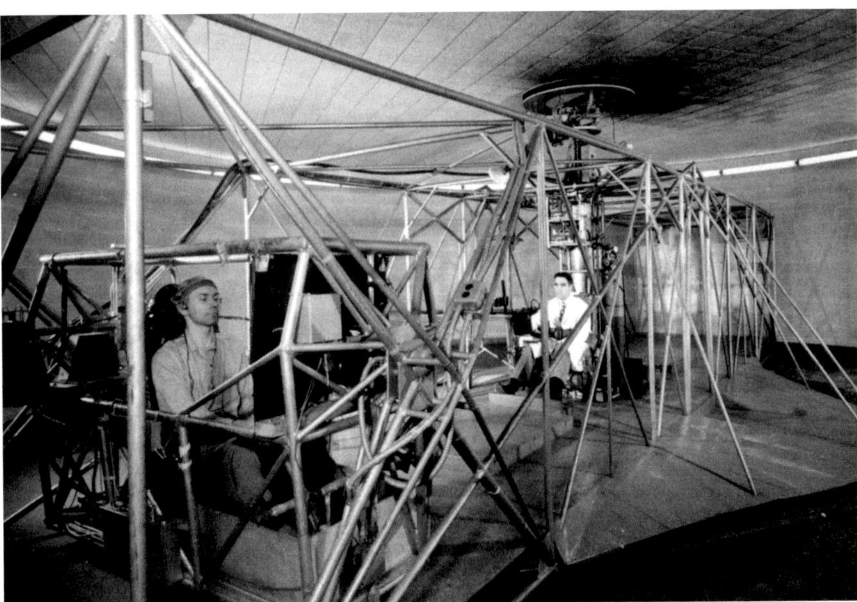

Fig. 2.3 The centrifuge was an essential part of this research effort. Seen here at the right is EH Wood conducting and monitoring the study, while the study participant (the subject, often a cardiology fellow or research associate) is seen on the left. (Used with permission of Mayo Foundation)

analysis of biplane LV videoangiograms (Fig. 2.4) [8]. A simple analogy to this method is to measure by border recognition the shortest and longest diameters of a Pringles potato chip, calculate its cross-sectional area, and then sum the derived areas of all chips to determine the volume of a stack of chips. The LV measurements are more challenging in that each LV chip perpendicular to the LV long axis differs in size from other chips and changes in size throughout each cardiac cycle. This validated method required no additional procedures or time, contrast media, or radiation and became routine for LVEF measurement in the cath lab.

Hugh Smith explored a method for measuring SVG blood flow, in ml/min, in the cardiac cath lab. In an animal model SVG, blood flows measured by simultaneous videodensitometic and electromagnetic flowmeter methods in the EH Wood lab showed good correlation [9]. With Bob Frye's support, SVG flows were determined from videoangiograms from the cath lab. To determine SVG volume, orthogonal films of contrast-filled SVGs were obtained, and the biplane source to film distances were measured to correct for the magnification inherent in divergent X-ray beams from a point source. Small (0.3–0.4 ml) injections of contrast media were then video recorded, and flows were determined from indicator dye curves in this SVG of known volume [10]. While videodensitometry was theoretically possible in the cath lab, two important lessons were learned. First, it was difficult to control all

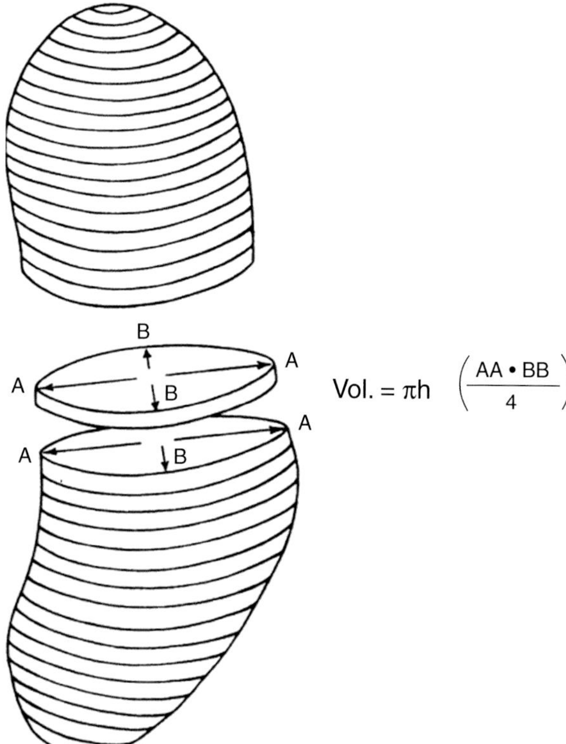

Fig. 2.4 Analysis of left ventricular function was optimized by the development of computer analysis based upon border recognition and then measuring volumes for each slice of two diameters (**a** and **b**) and summing them. (From Chapman CB et al., Use of Biplane Cinefluorography for Measurement of Ventricular Volume, Circulation 18, December 1958; used with permission)

variables in a clinical setting to the extent they can be controlled in an animal lab, and small patient movements, such as breathing, could alter the background radiation density and skew the dye curves. Second, unlike LV videometry, videodensitometric flow studies required additional contrast media injections, radiation, and time. Accordingly, these studies were used in research protocols but not routine clinical procedures.

There were tangential outcomes from these studies. Smith benefitted significantly from the rich technical and intellectual research milieu in Earl Wood's lab, but missed patient care. He had scrubbed in in the cath lab for videodensitometry studies and greatly enjoyed the experience. When Bob Frye offered Hugh a position in the laboratory in early 1972, he happily accepted – a career-changing decision. Hugh, like Gerry Gau, was a Canadian, who received his medical degree and internal medicine and early cardiology training in Manitoba. He came to Wood's lab at Mayo Clinic after completing 2 years of pulmonary vascular physiology research under John Butler and Claude Lenfant at the University of Washington. Hugh would succeed Bob Frye as director of the adult section of the cath lab in 1975 when Bob was appointed chair of the Cardiology Division. Hugh was an excellent communicator, mentor, and leader. It was his guidance that propelled the cath lab forward during the late 1970s and well into the 1980s and Hugh took on the most difficult cases in the lab and had a gift for translating his technical skills to those he trained. He inspired others around him to always do their best. Others in the lab will remember his good humor and some of the pranks he pulled.

A modest but very important early technical transfer from the Wood lab involved percutaneous arterial access. In the early 1970s, most laboratories used a Cournand needle with obturator to puncture the femoral artery from a near-vertical angle (the Seldinger approach). The obturator was removed, and with slow withdrawal of the needle, the appearance of pulsatile blood flow indicated when the needle bevel was in the lumen. This worked well, but frequently, both anterior and posterior arterial walls were punctured, requiring a longer duration of manual pressure to achieve hemostasis post procedure. Instead, the cath lab adopted a thin-walled 18-gauge needle with a very sharp and unique short curved "Wood" bevel without an obturator. This was advanced using a shallow attack angle nearly parallel to the long axis of the artery to puncture the arterial anterior wall with the short bevel totally within the lumen, without posterior arterial wall puncture. This seemingly modest technical adaptation assumed greater clinical significance in later years when angioplasty and thrombolytic therapy requiring the use of aspirin, heparin, and thrombolytic agents made postprocedure femoral artery hemostasis a greater challenge.

In these early days of coronary angiography and coronary bypass surgery, there were many more questions than answers, and Bob Frye encouraged all fellows to ask questions and seek answers. He was open to new ideas, techniques, and their critical evaluation and led by example. Several cardiology fellows and staff worked with Erik Ritman and the Wood lab in collaborative studies with the cath lab to develop novel computer-based measures of global and regional ventricular performance.

Jean Dumesnil was one of the earliest research fellows to work under Erik Ritman's direction in this area. A native of Quebec, Canada, he examined the quantitative regional LV function from clinical video-recorded angiograms [11], employing a new measure – the peak rate of regional LV systolic wall thickening. This was determined from the computerized border recognition (videometry) of regional LV endocardial and epicardial surfaces in 60 per-second video-recorded images. These were quantitated and correlated with clinical and electrocardiographic evidence of prior infarction. His work was extended to document changes in these regional wall metrics after sublingual nitroglycerine administration [12]. In 1974, Jean returned to Laval University in Quebec for a very productive career in academic cardiology with emphasis on left ventricular function and valvular heart disease.

James "Jim" Chesebro had obtained his MD degree and internal medicine training at the University of Rochester, New York, and moved to "the other Rochester" for his cardiovascular fellowship training at Mayo Clinic. He was a dogged researcher, rarely seen anywhere on the Mayo Clinic campus without 5–10 bulging manila folders under his arm. He lived and breathed cardiovascular research to the extent that his first English sheepdog was named Mobitz 1. It was no surprise to his colleagues, when years later, the successor Chesebro sheepdog was named Mobitz 2. Jim, working with Erik Ritman, using videometric peak rate of myocardial wall thickening, reported the important finding that the preoperative regional wall thickening response to nitroglycerine was a reliable predictor of the postoperative regional response after bypass grafting [13] and to late postoperative SVG flows [14].

Martin G. St. John Sutton, a research fellow from Guy's Hospital in London, examined the correlation between left main and proximal left anterior descending artery disease and peak rates of systolic anterior wall thickening and diastolic wall thinning in 70 patients. In all patients with ischemic heart disease, the peak rates of systolic wall thickening and diastolic wall thinning were significantly ($P < 0.01$) less than normal. There was no correlation between the severity of stenosis and peak rates of systolic wall thickening, but there was a significant ($P < 0.01$) reduction in peak rates of diastolic wall thinning for coronary lesions greater than 90%, indicating that diastole is a more sensitive regional myocardial function correlate of ischemia than systole [15]. Martin also examined the correlation between symptoms of dyspnea, angina, and syncope and global and regional ventricular function in 18 patients with idiopathic hypertrophic subaortic stenosis (IHSS). No correlations between dyspnea and syncope and any ventricular function parameters were identified. However, in patients with angina (but normal coronary arteries), anterior peak rates of systolic wall thickening and diastolic wall thinning were significantly less ($P < 0.001$) than in patients without angina [16]. Martin was known for working well into the evening on his research projects. Just how far into the evening was not really understood until one night at 1:00 AM, Hugh Smith received a phone call from Mayo Clinic Security staff stating they had heard a noise and seen a light on in the cath lab. Upon investigating they found a young man "with an accent." They reported that he gave his name as Martin Sutton and asked if Dr. Smith knew him? He did but apparently not that well.

Valentin Fuster joined the Mayo Clinic cardiovascular staff in 1971, around the time that he edited a textbook on cardiovascular disease. A native of Barcelona, Spain, and a national junior tennis champion, he received his medical degree and medical internship training from the University of Barcelona, then moved to Edinburgh, Scotland, where he completed a 3-year cardiovascular research program under the direction of Dr. Desmond Julian. He received his PhD degree in Edinburgh for his platelet research work, his thesis describing the function of platelet factor 4. At Mayo Clinic, Valentin quickly gained NIH funding and developed a very productive platelet research program exploring the interactions between platelets and arterial intima and the role of intracoronary artery thrombus and coronary occlusion in myocardial infarction. Jim Chesebro joined him in this research. In 1975, Valentin and Bob Frye reported on the angiographic patterns in 300 patients early in the onset of acute coronary syndromes, noting that total occlusion of at least one coronary artery was generally present in patients with myocardial infarction [17]. This presaged the need to develop strategies for primary infarct angioplasty.

Around this time there was growing awareness and disappointment that nearly one-half of patients undergoing coronary bypass surgery had at least one SVG occlusion. Based upon the platelet research work in Valentin Fuster's lab, Jim Chesebro and his cath lab colleagues wrote an NHLBI grant proposal for a prospective, randomized, placebo-controlled, double-blind trial of the effect of two antiplatelet agents – aspirin and dipyridamole – on SVG patency. The key endpoints were SVG patency at early and 1-year postoperative angiography. This grant application was, for unknown reasons, referred within NIH from NHLBI to the new drugs and devices program for review; funding was declined because neither aspirin nor dipyridamole were new drugs! Following communications back and forth, NIH acknowledged the problem, but noted that all current funds were committed, and encouraged Jim Chesebro to apply promptly to NHLBI for the next funding cycle. Jim was quite discouraged, but Bob Frye somehow found funds to get the study going without delay.

At the next NIH funding cycle, Chesebro and Smith were requested to appear at NIH for a reverse site visit. They outlined the study, and it was quickly clear that the NIH reviewers were convinced of the clinical need for such a study and were comfortable with the trial design and that the Fuster antiplatelet studies showed that aspirin and dipyridamole were excellent candidate drugs. However, the reviewers openly questioned the investigators' ability to recruit the 400 patients for the 800 postoperative angiograms outlined in the grant proposal. This is where Bob Frye's interim funding had been so helpful. Hugh and Jim informed the NIH committee that they had already enrolled and completed early post-op angiographic studies on nearly 25% of the target patient numbers during the several months of delay. This was quite a surprise to the NIH review committee, and their questions turned to how our enrollment had been so successful. This was due in part to the great care that Jim took in explaining the study to patients and the rapport that he established. But it was also a testimony to our patients, who understood the need for this research and agreed to participate despite their early postoperative discomfort and prospects of two more invasive cardiac procedures. Jim and Hugh knew they would be funded when Dr. Lawrence "Larry" Cohen, the chair of the NIH review committee, concluded, tongue in cheek, that perhaps if NIH delayed funding again, the study could be completed without any NIH resources!

NIH funding did come. At study completion, of 407 randomized patients, 360 (88%) underwent early (median 8 days) postoperative angiography. Only 8% of treated patients had one or more graft occlusions versus 21% in the placebo group, and this significant benefit persisted across more than 50 clinical and angiographic subgroups [18]. The subsequent 1-year follow-up angiographic study confirmed the sustained benefit of the aspirin and dipyridamole regimen, with 22% of patients in the treated group with one or more occlusions versus 42% in the placebo group (Fig. 2.5) [19]. These two NEJM reports were of fundamental importance and led to adoption of antiplatelet therapy for postoperative bypass patients worldwide and widespread extension of this therapy in some form to virtually all patients with coronary artery disease.

The primary mission of the cath lab was then, and is now, the provision of accurate anatomic and physiologic assessment of congenital and acquired cardiovascular disease in a safe and timely manner. It was evident in the early 1970s that a large population of patients with coronary atherosclerosis had symptoms inadequately managed by medication, leading to huge increases in coronary angiography numbers. This increased clinical workload significantly impacted staff and practices, which were magnified by key personnel losses. During this period, Gerry Gau rotated out of the cath lab as his other areas of interest had grown significantly and were now taking up his focus. The Mayo Clinic ECG lab provided computer-based ECG interpretation telephonically to a growing number of regional clinics and hospitals, and Gerry was spending increased time providing on-site technical and clinical consultation. The excellent relations that he developed helped pave the way for the large regional Mayo Clinic Health System formed two decades later. He was also the founding director of the Cardiovascular Health Clinic, providing needed analysis and advice to

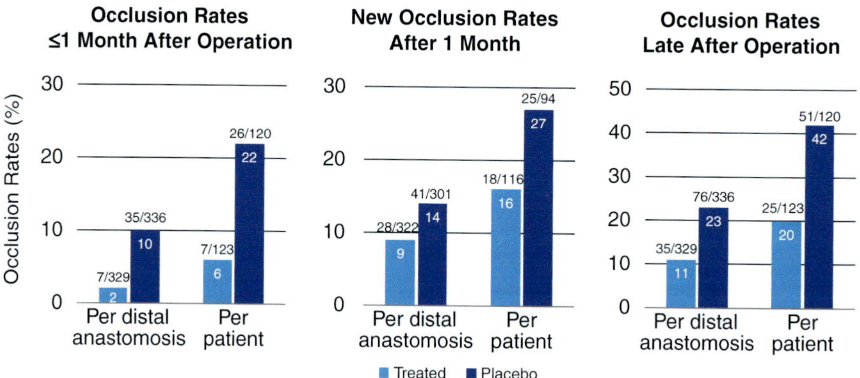

Fig. 2.5 Vein graft occlusion rates in this RCT documented a marked improvement in vein graft patency per distal anastomoses; occlusion rate with ASA and Persantine was 11% versus 23% for control, while per patient it was 20–42%. (From Chesebro et al. [18]; used with permission)

patients regarding modifiable coronary disease risk factors, a practice that was growing rapidly.

Invasive cardiologists were in great demand nationally, and Barry Rutherford was recruited by his friend and former Mayo Clinic colleague, Ben McCallister, to join his burgeoning cardiology practice in Kansas City.

Ron Vlietstra joined the cath lab staff in January 1977 and his impact was immediate. He was technically skilled and a hard worker, with a quick sense of humor and an infectious laugh. A New Zealander and University of Otago graduate, he was well trained in clinical cardiology in New Zealand and in Leeds, England, and had a deep interest in both cardiac catheterization and the pacemaker practice. He had also spent a year working in basic pharmacology with John Blinks, a leading researcher in myocardial calcium transport. Ron's intellectual curiosity, high energy, and enthusiasm led to numerous clinical studies and publications, particularly in pharmacologic procedures in the cath lab, and new interventions, such as coronary angioplasty. He directed a prospective randomized placebo-controlled trial of intravenous verapamil on left ventricular function [20, 21] and conducted and published many thoughtful analyses of the CASS database. He was articulate in speech and writing, and this clarity extended to medical graphics. Working with John Desley and Bill Westwood, Mayo Clinic medical illustrators, he published drawings of the angioplasty process [22] that were clear, immediately understandable, widely copied, and used by others in cardiology teaching conferences nationally, sometimes without attribution (Fig. 2.6a, b).

In the 1970s, there was growing awareness that Prinzmetal or "variant" angina, usually occurring at rest, could be caused by coronary artery spasm. This was occasionally witnessed in the cath lab, occurring spontaneously in normal-appearing coronary arteries, and associated with chest pain and ischemic ECG changes. Could this phenomenon be reliably and safely provoked and documented in clinically suspected cases? Ron Vlietstra had met with Fred Heupler at Cleveland Clinic and learned of his use of graded doses of intracoronary ergonovine to provoke and

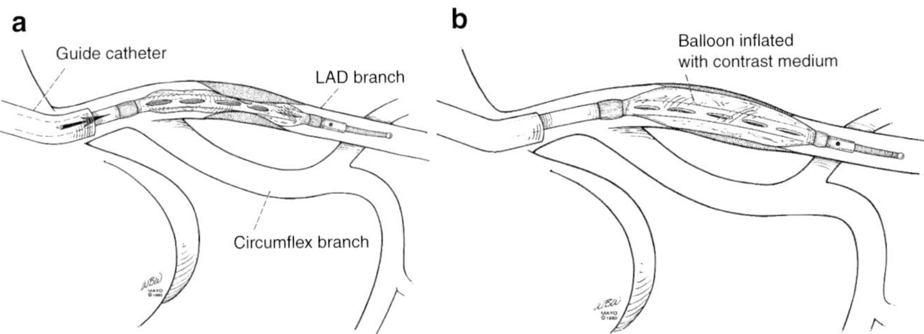

Fig. 2.6 (**a**) (Left panel) Medical illustrations created by John Desley of Medical Graphics depicted actual balloon dilatation equipment used – the stenosis in the left anterior descending coronary artery to be treated; (**b**) (Right panel) An illustration of the actual balloon dilatation. (Used with permission of Mayo Foundation)

uncover this spasm propensity. Ron initiated this approach in the cath lab for the small but increasing minority of patients referred for evaluation of this entity.

In the late 1970s, David Pritchard joined the cath lab staff. He came to Mayo Clinic from Brisbane, Australia, via further training at Green Lane Hospital in Auckland, New Zealand, where he gained additional experience in invasive cardiac imaging from Peter Brandt, radiologist. He contributed significantly to the clinical and educational practice in the cath lab until 1979 when he received an offer to return to Australia. Our sense of loss at Dave's departure was lessened by the knowledge that in 1984, he, along with a cardiac surgical colleague, established the first comprehensive cardiology and cardiac surgical practice in Queensland, the third in Australia.

A key addition during this time was Geoffrey Hartzler who was born in Indiana and entered medical school at the University of Indiana. As a freshman, he worked monitoring ECG telemetry and responding to cardiac arrhythmias. He was awarded a 3-month summer externship at Mayo Clinic where, by coincidence, he worked with David Holmes, another extern, in the ECG lab. Both would subsequently complete their internal medicine and cardiology training at Mayo Clinic, join the cardiology staff in 1977, and play important roles in the field. Hartzler was unusually creative, with considerable technical interest and skill in invasive electrophysiology, cardiac catheterization, and angiography, and he spent time in both laboratories. He developed and implemented approaches for catheter-based endocardial mapping, burst pacing for termination of refractory arrhythmias, intraoperative endocardial mapping for surgical obliteration of Wolff-Parkinson-White bypass tracts in patients with supraventricular tachycardia, and catheter ablation of ectopic foci of ventricular tachycardia. In 1976, he had met Andreas Gruentzig when the latter presented his work on coronary angioplasty in canines, and this experience sparked Hartzler's interest in new horizons in coronary artery disease.

In these times of rapidly evolving technology and knowledge, there was tremendous enthusiasm and industry in the laboratory and close interactions between practice, education, and research. The teamwork between colleagues with uniquely different skills and training and the willingness to help each other with new or unusual situations in the procedure room or with schedule conflicts was evident. These relationships were very helpful in dealing with the tensions that are an intrinsic part of new or different invasive procedures, unstable coronary syndromes, and cardiac emergencies. Ron Vlietstra, Hugh Smith, and Bob Frye also found that a friendly but very competitive game of racquetball several times per week helped. Despite the welts from wayward racquetballs, they always seemed more relaxed after a spirited game.

In the 1960s, caseloads of two to three procedures per staff member per day had, by 1970, more than doubled. The pace had also increased, and the described urgency in scheduling unstable or hospitalized patients for angiography extended to the review of angiographic cine films and reports as well. The existing practice of completing all procedures, reviewing all angiograms, and dictating reports did not meet clinical needs. Of interest, during this time, the cath lab explored the use of 16-mm film as archival media; however, this was short lived, and the lab joined the rest of the entire field to use 35-mm film. The catheterization reports dictated late in the day were transcribed, then reviewed and signed by the angiographer between cases the next morning. Any question or concern about findings or transcription error required reviewing the cine film again. Consequently, some cine films and reports did not leave the lab until the following mid-day. For many clinical situations, this was not soon enough.

Hugh Smith and Bob Frye discussed possible solutions. Hugh, with Bob's oversight and support, developed with Don Cravath, an EH Wood lab programmer, an interactive computer graphic standardized coronary artery "tree" (Fig. 2.7). This was displayed on a computer monitor adjacent to each Tagarno cine film projector. Angiographic findings were entered into the report in real time while reviewing the film and appeared both graphically and as text in the report. The report was reviewed, checked for accuracy, and signed while the angiogram was in front of the angiographer. Consequently, both the report and cine film became available immediately. Templates such as these formed the basis for standardized coronary angiography reports and evaluations in virtually all subsequent studies in the field.

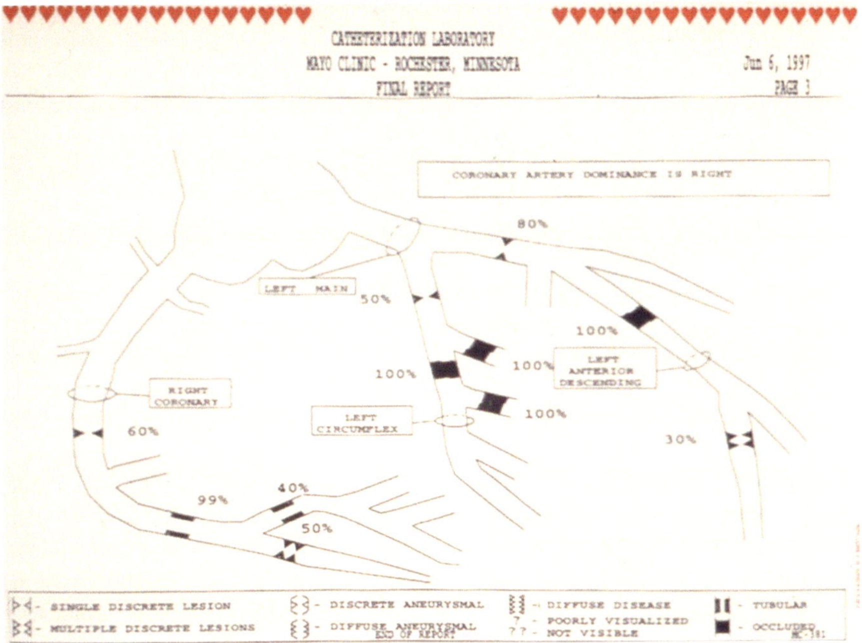

Fig. 2.7 The development of an interactive computer graphic standardized coronary arterial tree was an important addition which optimized standardization of data and facilitated collection of data useful for analysis to address clinical questions. Such interactions have been standard in randomized clinical trials for patient inclusion and analysis of outcome. Author's note: Faded computer-generated graphic coronary angiogram report from a 25 year-old Mayo Clinic paper patient record. All paper records, including these reports, were replaced some two decades later by a comprehensive electronic medical record system. The computerized coronary angiographic data bases of both record systems continue to support longitudinal clinical studies and analyses

There was another less immediate but very significant benefit to this computer reporting process. The existing laboratory-printed report filing system did not facilitate any systematic review of coronary angiographic data, so manual retrieval and review of all angiograms or reports was necessary to locate those patients with, for example, left main stenosis greater than 80% or left ventricular ejection fractions less than 40%. Going forward, the digitized coronary angiographic findings could now be stored in a "machine-readable" format, greatly facilitating selection, retrieval, and analysis for clinical research studies. The laboratory staff now had to learn a new skill – interfacing with a computer system for angiographic reporting. This was felt to be a modest inconvenience; however, it was discovered that Bob Frye had been quietly coming in on weekends for the past few months to retroactively report all prior coronary angiograms in this new computer format, such that the computer-retrievable coronary angiographic database and length of clinical follow-up was greatly improved.

This valuable database was also available to Dr. Lila Elveback, a wise Mayo Clinic statistician with strong involvement in cardiovascular disease research, and both Lila and the computer database were critical to many published studies. Cardiology staff and fellows all learned valuable lessons from Lila about clinical trial design, patient numbers and statistical power, the pros and cons of various statistical measures, and confidence limits. All remember a sign on the wall above her desk, in deliberately fuzzy print, that read: "STATISTICS – I know that you think you know what I said, but what you don't realize was that what I said was not what I meant," and that a "P" value is not meaningful unless it was reflective of significant clinical meaning: precepts which remain a caution to us all.

Coronary artery disease does not have a single, stereotyped clinical presentation but may present anywhere along a broad spectrum of clinical and angiographic subgroups. Cardiologists worldwide in the early 1970s were facing the challenges of determining for each unique patient whether they required angiography, and following angiography, whether medical or surgical therapy offered the best short- and long-term outcomes. Mayo Clinic staff felt the need to stay on top of this rapidly evolving field of coronary angiography and coronary artery bypass surgery. The weekly cath lab conferences provided a forum for sharing "new" knowledge. Correlations between clinical and angiographic findings and indications for and outcomes of medical and surgical therapy were frequent topics. Two Mayo Clinic cardiac pathologists, Simon Lie and Bill Edwards, continued a long-standing Mayo Clinic tradition of providing instructive pathology on a regular basis. Presentations by visiting professors were regularly scheduled. A Harvard lab logbook for interesting cases was kept in the cath lab office, and lab staff entered the name, clinic number, date, and significant findings of their unusual and controversial cases. These were presented regularly, were instructive, and often led to spirited discussions. Many appeared in the literature as case reports or as the propositus of a series of similar cases. These weekly conferences were regularly attended by more than 80 cardiologists, cardiac surgeons, and related specialists, fellows, and technicians. The thoughtful, vigorous discussions and unanswered questions that characterized these conferences frequently prompted clinical studies.

These sessions were a challenge for the fellows as they were responsible for running the Tagarno, a multi-knobbed control machine for projecting the long rolls of cine films used for clinical decision-making and were a focus for case discussions. One of the authors (DRH) remembers quite vividly an experience early on in his training when he was the upfront person identified to show the films. In setting up the "Tage," either inadvertently or nervously, he set it up in such a way that when turning it on, the very long spool of cine film unrolled freely on the floor in front of him and the entire auditorium of cardiologists, surgeons, and other participants. Lesson learned, but in a painful and rather embarrassing way.

Recalling the protracted uncertainty and controversy regarding the Vineberg procedure, most Mayo Clinic cardiologists and cardiac surgeons were determined not to repeat this experience with respect to coronary artery bypass surgery (CABG). Consequently, as the number of patients undergoing CABG surgery escalated, questions arose about its objective benefits relative to medical therapy and which clinical and angiographic patient subgroups benefited most from each therapy. The cath lab under Bob Frye's direction was both a critical intellectual and clinical resource for the landmark, NIH-funded, multicenter Coronary Artery Surgery Study (CASS), in which prospectively randomized patients and a non-randomized cohort were evaluated before and for many years following medical or surgical therapy. This study, launched in 1973, randomized its first patients to medical or surgical therapy in 1975. Importantly, a large ($n > 24{,}000$) group of randomizable but not randomized patients were included in a registry and served as the universe or usual clinical context against which the results of the randomized study could be compared. Long-term follow-up of the randomized and the randomizable, but not randomized groups, continues to this day, and more than 60 papers have been published from the CASS database, many by Mayo Clinic Cath Lab staff and colleagues. Between 1975 and 1979, 780 patients with stable coronary heart disease were randomized to receive CABG surgery ($n = 390$) or medical ($n = 390$) therapy. The 5- and 10-year follow-up did not show any significant differences in survival between treated groups (82% vs 79%, $P = $ NS). However, by 10 years, there was a significant survival benefit (79% vs 51%, $P = 0.01$) of CABG in those patients (25% of the total randomized patients) with initial LVEF < 50% [23] (Fig. 2.8a–c). The average annual crossover rate to CABG of patients initially assigned to medical therapy was 4.7%. Importantly, outcomes in the large non-randomized patient group were essentially similar to the randomized group. This trial set the stage for entire multiple generations of randomized clinical trials comparing CABG with either medical therapy or percutaneous coronary interventions, or both.

A vulnerability of long-term trials is that over time, study patients are lost to follow-up and evidence of differences between treatment groups may become lost or impaired. It became evident during the CASS trial that Mayo Clinic had a consistently higher (>10%) rate of successful patient follow-up than other participating centers, which could not be explained by demographic factors. Mayo Clinic's CASS data coordinator, LaVonne Hammes (previously a cath lab technician), and her team had developed uniquely successful ways of staying in touch with the CASS patients. LaVonne provided a workshop on these methods to the coordinators of the other

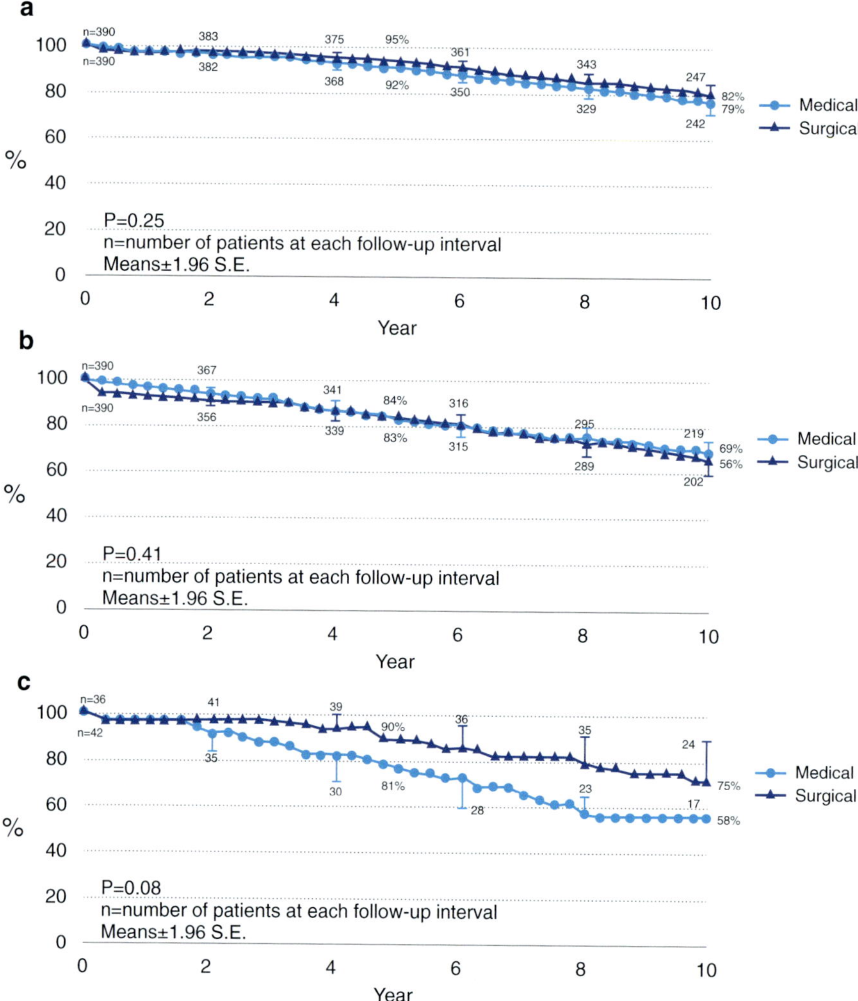

Fig. 2.8 The CASS trial randomized patients with coronary artery disease to either medical or surgical (CABG) therapy. (**a**) At 10 years of follow-up in the randomized patients, there was no significant difference in survival between the two strategies of care. (**b**) At 10 years of follow-up, there was also no significant difference in the percentage of patients free of death and myocardial infarction between the two strategies of care. (**c**) Life table plots of patients with an ejection fraction <0.50 and three vessel coronary artery disease. This documents a trend (0.008) with better survival with coronary bypass graft surgery (75% vs 58%). (From Alderman et al. [22]; used with permission)

national CASS-participating centers at an annual CASS working meeting. In the 1980s, this skilled team provided vital data support to the Mayo Clinic angioplasty registry, which served as the template for several national collaborative registries and trials of evolving coronary interventional procedures.

While selective coronary angiography and percutaneous coronary angioplasty procedures dominated the cath lab schedule in the 1970s, Mayo Clinic, as a major national medical center, had many patients referred with unexplained or undiagnosed cardiac problems. Accordingly, the cath lab staff had to anticipate the unusual and be creative in their thinking and the procedures they employed to define the problem or provide therapy. This creativity extended to the use of other imaging modalities, including echocardiography, an emerging, valuable, noninvasive diagnostic tool. Jamil Tajik and Jim Seward, later recognized internationally as echocardiographic pioneers, were junior staff cardiologists in the congenital heart part of the cath lab. The strong collaborative team culture and proximity of colleagues with different skill sets complemented each other and provided the necessary creativity in the cath lab to meet these challenges. Accordingly, there were many cath lab "firsts," in which procedures were performed for the first time worldwide, new syndromes were described, or unique collaborative efforts between cardiac imaging disciplines were developed, which significantly advanced our knowledge and care of patients with cardiac disease. Four illustrative examples are provided that enable the reader to understand how these occurred and their broad clinical impact.

1. A patient was referred to the cath lab with tamponade several days following urgent coronary bypass surgery. Five traditional "blind" pericardiocentesis attempts had been made with an approach in the classic fourth left parasternal intercostal space, but no pericardial fluid was aspirated and the signs and symptoms of tamponade – tachycardia, hypotension with narrow pulse pressure, and dyspnea persisted. Jim Seward and Hugh Smith, using a combined echocardiographic and fluoroscopic approach, confirmed the significant hemodynamic impact of a tense-loculated effusion involving the entire posterior aspect of the left ventricle, with no part of the effusion anteriorly. Using a 7-inch spinal anesthesia needle with sheath and rotating the patient 45° to the left in the cath lab cradle, the needle was advanced under echocardiographic guidance from the left chest at the apex posterior to the LV into the effusion. The dark nonclotting blood spurted from the sheath under high pressure, and within 1 minute, the pulse rate had slowed, the blood pressure and pulse pressure rose to normal levels, and the patient noted profound relief. This experience prompted a review of the literature on the reported success and complication rates of traditional non-image-guided pericardiocentesis. Ultrasound-guided pericardiocentesis was then performed in the next 40 consecutive patients. In sharp contrast to traditional methods, no complications occurred. Routine ultrasound guidance for pericardiocentesis was recommended [24], and subsequently became the standard therapy which continues to this day.

2. A patient was referred for an invasive cardiac evaluation for severe dyspnea, lightheadedness, and near syncope, but no clinical or echocardiographic abnormalities had been previously found. A psychosomatic diagnosis had been entertained, but the patient described his symptoms in a calm, objective way. He noted that they were much worse when standing and that while golfing on hot days, he

found that squatting helped. Hugh Smith began the study in room 75. All supine hemodynamic studies were normal, and indocyanine green dye curves and angiography from an inferior vena cava contrast injection provided no evidence of any shunt (Fig. 2.9). However, when the patient's torso was propped up to 45° while still supine on the cath lab table, a moderate right-to-left shunt at atrial level was documented by both arterial oxygen desaturation and dye curve findings. When standing by the catheterization table, his symptoms occurred, and arterial desaturation and dye curves were now consistent with a very large right-to-left shunt at atrial level. However, it was not possible in this procedure room to perform and record an angiogram with the patient standing. After discussion with the patient, he walked with support and a sterile, gloved hand over his femoral vein catheter to room 73 where the Elema-Schonander radiographic system allowed for an upright, large-film angiogram. Contrast media injected again at the inferior vena cava level now showed prompt and extensive filling of the left atrium consistent with a large right-to-left shunt (Fig. 2.10). A large atrial septal defect (ASD) was surgically repaired. A large Eustachian ridge on the posterior wall of the right atrium, normally present in utero but regressing after birth, appeared to deflect blood flow from the inferior vena cava across the ASD. He remained active and asymptomatic for many years of follow-up. Over the next few years, Mayo Clinic cardiologists and cardiac surgeons, now aware of this unusual entity, identified another six patients with this unique cardiac problem. Jim Seward reported this entity for the first time, with the recommended diag-

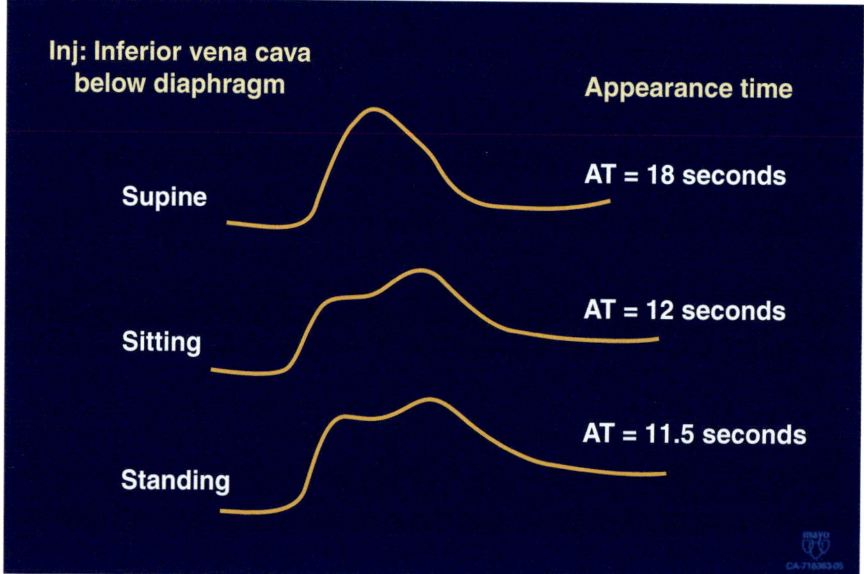

Fig. 2.9 In this patient with postural symptoms, indocyanine green dye is injected into the IVC in a supine position documenting no right-to-left shunt. However, when sitting and/or standing, a large shunt is documented soon to be labelled as "platypnea-orthodeoxia."

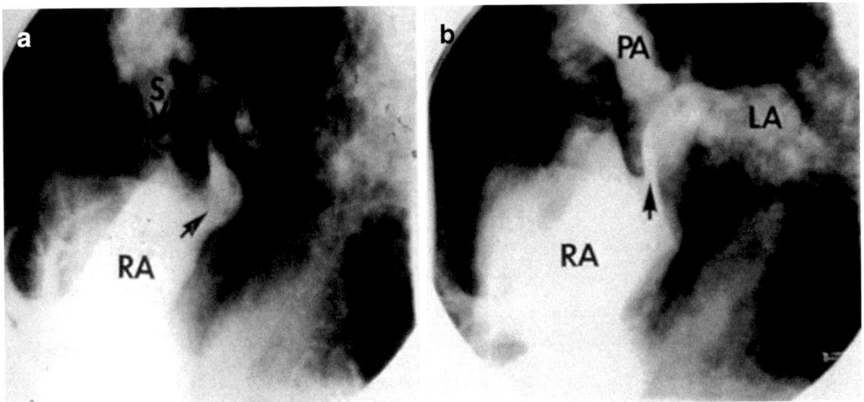

Fig. 2.10 (**a**) In the supine position, a modest amount of contrast media (arrow) is seen entering the LA. (**b**) In the upright position, a large RA to LA (arrow) is now demonstrated

nostic approach and documented findings in seven patients with platypnea-orthodeoxia, a rare and poorly understood syndrome of orthostatic accentuation of a right-to-left shunt, usually across a patent foramen ovale [25].
3. Right ventricular endomyocardial biopsy was employed in the cardiac cath lab in the 1970s, generally via a right jugular vein approach. Initially, it was used to identify active myocarditis and restricted processes, such as amyloid, unexplained dilated cardiomyopathy, and later, for immune rejection in cardiac transplant patients. The clinical and pathological correlations of the first 100 consecutive patients were published [26]. Hartzler documented cardiac Fabry's disease in one case and creatively used the bioptome catheter to retrieve a bullet lying free in the right ventricular cavity in another (Fig. 2.11a, b, and c).
4. A new staff member, Ian Clements, worked with Ron Vlietstra to validate a new radionucleotide method for measuring peripheral circulatory dynamics in humans. The old, established method was to use Whitney strain gauge plethysmography, but this was very sensitive to muscle contraction and tissue fluid accumulation. They used the subject's red cells labelled with technetium-99m pertechnetate (Tc-99m) for blood pool imaging and forearm strain gauge plethysmography devised by Mayo Clinic researcher, John Shepherd, and found excellent correlations ($r = 0.98$ and $r = 0.96$) for static and stepwise volume changes. Using the two methods together, it was possible also to quantify tissue fluid accumulation [28].

These four examples help provide insight into the spectrum of the invasive cardiology practice, the innovative and collaborative nature of the cath lab staff, and their impacts broadly on cardiac care in the 1970s.

In 1975, Bob Brandenburg stepped down as chair of the Cardiology Division, and Bob Frye was selected as the next chair. At Mayo Clinic, the Personnel Committee of the Board of Governors makes this determination but only after

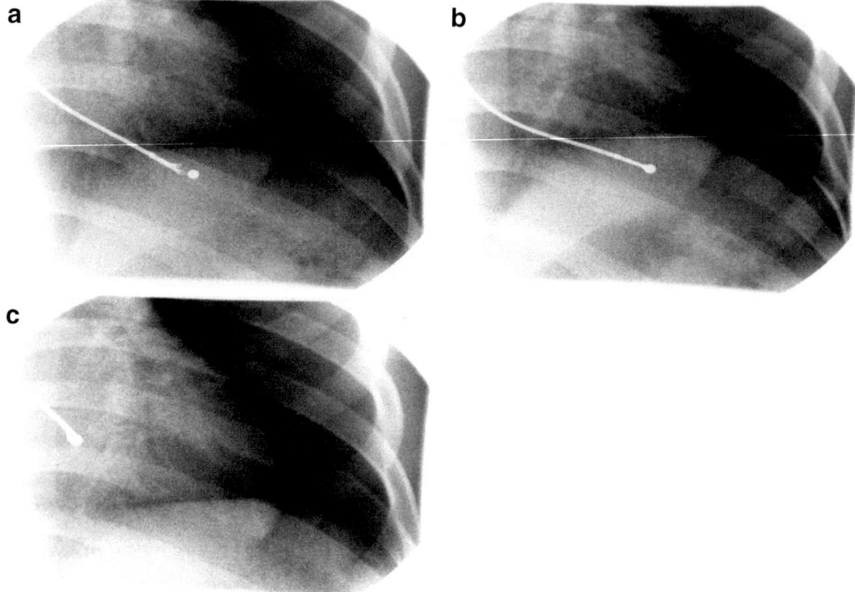

Fig. 2.11 (**a**) Prior to removal of the pellet in the right ventricular apex. (**b**) The bioptome grasps the pellet. (**c**) The AHA moment. (From Hartzler et al. [27]; used with permission)

thoughtful interviews with all members of the division. Thus, chair selection indicates strong support "above and below." In Bob's case, this was easy, as his leadership skills, much appreciated by his cath lab colleagues, were broadly recognized in the division. Bob appointed Hugh Smith to succeed him as cath lab co-director.

Throughout the 1970s and early 1980s, the clinical demand for invasive cardiologists nationally far outstripped supply. With a minimum of 3 years of cardiology training for national subspecialty board certification and many academic centers now offering a fourth year of invasive cardiology training, the supply was very slow in catching up to demand. The Mayo Clinic Cath Lab was not immune to this problem and had sustained some internal and external staff losses (Gau, McCallister, Rutherford, and Pritchard). During this time period, all current cath lab staff had received offers to join private practice groups with compensation levels substantially above their Mayo Clinic salary. Several excellent Mayo Clinic cardiology fellows with solid invasive cardiology skills, clinical acumen, and temperament had chosen to join private practices with large fee-for-service compensation levels. The development of coronary angioplasty and its use, with or without direct coronary artery infusion of thrombolytic agents for patients with unstable angina or evolving infarction, had greatly increased the lab's 7-day, 24-hour call schedule. For several years, these on-call duties were shared between only three, sometimes two, invasive cardiologists skilled in these procedures. In addition, there was increased radiation exposure inherent in angioplasty and intracoronary thrombolytic therapy, with the operator in close proximity to radiation sources for protracted periods. Although the lab staff wore lead aprons, thyroid collars, and lead glasses, they received calls from the radiation safety officer that their radiation badges had exceeded safety thresholds. Additional cath lab staff was needed.

Hugh Smith discussed this with Bob Frye, who fully understood the situation, as he had, despite his new clinical and administrative duties as Cardiology Division chair, continued to rotate part time in the laboratory for several years to help meet clinical demands for invasive cardiology. Raising the compensation for a subgroup of cardiologists might seem like an easy decision, but Mayo Clinic's use of salary rather than productivity-based compensation was critical to maintaining the ideal balance between practice, education, and research. Hugh Smith well recalled his staff orientation meeting a decade earlier with a senior administrator who explained that Mayo Clinic consultants could provide their very best, most ethical care "free from perverse financial incentives." This was broadly appreciated by Mayo Clinic staff, and importantly, by Mayo Clinic patients. Further, a common salary across a specialty provides a sense of equity and underpins the collaborative and collegial approach so characteristic of Mayo Clinic. Nevertheless, the cath lab was operating at minimum staffing levels, and while it was meeting clinical demands, research and education were negatively impacted.

Bob Frye made a recommendation to the institutional compensation committee, and it was accepted. This had a salutary effect. The cath lab staff recognized that this was a major departure from the established Mayo Clinic compensation model, and while less than most offers in private practice, it narrowed the gap, and there were other significant benefits that Mayo Clinic provided that private practice could not offer. Importantly, Mayo non-cath lab cardiologists understood these workloads and recruiting challenges and did not begrudge this compensation difference. Bob Frye's advocacy, institutional flexibility, and approval were important to the recruitment and retention of a new cadre of outstanding young invasive cardiologists. Ron Vlietstra and Geoffrey Hartzler joined the cath lab staff in 1977, and David Holmes joined in early 1980, all at the start of internationally recognized, stellar careers. The FTEs in the adult section of the cath lab increased from 1.47 in 1976 to 1.81 in 1978 to 2.15 in 1980. These increased staffing levels may seem modest, but they were palpable and welcome, as they enabled restoration of a more optimum balance between clinical practice, education, and research in the cath lab. The year 1977 was auspicious in cardiology for the inventive application of a catheter technique to open coronary stenosis. Andreas Gruentzig (or, in German, Grüntzig), in Zurich, Switzerland, had developed a double-lumen balloon catheter for treating femoral and iliac stenosis in 1974, and, by 1977, had performed more than 250 such procedures with a primary success rate of 84% [26].

Gruentzig then turned his attention to the coronary arteries. Through a pre-shaped Teflon-guiding catheter, he introduced a thin double-lumen catheter into the left or right coronary arteries. One lumen served for pressure measurement or contrast injection and the second for inflation of the sausage-shaped balloon located near its tip. Using a compressor-driven fluid pressure of 5–6 atmospheres, the balloon could be inflated to a diameter of 3.0–3.8 mm.

Amazingly, after canine, postmortem, and intraoperative studies, the first successful patient, a 38-year-old man, with a severe stenosis of the LAD, was treated on September 16, 1977. Presentation of this case and three more at the November 1977 AHA [5] meeting and later in a letter to the *Lancet* [29] aroused great interest in many and skepticism in an equal amount of others.

Gruentzig reported on eight successfully treated patients at a conference held in Frankfurt in February 1978, a meeting attended by Carlos Harrison, Mayo Clinic clinician and researcher [30]. Carlos returned to Rochester and told us of this exciting development, and he strongly encouraged Vlietstra to visit Gruentzig during an upcoming April trip to Europe.

Vlietstra spent 2 days with Gruentzig, making ward rounds on both adult and pediatric patients, meeting Gruentzig's chief, Hans Peter Krayenbuhl, and most importantly, reviewing angiograms of many of his early coronary angioplasty patients. Gruentzig was nothing less than brilliant in his recounting of how he had designed a workable catheter system and the challenges he had faced and overcome in applying it to patients. Even at that early stage, he expressed an interest in working in the United States, where he believed his research could better thrive and achieve more widespread acceptance.

On returning to Rochester, Vlietstra shared what he had learned with Hugh Smith, Bob Frye, and Geoff Hartzler, as well as presented slides, given to him by Gruentzig, at Thursday morning conferences. This was received enthusiastically by some, but others questioned its value. To wit, we already had an excellent means of dealing with coronary artery obstructions (CABG); how could rigid, even calcified, lesions be opened with such a tiny balloon, where does the plaque go, and what are the hazards of such "invasiveness" within the coronary tree were among the many questions asked.

It was clear that for Mayo Clinic clinicians and surgeons to embrace such a radical step, more information was needed. Several measures were taken to assuage these concerns. Because the greatest experience with balloon angioplasty was in patients with peripheral vascular disease, we proposed a randomized trial comparing angioplasty with surgery in patients with focal femoral artery disease. We believed that, if positive, such a trial would address many of the issues raised by skeptics. However, the Cardiovascular Research Committee turned down the proposal on the grounds that not enough was known about the advantages and disadvantages of this new experimental method. Catch 22! Pat Sheedy and Tony Stanson of the Department of Radiology pushed ahead, however, and performed peripheral arterial angioplasty on carefully selected patients whose clinical condition merited it.

In 1979, Ron Vlietstra, Geoff Hartzler, and Hugh Smith developed protocols for treating selected patients with focal lesions with the new technique. They required overview by two senior members of the cardiovascular staff and agreement by at least one of the cardiac surgeons (who would provide backup). These protocols were approved by the Cardiovascular Division Clinical Practice Committee and subsequently the Clinical Practice in the Department of Internal Medicine. Much of the detail that went into these proposals is outlined by Bruce Fye in his book *Caring for the Heart* [30].

There was still much concern expressed by Mayo Clinic clinicians about proceeding with such a novel approach, and potential candidates were not referred for treatment. However, a very suitable candidate was referred from an Iowa cardiologist, Dr. Hugo Koo, to Geoff Hartzler specifically for this indication. On October 9, 1979, Geoff and Hugh performed Mayo's first case. This is how Hugh Smith recalls the details.

The decision to perform this angioplasty was not straightforward. While Ron Vlietstra, Geoff Hartzler, and Hugh Smith had worked on the angioplasty protocols and technical details together, it was Ron Vlietstra who had spearheaded our entire angioplasty effort, met with Gruentzig, and obtained the guide and dilation catheters, pressure gauges, and all the Mayo approvals to proceed. However, Ron was away at a medical meeting in Toronto. For the past few months, we had reviewed all coronary angiograms to determine if any patients met the rigorous clinical and angiographic criteria that we had established, and this patient was the first to meet them all. He had a severe (95%) eccentric tubular stenosis (Fig. 2.12) of the mid-left anterior descending (LAD) coronary artery, with the downstream LAD, right, and left circumflex coronary arteries nearly normal. His angina had accelerated over 2 months from onset to daily occurrence (class 3), with modest effort despite good medication. He was unable to perform his physically demanding work, and CABG surgery was clearly indicated. Dr. Francisco Puga, a cardiac surgical colleague, had examined the patient and medical records, concurred with this assessment, and agreed to stand by.

The primary Mayo Clinic value "the needs of the patient come first," first articulated by William J. Mayo in 1910, influenced our decision, and we began the procedure shortly after 7:30 AM. Geoff Hartzler was the operator, directing the catheters and the procedure, and Hugh Smith assisted, handling the syringes for injections of contrast media (diluted to reduce viscosity and improve flow in small lumens of the four French dilation catheter) and pressure gauge to guide balloon inflations.

Femoral artery entry and advancement of the #9 French guide catheter to the left main ostium went easily, and the #4 French dilation catheter was advanced through the guide catheter to the left main coronary artery. After several passes, the dilating catheter negotiated the bend anteriorly into the LAD and moved easily to the stenosis but could not pass entirely through. Several inflations were made in its proximal portion, the dilating catheter was withdrawn, and the small guide wire fixed to the tip of this first generation Gruentzig catheter was reshaped and advanced again to the LAD lesion. After one or two inflations in the proximal part, the catheter advanced so that the 20-mm-long balloon straddled the stenosis, and two inflations were made. The dilute contrast-filled balloon, initially indented by the stenosis at low pressure, increased to its full cylindrical shape as the inflation pressure increased, suggesting successful stenosis effacement. The initial arterial pressure downstream from the stenosis had doubled from the low 30s to mid-70s, becoming more pulsatile, and a reverse thermodilution catheter in the coronary sinus showed a 20% increase in flow (Fig. 2.12b). The coronary sinus drains a watershed from more than the LAD, so the flow increase within the dilated LAD would be greater than the % increase recorded.

The balloon catheter was withdrawn, and angiography with non-diluted contrast medium confirmed nearly complete elimination of the stenosis (Fig. 2.12b). The patient, mildly sedated and pain free throughout, had been closely watching on the monitor. Seeing the now unobstructed LAD, he was elated and announced that, as a public works supervisor, he knew "we had cleared the pipe" and offered to buy the entire team a round of drinks in his hometown saloon.

We heard congratulations coming from the small recording area and doorway of the procedure room and became aware for the first time that 8–10 staff and fellows had come in to observe this procedure. Our own elation was short lived, as we each

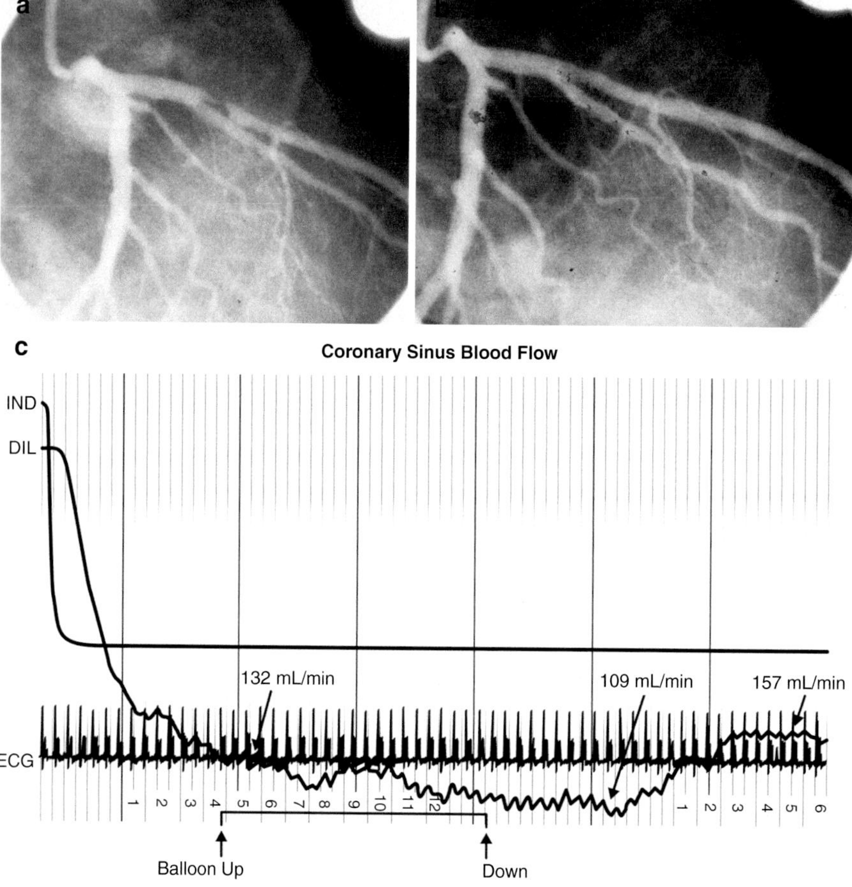

Fig. 2.12 (**a**) Baseline coronary angiogram of the first patient to undergo PTCA at Mayo Clinic documenting a severe stenosis in the middle LAD. (**b**) After dilatation, there is normalization of the angiographic appearance of the stenosis. (**c**) During dilatation, there is an increase in the pressure downstream from the stenosis and a 20% increase in flow measured by using thermodilution catheter assessment in the coronary sinus. (From Hartzler et al. [27]; used with permission)

had three or four more invasive diagnostic procedures to perform that day. The patient was dismissed to home 2 days later, returned to a full work schedule, and was asymptomatic; a follow-up stress test was now normal and a 10–20% residual stenosis was noted at follow-up angiography. He remained active and asymptomatic for many years [31].

Hartzler, Smith, and Vlietstra combined on another three cases through the rest of 1979, all successful. They presented their results at the second Gruentzig teaching course held in Zurich in early January 1980. David Holmes joined the team during those months and quickly showed the qualities that would lead him to become another world leader in interventional cardiology, all of us standing on the shoulders of giants who had come before.

References

1. Dimond EG, Kittle CF, Crockett JE. Comparison of internal mammary artery ligation and sham operation for angina pectoris. Am J Cardiol. 1960;5:483–6.
2. Favaloro RG, Effler DB, Groves LK, Sheldon WC, Sones FM Jr. Direct myocardial revascularization by saphenous vein graft. Present operative technique and indications. Ann Thorac Surg. 1970;10(2):97–111.
3. Sones FM Jr, Shirey EK. Cine coronary arteriography. Mod Concepts Cardiovasc Dis. 1962;31:735–8.
4. Gruentzig A, Myler R, Hanna E, Turina M. Coronary transluminal angioplasty (abstr). Circulation. 1977;56(Suppl 3):84.
5. Judkins MP. Selective coronary arteriography. I. A percutaneous transfemoral technic. Radiology. 1967;89(5):815–24.
6. Johnson LW, Lozner EC, Johnson S, Krone R, Pichard AD, Vetrovec GW, et al. Coronary arteriography 1984-1987: a report of the registry of the Society for Cardiac Angiography and Interventions. I. Results and complications. Catheter Cardiovasc Diagn. 1989;17(1):5–10.
7. Ritman EL, Sturm RE, Wood EH. Biplane roentgen videometric system for dynamic (60-sec) studies of the shape and size of circulatory structures, particularly the left ventricle. Am J Cardiol. 1973;32(2):180–7.
8. Smith HC, Sturm RE, Wood EH. Videodensitometric system for measurement of vessel blood flow, particularly in the coronary arteries, in man. Am J Cardiol. 1973;32(2):144–50.
9. Smith HC, Frye RL, Donald DE, Davis GD, Pluth JR, Sturm RE, et al. Roentgen videodensitometric measure of coronary blood flow. Determination from simultaneous indicator-dilution curves at selected sites in the coronary circulation and in coronary artery-saphenous vein grafts. Mayo Clin Proc. 1971;46(12):800–6.
10. Dumesnil JG, Ritman EL, Frye RL, Gau GT, Rutherford BD, Davis GD. Quantitative determination of regional left ventricular wall dynamics by roentgen videometry. Circulation. 1974;50(4):700–8.
11. Dumesnil JG, Ritman EL, Davis GD, Gau GT, Rutherford BD, Frye RL. Regional left ventricular wall dynamics before and after sublingual administration of nitroglycerin. Am J Cardiol. 1975;36(4):419–25.
12. Chesebro JH, Ritman EL, Frye RL, Smith HC, Rutherford BD, Fulton RE, et al. Regional myocardial wall thickening response to nitroglycerin. A predictor of myocardial response to aortocoronary bypass surgery. Circulation. 1978;57(5):952–7.
13. Chesebro JH, Ritman EL, Frye RL, Smith HC, Connolly DC, Rutherford BD, et al. Videometric analysis of regional left ventricular function before and after aortocoronary artery bypass sur-

gery: correlation of peak rate of myocardial wall thickening with late postoperative graft flows. J Clin Invest. 1976;58(6):1339–47.
14. St John Sutton MG, Frye RL, Smith HC, Chesebro JH, Ritman EL. Relation between left coronary artery stenosis and regional left ventricular function. Circulation. 1978;58(3 Pt 1):491–7.
15. Sutton MG, Tajik AJ, Smith HC, Ritman EL. Angina in idiopathic hypertrophic subaortic stenosis. A clinical correlate of regional left ventricular dysfunction: a videometric and echocardiographic study. Circulation. 1980;61(3):561–8.
16. Fuster V, Frye RL, Connolly DC, Danielson MA, Elveback LR, Kurland LT. Arteriographic patterns early in the onset of the coronary syndromes. Br Heart J. 1975;37(12):1250–5.
17. Chesebro JH, Clements IP, Fuster V, Elveback LR, Smith HC, Bardsley WT, et al. A platelet-inhibitor-drug trial in coronary-artery bypass operations: benefit of perioperative dipyridamole and aspirin therapy on early postoperative vein-graft patency. N Engl J Med. 1982;307(2):73–8.
18. Chesebro JH, Fuster V, Elveback LR, Clements IP, Smith HC, Holmes DR Jr, et al. Effect of dipyridamole and aspirin on late vein-graft patency after coronary bypass operations. N Engl J Med. 1984;310(4):209–14.
19. Vlietstra RE, Farias MA, Frye RL, Smith HC, Ritman EL. Effect of verapamil on left ventricular function: a randomized, placebo-controlled study. Am J Cardiol. 1983;51(7):1213–7.
20. Patton JN, Vlietstra RE, Frye RL. Randomized, placebo-controlled study of the effect of verapamil on exercise hemodynamics in coronary artery disease. Am J Cardiol. 1984;53(6):674–8.
21. Vlietstra RE, Holmes DR Jr, Smith HC, Hartzler GO, Orszulak TA. Percutaneous transluminal coronary angioplasty: initial Mayo Clinic experience. Mayo Clin Proc. 1981;56(5):287–93.
22. Alderman EL, Bourassa MG, Cohen LS, Davis KB, Kaiser GG, Killip T, et al. Ten-year follow-up of survival and myocardial infarction in the randomized coronary artery surgery study. Circulation. 1990;82(5):1629–46.
23. Callahan JA, Seward JB, Tajik AJ, Holmes DR Jr, Smith HC, Reeder GS, et al. Pericardiocentesis assisted by two-dimensional echocardiography. J Thorac Cardiovasc Surg. 1983;85(6):877–9.
24. Seward JB, Hayes DL, Smith HC, Williams DE, Rosenow EC 3rd, Reeder GS, et al. Platypnea-orthodeoxia: clinical profile, diagnostic workup, management, and report of seven cases. Mayo Clin Proc. 1984;59(4):221–31.
25. Nippoldt TB, Edwards WD, Holmes DR Jr, Reeder GS, Hartzler GO, Smith HC. Right ventricular endomyocardial biopsy: clinicopathologic correlates in 100 consecutive patients. Mayo Clin Proc. 1982;57(7):407–18.
26. Clements IP, Strelow DA, Becker GP, Vlietstra RE, Brown ML. Radionuclide evaluation of peripheral circulatory dynamics: new clinical application of blood pool scintigraphy for measuring limb venous volume, capacity, and blood flow. Am Heart J. 1981;102(6 Pt 1):980–3.
27. Hartzler GO, Smith HC, Vlietstra RE, Oberle DA, Strelow DA. Coronary blood-flow responses during successful percutaneous transluminal coronary angioplasty. Mayo Clin Proc. 1980;55(1):45–9.
28. Gruntzig A. Transluminal dilatation of coronary-artery stenosis. Lancet. 1978;1(8058):263.
29. Gruntzig A, Senning A, Siegenthaler W. Third symposium on ischemic heart disease 1978:325–343.
30. Fye W. Caring for the heart, vol. 672. New York: Oxford University Press; 2015.
31. Cobb LA, Thomas GI, Dillard DH, Merendino KA, Bruce RA. An evaluation of internal-mammary-artery ligation by a double-blind technic. N Engl J Med. 1959;260(22):1115–8.

Chapter 3
1980s: Expanding the Practice

David R. Holmes Jr., Hugh C. Smith, and Ronald E. Vlietstra

The 1980s Quadrennial Review reiterated and emphasized that the major function of the cardiac laboratory was to obtain the data needed for the accurate anatomic and physiologic assessment of both congenital and acquired cardiovascular disease. In addition to that fundamental mission, interventional therapeutic procedures were to become an increasingly major part of the practice requiring new imaging modalities and recording equipment, expanded skill sets, and an increasing interchange with multiple stakeholders including CV surgery, the CCU, echocardiographers, hematology, and basic scientists among others. Topics of interest expanded greatly (Table 3.1).

The background of this transformational technology and approaches had been laid by Seldinger, Sones, Dotter, Judkins, and Zeitler (Fig. 3.1), each of whom had set the stage with their investigations, development of new technology, implementation of new approaches for coronary angiography, and treatment of peripheral arterial disease. These efforts blossomed with the involvement of Andreas Grüntzig, initially in the peripheral arterial field where he had been trained as an angiologist and then its subsequent migration to the coronary arterial arena. Using equipment initially hand modeled and fabricated on a kitchen table in Zurich, a series of peripheral and coronary artery prototypes were developed and then tested in animal models. Following that, the classic, iconic picture from the 49th Scientific Sessions of the American Heart Association in 1976 shows Dr. Grüntzig describing his

D. R. Holmes Jr. (✉)
Department of Cardiovascular Diseases, Mayo Clinic, Rochester, MN, USA
e-mail: Holmes.david@mayo.edu

H. C. Smith
Mayo Clinic (retired), Rochester, MN, USA

R. E. Vlietstra
Mayo Clinic (retired), Rochester, MN, USA

Watson Clinic (retired), Lakeland, FL, USA

D. R. Holmes Jr., R. L. Frye (eds.), *The Mayo Clinic Cardiac Catheterization Laboratory*, https://doi.org/10.1007/978-3-030-79329-6_3

Table 3.1 Expanding the focus of interest and personnel

Angioplasty in multivessel disease	New staff members, and Fred Bove returns to Temple
New interventional catheters	Changing the drug protocols for angioplasty
Intracoronary thrombolytics and the TIMI trials	Angioplasty in total occlusions
Angioplasty following thrombolytics in acute MI	Angioplasty in venous grafts
Angioplasty as the primary approach in acute MI	Contrast materials and renal complications
The revival of transseptal catheterization	Balloon angioplasty for restenosis
David Holmes takes over from Hugh Smith as adult Director in the lab	Valvuloplasty
The BARI trial	Complete versus incomplete revascularization
Drug assessment for primary pulmonary hypertension	The elderly and angioplasty
Working with GE to improve imaging systems	Angioplasty of internal mammary grafts
Starting coronary atherectomy, including pathology findings	The start of Rob Schwartz laboratory work
Introducing coronary stents, the Roubin stent	Laser atherectomy

experience with coronary dilations in a canine model (Fig. 3.2). The subsequent events have been elegantly and fully described in the history of coronary angioplasty [1] which resulted in the first successful dilation procedure to treat an isolated single-vessel proximal LAD stenosis in a 38-year-old man on September 16, 1977, in Zurich, Switzerland (Fig. 3.3). This first successful procedure was then described in a LANCET communication, and interest expanded exponentially. There were multiple consequences of this, including new strategies of care, new devices, new applications in noncardiac fields, and, very importantly, new approaches for communication and education. Dr. Grüntzig was inundated by requests to visit and observe procedures. Dr. Vlietstra was one of such individuals who visited, made rounds, and reviewed cases during 1978–1979. These requests, however, became overwhelming, resulting in the organization and introduction of meetings in Zurich that included pioneers in the field, medical industry, cardiologists interested in learning the procedures, cardiovascular surgeons, hospital administrators, and regulatory agencies among others. The meetings/courses were based on the centerpiece of live cases performed with the chance to interact with the audience as well as the faculty. This approach to education with presentation of patients being treated online during the courses revolutionized the field and has become standard for many local, regional, and international conferences since then. The Zurich trip was a pilgrimage of sorts and fostered networking with the other stakeholders as well as the development of new technology, innovation, and research.

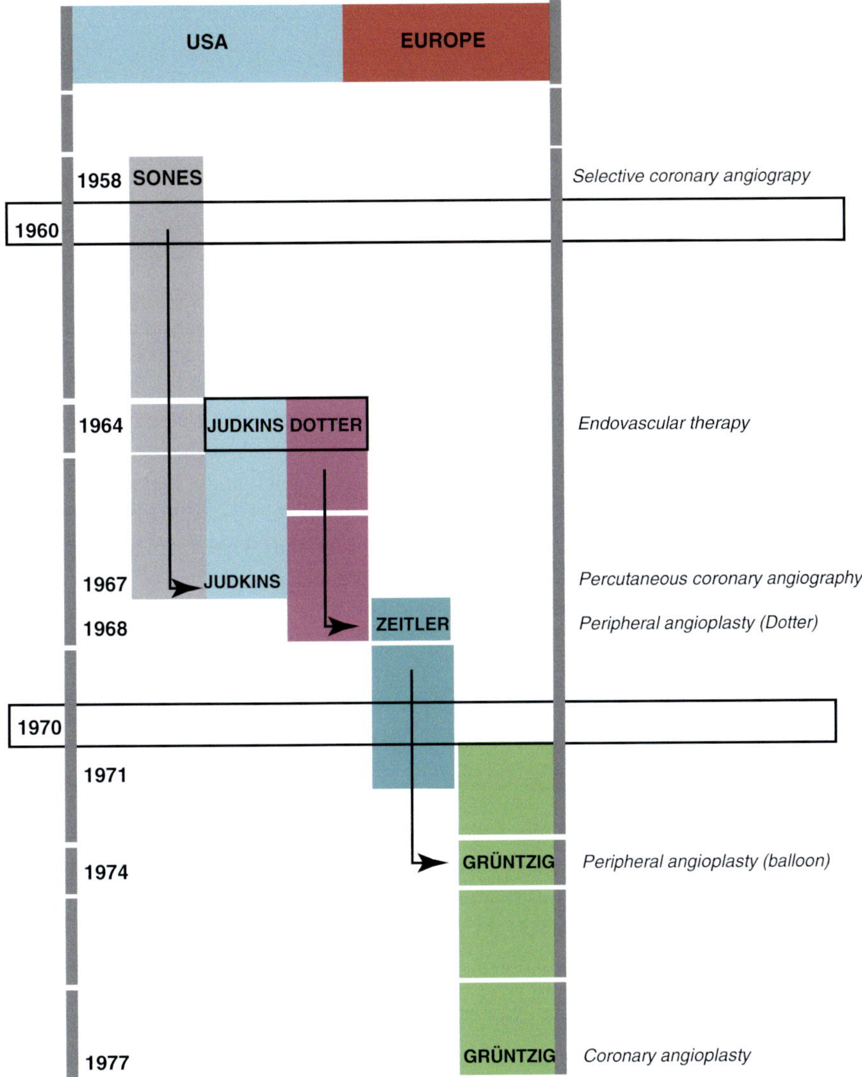

Fig. 3.1 The historical background of percutaneous strategies that had been developed by pioneering approaches and pioneers in both USA and Europe resulted in the eventual field of percutaneous revascularization strategies

The setting was iconic—Zurich, Switzerland, where Dr. Grüntzig might arrive to the hospital on his motorbike. The auditorium with theater seating focused on the screens which transmitted live cases. Dr. Hans Peter Krayenbuehl, Chair of Cardiology, hosted the meeting, but seemed discomfited by this large audience

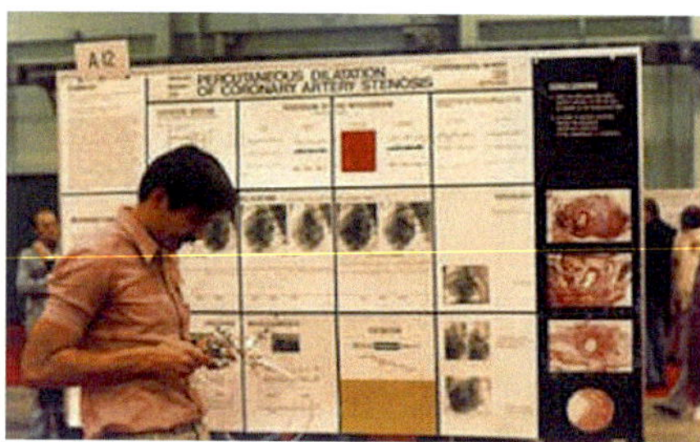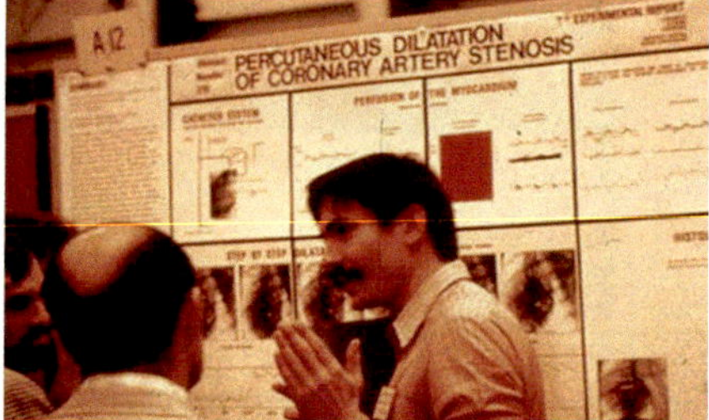

Fig. 3.2 This iconic figure of a poster with a description by Grüntzig of the effects of dilatation in a dog model has been reproduced multiple times. It set the stage for the development of this transformation technology and attracted substantial interest. (Used with permission of Mayo Foundation)

coming to learn from his junior colleague (Fig. 3.4). In the very earliest days, members of the audience presented their own case series which were then written by hand on the blackboard and added to the tally. Mayo Clinic had a presence at some of the earliest meetings with Drs. Smith, Vlietstra, and Hartzler. David Holmes, the newest addition to the Mayo Clinic cardiac laboratory staff, back from the US Navy, participated in a subsequent Zurich meeting and presented an update of Mayo Clinic cases (Fig. 3.5). He then presented the world's first basilar artery angioplasty. The patient, a Montana rancher, was severely symptomatic, with more than 20 drop attacks due to vertebrobasilar artery insufficiency. He had lost his driver's license due to auto accidents caused by transient losses of consciousness and was referred to Dr. Thoralf Sundt, Mayo Clinic Chair of Neurosurgery. The patient was found to have a severe basilar artery stenosis, an underdeveloped circle of Willis (Fig. 3.6), and was not a candidate for a surgical procedure that had been pioneered by Dr. Sundt. To relieve the incapacitating symptoms, Drs. Sundt and Smith then planned basilar artery angioplasty, a procedure never previously reported. This was performed by Sundt and Smith in the neurosurgical suite at St. Mary's Hospital, with the patient anesthetized in an upright sitting position for surgical exposure of the vertebral artery above the spinal atlas. The dilating catheter was introduced through the exposed vertebral artery and advanced to the basilar artery, under fluoroscopic guidance that was marginal, at best (Fig. 3.6b). Radiologic imaging, provided by and dependent on a small portable C-arm unit wheeled into the surgical suite, did not have image intensification, and the basilar artery lies between radiologically dense petrous portions of the skull, all of which led to suboptimal imaging. The procedure which used a fixed wire DG 20–30 and 3.0-mm balloon catheter inflated three times to 6 atmospheres followed by three further inflations with a 3.7-mm balloon was successful (Fig. 3.6c) [2] with a residual hazy lumen but normal flow.

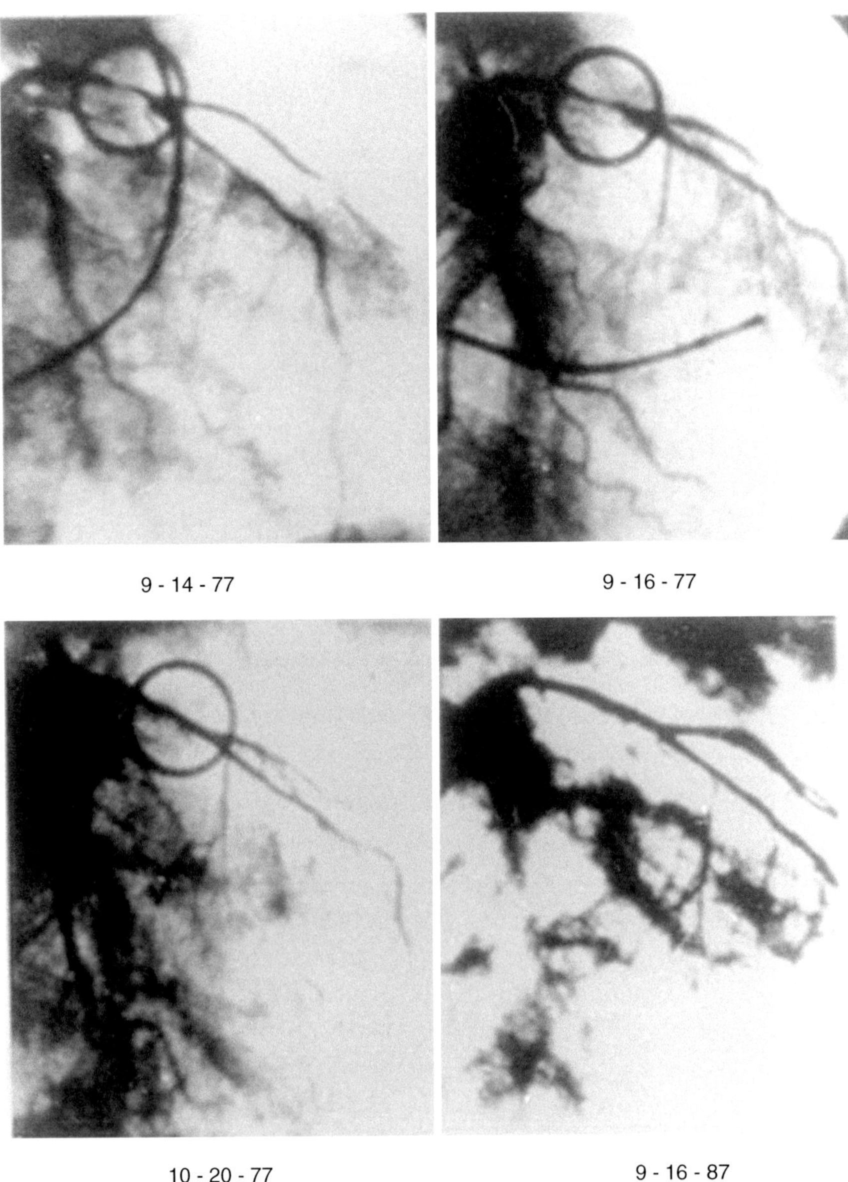

Fig. 3.3 Angiograms of the first dilatation performed by Andreas Grüntzig, September 16, 1977. As can be seen, a proximal LAD lesion was dilated, leading to lasting results seen on a follow-up angiogram in 1987. (Used with permission of Mayo Foundation)

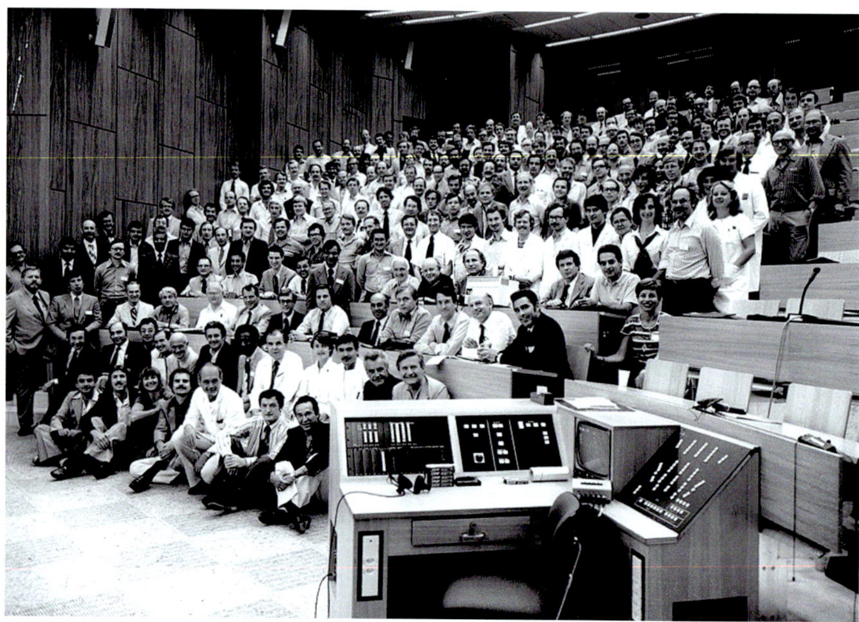

Fig. 3.4 Subsequent meetings in the same theater setting became increasingly popular. These pictures documented the presence of the earliest pioneers Sones, Judkins, Amplatz, Myler, and Stertzer among others along with Grüntzig. (Used with permission of Mayo Foundation)

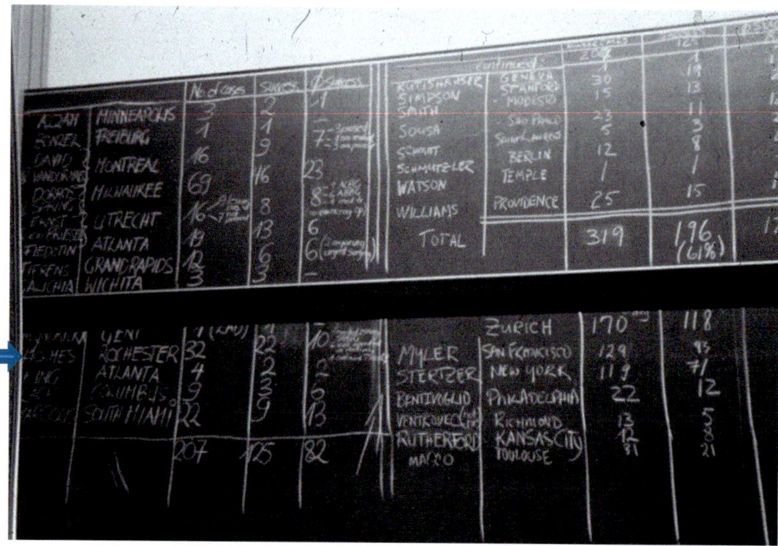

Fig. 3.5 The blackboard here which was positioned on the dais during early Zurich meetings captured early cases allowing the audience to follow then the result of multicenter experiences. As seen (*arrow*) Holmes presented Mayo Clinic's first 32 cases. (Used with permission of Mayo Foundation)

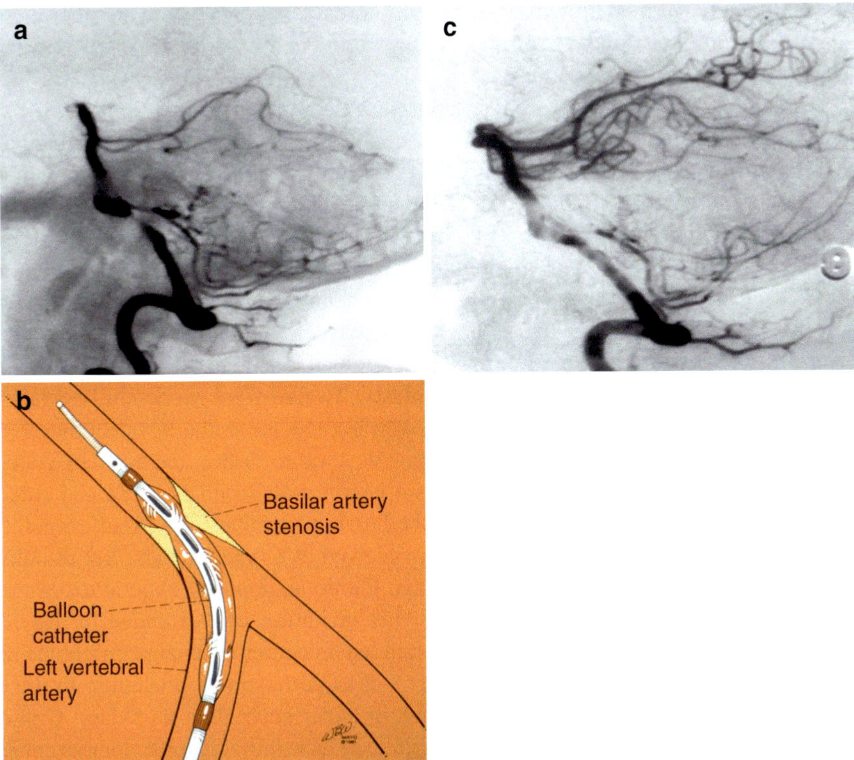

Fig. 3.6 (**a**) Angiography documenting the severe basilar artery stenosis in this patient which was responsible for multiple clinical drop attacks. (**b**) Diagram illustrating the placement of the balloon dilatation catheter through the exposed vertebral artery. (**c**) Following dilatation, the lumen had been significantly improved. The haziness of the residual was similar to that sometimes seen with PTCA in the coronary arteries. (From Sundt et al. [2] Used with permission of Mayo Foundation)

Interesting sidelights included the fact that Holmes was on call following the procedure. Later that day after the procedure was finished and the patient had been returned to his intensive care room, Holmes was called urgently to evaluate the patient who had become quadriplegic (the definition of "a rich emotional experience"—REE). Intravenous heparin had been stopped because of surgical site oozing, but was promptly restarted along with verapamil. The quadriplegia, fortunately, was transient, a relief to all. The patient remained active and asymptomatic for a dozen years, and sent follow-up postcard reports to Drs. Sundt and Smith annually. Six more cases were performed and most were successful. However, in a small number of patients, procedural complications developed which were usually fatal, as the basilar artery supplies vital midbrain structures and basilar angioplasty, unlike with coronary artery angioplasty, does not have a rapid surgical backup option or, more often, no surgical option at all. Accordingly, it was recommended that this procedure be performed only in severely symptomatic patients where no other therapeutic options exist and in settings where excellent fluoroscopic systems were available to guide the procedure.

Although enthusiasm for coronary angioplasty continued to grow in the USA, it received a very uneven reception in other countries. Dr. Ed Varnauskis, Principal Investigator of the European Coronary Surgery Study (ECSS), visited Mayo Clinic in 1981 to compare ECSS and Coronary Artery Surgery Study (CASS) trial methods and outcomes with Bob Frye and other Mayo Clinic CASS colleagues. While at Mayo Clinic, he observed an angioplasty procedure by Hugh Smith in which a totally occluded LAD was successfully dilated, and invited Smith to the Sahlgrenska Institute in Gothenburg, Sweden, to teach angioplasty to their invasive cardiologists. Over a 2-week period at the Sahlgrenska Institute, 15 patients with severe single-vessel disease underwent coronary angioplasty. Twelve were successfully dilated and there were no major complications. Hakan Emanuelsson, the Swedish invasive cardiologist, and an interventional radiologist were quite skilled and assisted Smith on the first five procedures, the next five as operator with Smith assisting and guiding, and the final five with Smith not scrubbed in, but advising. This experience, the first in Sweden, was reported and warmly received at Grand Rounds. Six months later, Smith was invited to present the Mayo Clinic angioplasty experience at the Royal Infirmary in Edinburgh, Scotland. This invitation was extended by Royal Infirmary invasive cardiologists who had attended an earlier Grüntzig conference in Zurich, but had been unable to obtain approval to perform this procedure in their own institution. Smith presented the Grüntzig experience, then the Mayo Clinic experience, by now more than 40 cases, with excellent initial results, angiographic follow-up showing a 20% restenosis rate, and clinical follow-up showing very good symptomatic results in three-fourths of the patients, dating back to the first Mayo Clinic patient, 18 months earlier.

Initially, this was warmly received and there were many questions. However, Sir Michael Oliver, an esteemed national leader in the biochemical and lipid aspects of atherosclerosis, was invited to provide concluding remarks. From the top row of the very steep lecture hall, he commented that in his many years, he had seen medical fads come and go, and opined that angioplasty would be a fad, not supported by longer-term outcomes. Both Smith and his gracious hosts were not optimistic that angioplasty would soon be underway at the Royal Infirmary.

In contrast to this experience, in the USA, a workshop on percutaneous transluminal coronary angioplasty sponsored by the Cardiac Diseases Branch of Heart and Vascular Diseases at NIH was held June 15–16, 1979, less than 2 years after the first successful global experience performed by Dr. Grüntzig (Fig. 3.7). This workshop attended by both Drs. Vlietstra and Hartzler included clinical results, myocardial perfusion, left ventricular function following PTCA, equipment and technical issues, histologic studies, discussion about future research and standardization of the technique, and endpoints. Dr. Michael Mock, Chief of Cardiac Diseases Branch Division of Heart and Vascular Disease of the NHLBI, was one of the conference directors. After each section, there was group discussion followed by recommendations. Out of this came the recommendation that a NHLBI Registry be formed with

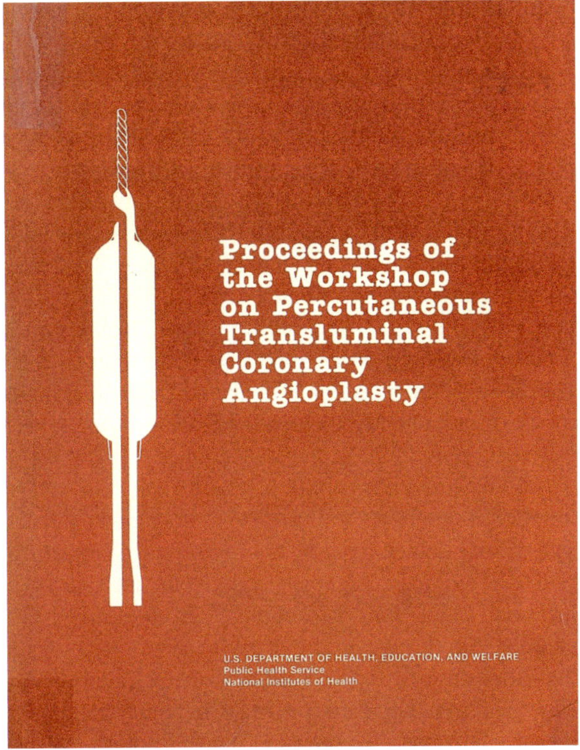

Fig. 3.7 Less than 2 years after the first successful angioplasty by Grüntzig, the National Institutes of Health (NIH) recognizing the potential importance of this transformation technology held a workshop devoted exclusively to it

standard data forms and follow-up and would enroll consecutive patients undergoing treatment. Lloyd Fisher, PhD, the Director of the Coordinating Center for Collaborative Studies in Coronary Artery Surgery and the University of Washington in attendance at the meeting, was instrumental in designing baseline and follow-up data forms for this NHLBI National Registry on Percutaneous Transluminal Coronary Angioplasty Registry.

Both Fisher and Mock subsequently joined the staff of the Cardiovascular Division at Mayo Clinic as superb thought leaders, scientists, physicians, and colleagues and served as advocates for the procedure and for scientific research related to it, participating fully in their roles in the NHLBI Registry and Bypass Angioplasty Revascularization Investigation (BARI) trial. The summation of the meeting was given by Andreas Grüntzig in 1979: "To summarize, my early impression over the last 2 years is that if the patient really needs something other than medical treatment…and if I can demonstrate by an objective measure like thallium or stress tests that this patient has ischemia and a lesion which looks like it can be dilated, then I feel comfortable in doing the procedure." That thought resonated with people in the meeting and throughout the cardiovascular medical community at large. It continues to resonate to this day as we focus on the importance of treatment focused on lesions which produce ischemia. It forms the basis for the subsequent randomized clinical trials up to the future including the ISCHEMIA trial.

In the early 1980s, angioplasty was rapidly evolving. The small fixed guide wire on the early Grüntzig dilating catheters was replaced by a separate guide wire over which the dilating catheter could be introduced. This greatly enhanced the operator's ability to negotiate tight bends and eccentric stenoses in the coronary arteries. Commensurate with technical advances and growing experience and skill, angioplasty outcomes steadily improved. Consequently, the strict initial angioplasty selection criteria were being progressively relaxed and expanded, and the population of patients being considered for angioplasty continued to grow. Fortunately, the cardiac catheterization laboratory, which had experienced a relative shortage of invasive cardiologists for much of the 1970s, had been greatly bolstered by the additions of Vlietstra and Hartzler in 1977 and Holmes in early 1980. They were closely followed by Guy Reeder, Fred Bove, and John Bresnahan, all superb cardiologists with solid technical skills. With the addition of an increasing number of colleagues, robust discussions were common as were strongly held opinions which sometimes were held even in the absence of science.

At this time, Mayo Clinic cardiology staff rotated on 3-week (or multiples thereof) assignments to the various outpatient, inpatient, and laboratory services. The cardiac catheterization laboratory had changed from an exclusively diagnostic role to a combined diagnostic and therapeutic role. Aware of the pace of change and increased complexity and clinical responsibilities that the invasive practice now entailed, Smith requested that all invasive cardiology staff commit at least 50% of their time annually to the cardiac catheterization laboratory practice, so they could stay "on top of their game." He had anticipated some resistance to this, as there were other exciting developments during this period, particularly in echocardiology and nuclear cardiology, but this construct was broadly supported. Several catheterization laboratory colleagues indicated their preference that intervals between cardiac laboratory assignments should not exceed 9 weeks—a reflection of the fact that technical innovations and strategies were changing so frequently.

As has been widely described, PTCA was initially felt to be suitable for patients with proximal, nontortuous, noncalcified, subtotal lesions in patients with stable angina who would be potential candidates for CABG. Of interest, this included patients with LMCA disease, and Mayo investigators performed PTCA in that setting typically with excellent results (Fig. 3.8a, b). The potential size of the patient population, using those angiographic criteria that might be suitable, was investigated by Mayo Clinic investigators using those descriptors in the CASS randomized clinical trial in which Mayo Clinic had enrolled and randomized patients. Using those criteria, it was felt that only approximately 5% of patients would be candidates for this new technique—percutaneous transluminal coronary angioplasty (PTCA) [3].

However, the field of coronary intervention had moved well beyond that initial "constriction" of potential numbers of patients who might benefit. It must be remembered that during this early phase of introduction, complications were not infrequent, related to either difficult anatomy, patient comorbidities, or the first-generation devices routinely available at that time which tended to be rigid, bulky, and nonsteerable. An interesting conversation is vividly remembered by Holmes

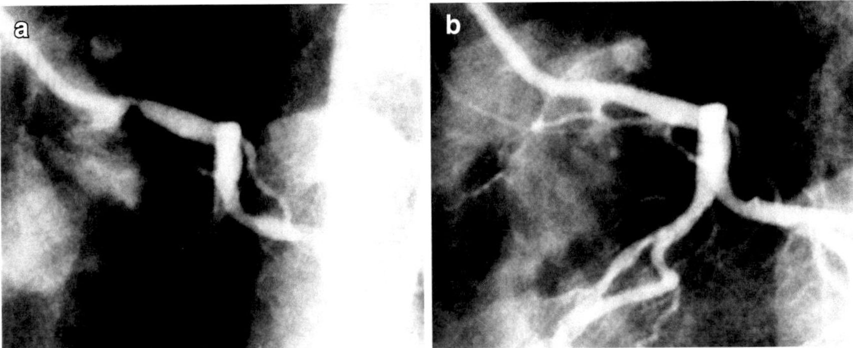

Fig. 3.8 (**a, b**) The initial dilatation criteria included proximal, nontortuous, noncalcified, subtotal lesions. These criteria would have been seen with ostial or mid-shaft LMCA lesions. As can be seen, this ostial LMCA stenosis could be treated although downstream LAD lesions were often co-existent (**a** pre) (**b** post). (From Vlietstra RE, Holmes DR. PTCA, 1987 use with permission of Mayo Foundation)

during his early experience with a complication and resultant poor outcome. After such cases, analyses of the procedure and approaches to mitigate the issues in other cases were typically discussed. After all this time, Holmes remembers in the meeting with Smith following that specific procedure the rather straightforward comment from Smith "that if you can't stand the heat, then it is best to stay out of the kitchen"—a thought which continues to resonate to this day. The evolution from a primarily diagnostic focus in the 1970s to a mixed diagnostic and interventional focus in the 1980s was accompanied by increased invasiveness and complexity, patient benefits and risks, and operator stress. Catheterization laboratory staff in the 1980s had to "up their game." There was intense interest in the field in complications. In the initial NHLBI PTCA Registry from 1978 to 1981 of 1,155 patients, while death was infrequent at 1.2%, the composite of death, MI, or emergency CABG occurred in 8.8% of patients [4]. Subsequent technologic improvements, most prominently the introduction of stents in later decades, dramatically decreased the rates of emergent CABG, thereby improving outcome in the increasing number of patients being treated.

Adjunctive Therapy for PTCA

When Andreas Grüntzig set up his protocol for PTCA, he was concerned about coronary spasm and coronary thrombosis. For the former, he used liberal doses of nitroglycerin, both sublingual and by intracoronary injection. At Mayo Clinic, we had intravenous verapamil available and initially relied on that for preventing spasm; later we used oral calcium blockers instead to minimize the hypotension seen with intravenous administration. We were comforted by the fact that spasm seemed to be an uncommon occurrence, even though we had frequently used multiple guide wires and catheters when addressing complicated lesions and bifurcation disease.

The issue of coronary thrombosis was more problematic. In the early days of the NHLBI PTCA Registry, an acute occlusion occurred in approximately 10% of the cases. Sometimes angiography revealed the presence of a dissection, but, more often, acute thrombosis was suspected as the cause. In addition, the role of antecedent thrombus as a significant risk factor for complications developing during or early after PTCA was first published by Tom Mabin, an interventional fellow from South Africa. During his research experience, he reported on "the role of intracoronary thrombus in coronary occlusion complicating percutaneous transluminal coronary angioplasty" [5]. As part of his training, he had reviewed 238 consecutive patients undergoing PTCA and found that in patients with intracoronary thrombus present prior to dilatation, complete occlusion subsequently developed in 73%. This finding led the way to strategies to mitigate this problem, including more intense antiplatelet and anticoagulant therapies. Declan Sugrue, a fellow of the Royal College of Physicians and Surgeons of Ireland, another advanced invasive cardiology fellow in the cardiac laboratory, reported just 16 months later [6] on a subsequent 297 consecutive angioplasty patients without prior infarction in whom preprocedure antiplatelet therapy and 24-hour post-PTCA intravenous heparin were employed. Antecedent thrombus was present in 34 patients (11%), and abrupt occlusion occurred in 8 of these patients (24%), whereas, in the 263 patients without prior thrombus, complete occlusion during or immediately following the procedure occurred in 34 (13%). It was clear that patients with preexisting thrombus continued to be at greater risk from complete occlusion than patients without thrombus (24% vs 13%), but the incidence of complete occlusion (24%) in these at-risk patients was considerably reduced from the 73% occlusion rate noted prior to initiating a more aggressive antiplatelet and anticoagulation regimen.

These two published studies highlight several key characteristics of the cardiac laboratory during these times. First, the pace of change in the field was rapid, and there was ongoing critical evaluation of the procedure protocols and outcomes. Second, identification of procedural risk factors (such as antecedent intracoronary thrombus) led promptly to procedural changes aimed at mitigation. Third, the effectiveness of these mitigating procedural changes was critically examined and promptly reported, thus contributing to the global evolution and improvement in an important interventional technique. Finally, the performance of the procedures, their critical evaluation, and reporting on the effectiveness of these protocol changes on outcomes would not have been possible without significant contributions from the cardiac laboratory fellows. The cardiac laboratory was blessed by our ability to select outstanding national and international fellows from all over who applied for these coveted interventional fellowship positions, and all benefited greatly. Mabin and Sugrue are but two examples of the many fellows who have contributed to the laboratory's clinical and academic productivity. Mabin returned to South Africa, where he became a prominent pioneer in interventional cardiology and was the founding president of the South African Society of Cardiovascular Intervention (SASCI). Sugrue returned to Ireland and became Professor and Chair, Cardiology, Mater Misericordiae Hospital, and University College in Dublin, Ireland.

This experience reminds us of the mutual benefits of our educational programs, as summarized by William J. Mayo many years before. "Each day I go through the hospitals surrounded by younger men, they give me of their dreams, and I give them of my experience, and I get the better of the exchange." All cardiac laboratory consultants, working side by side with the fellows during a procedure, in post procedure analysis and report generation, and in manuscript writing, have had good reason to echo his words.

Grüntzig's initial protocol included heparin and dextran as prophylaxis against thrombosis. We continued with the former (to an APTT of twice normal) but, after an in-house-controlled comparison of dextran and saline, soon abandoned the latter. Mayo Clinic's good experience with aspirin and dipyridamole in CABG patients led us to prescribe those two drugs preprocedurally as well.

Looking back, up to 40 years later, it is still easy to remember the uncertainties that characterized much of what we faced in dealing with symptomatic, and sometimes acutely compromised, patients with coronary artery disease. What progress we achieved during those times was in great part due to the support and encouragement of our Mayo Clinic colleagues in and outside the cardiac laboratory in both cardiovascular and cardiovascular surgeries.

As the technology improved and as the number of operators trained increased, the number of patients expanded greatly. In addition, patient selection criteria broadened widely to include patients with unstable angina and myocardial infarction including STEMI and what was then termed "non-transmural myocardial infarction." Information on the shorter-term outcome of this latter group of patients had come from observations by Drs. N.P. Madigan and B. Rutherford at Mayo Clinic which had led to more aggressive strategies. While intracoronary thrombus had been recognized as the culprit in STEMI, early work from Mayo Clinic with Holmes and Fuster among others documented, for the first time in the literature, that it was also important as part of the pathophysiology of unstable angina and NSTEMI [7] (Fig. 3.9). Re-thrombosis during or following PTCA became more common once we started treatment of patients with acute myocardial infarction. In retrospect, some of these problems were aggravated by the frequent concomitant use of fibrinolytics and the lack of availability of more powerful antiplatelet drugs, such as abciximab, which was not widely available until the mid-1990s.

Recognition of the role of early and prompt revascularization in these latter two groups of patients, specifically STEMI, gave rise to the development of two major strategies of care, namely, thrombolytic therapy, initially with streptokinase and then with several selective fibrinolytic agents, versus PTCA alone. The first case of primary angioplasty at Mayo Clinic was performed in a young patient who had become trapped while spelunking in a cave in Forestville/Mystery Cave State Park

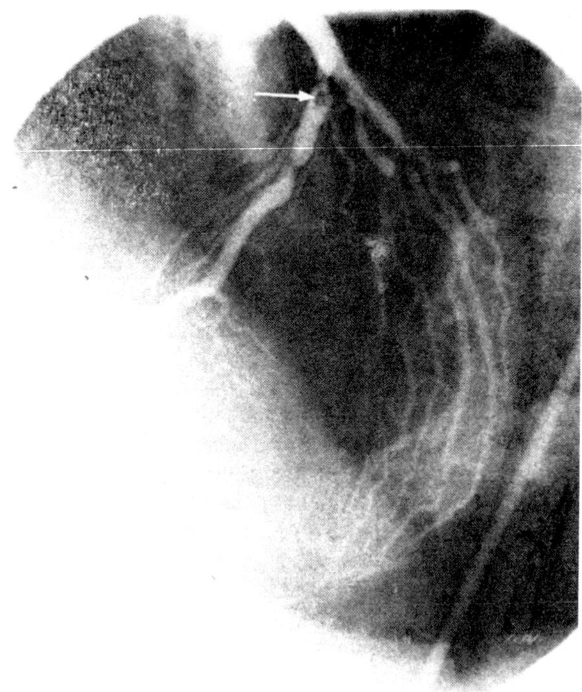

Fig. 3.9 Although thrombus was known to be an important element in STEMI, there was little information in patients presenting with other acute coronary syndromes. In a very early report from Mayo Clinic (Holmes and Fuster), intracoronary thrombus was documented in patients with unstable angina. Left anterior oblique coronary angiogram performed in a patient with an acute ischemic syndrome, but not a STEMI in whom intracoronary thrombus was identified proximal to severe lesion in the LAD. (From Holmes et al. [7]; used with permission)

and had developed chest pain consistent with a STEMI. Upon urgent arrival to the catheterization laboratory, the infarct-related vessel occlusion was successfully dilated without lytic therapy. Other strategies were developed in clinical practice and then studied in multiple randomized clinical trials. Combined therapy with lytic therapy followed by PTCA was common in patients in whom lytic reperfusion was not felt to have been initially successful based on incomplete improvement in ST elevation or in whom a complication such as recurrent chest pain and ECG changes had occurred, suggesting reocclusion of the infarct-related artery. There were robust discussions at local, regional, national, and international meetings about optimal treatment strategies. A review of the talk titles given by one of the authors during that decade attests to the widespread interest in the field (Table 3.2). An interesting sidelight was the development of debates concerning crucial issues such as PTCA versus thrombolysis and PTCA versus CABG. These debates have continued to offer opportunities for excellent discourse on not only science but also entertainment, although the former remains central. The opportunities in the field offered the potential for scientific study and evaluation in multiple clinical and registry studies including the NHLBI Thrombolysis in Myocardial Infarction trial. Mayo Clinic participated not only the randomized trials but developed a robust triage referral strategy for primary PTCA from the region which facilitated early access for patients presenting to outside hospitals which did not have interventional facilities. As part of that process, the "Mayo Randomized Clinical Trial of PCI Versus Thrombolysis" was designed, implemented, and subsequently published in NEJM.

Table 3.2 Lecture titles in the field delivered by Mayo Clinic physicicans

Controversies concerning optimal strategies for infarction
Acute infarction, Mayo Clinic, 1985
Techniques of reperfusion
Mechanical reperfusion alone or combined with lytic therapy, Hawaii, 1986
Streptokinase vs PTCA for myocardial infarction
Heart attack-counterattack
Thrombolysis in acute myocardial infarction: results of multicenter trials for streptokinase and t-PA, Orlando, FL
Results of PTCA after lytic therapy, Orlando, FL
PTCA—unstable angina, Hawaii, June 1986
PTCA during acute infarction, Dublin, Ireland, 1986
Reperfusion therapy during acute infarction
PTCA after thrombolysis, New Orleans, LA, March 1987
Thrombolytic therapies in myocardial infarction, Seattle, WA, April 1987
Thrombolytic therapy in AMI, Cape Town, South Africa, April 1987
Role of coronary angioplasty in acute myocardial infarction, Williamsburg, VA, April 1987
PTCA in acute myocardial infarction, Santa Barbara, CA, September 1987
Thrombolytic therapy, Milwaukee, WI, January 1988
What is the role of PTCA post-thrombolysis?, Dublin, Ireland, July 1988
Thrombolytic therapy in acute myocardial infarction: Update, St. Paul, MN, September 1988
Thrombolysis and myocardial infarction—1988: what should we be doing?, October 1988
PTCA in acute ischemic syndromes, October 1988
What is the best reperfusion strategy?, October 1988
Angioplasty in acute MI, Rockland, ME, February 1989
The conservative versus aggressive posture toward myocardial infarction, Anaheim, CA, March 1989
Update in the treatment of acute myocardial infarction, Minneapolis, MN, April 1989
Thrombolytic therapy, Austin, MN, and Rochester, MN, August 1989
Thrombolysis therapy in acute MI, Charles City, IA, October 1989
An interventionalist's view of thrombolysis, New Orleans, LA, November 1989

Leadership Changes

In 1984, Dick Weeks stepped down as Chair, Department of Internal Medicine, which comprised, at that time, more than 400 internists, and after the previously described rigorous Mayo Clinic leadership succession process, Bob Frye was selected as the next Department of Internal Medicine Chair. This announcement was warmly greeted by all cardiologists and internists, as Bob's quiet, inclusive, steady, and forward-looking leadership as the Cardiovascular Division Chair was broadly appreciated within the department and clinic-wide. This created an open Cardiovascular Division Chair position, and several weeks after Bob's appointment, Hugh Smith was selected to succeed Bob as the Cardiovascular Division Chair. Shortly thereafter, Hugh Smith appointed Holmes as Director of the adult section of the cardiac catheterization laboratory. He was a skilled and experienced interventional cardiologist, who had clearly benefited from the leadership training he had received in the US Navy. He had that unique blend of keeping his patients' safety and well-being paramount without being risk aversive and was willing to thoughtfully explore new and untested technologies that had the potential benefit to advance patient care. Importantly, he was a consistent advocate of the critical evaluation of these new technologies, both within the Mayo Clinic Cath Lab and in the laboratory's participation and leadership in national clinical trials and registries.

These leadership transitions were seamless and well received. This is the usual experience at Mayo Clinic. Unlike department leadership changes in many academic medical centers, where a "new broom sweeps clean," there were not wholesale committee, division and section chair changes based on academic political allegiances.

This did create some interesting administrative structures and relationships. Bob Frye, Internal Medicine Department Chair, continued his practice, education, and research in the Division of Cardiovascular Diseases, under the direction of Hugh Smith who continued his cardiovascular practice, education, and research in the Department of Medicine, under the direction of Frye. While theoretically, this might cause difficulties, this never happened. This is due, in large part, to the largely unspoken but powerful cohesive culture and team approach that guides the performance and behavior of all Mayo Clinic staff, including its leaders.

There was an interesting personal and humorous sidelight to these leadership announcements. Hugh took a phone call in his catheterization laboratory office between his first and second procedures from the Chair of the Personnel Committee of the Board and was informed of his selection as next Cardiovascular Division Chair. He was admonished that he could call his wife and let her know, but he was to not speak about this to anyone until an official announcement had gone out the following day. However, when he came back to his office between his second and third procedures of the day, his office door was darkened by brothers Dennis and John Bresnahan, both catheterization laboratory staff, and both between 6 foot 3 and 6 foot 4, standing side by side with big grins on their faces. They congratulated him on his new appointment, without divulging how they knew, and strongly recommended that he consider future cardiovascular consultant compensation on the basis of height! They all had a good laugh and went back to their caseloads, but Hugh was left with a strong reminder that there were few real secrets in a close-knit organization, and to never underestimate the power of the "grapevine."

Bob Frye had continued to work, at significant personal effort, in the cardiac laboratory after being named division chair, in large part because of the increasing invasive cardiology workload and lab staff shortage in 1975. Hugh Smith, however, stepped out of the laboratory, as in 1984 (unlike 1975) it had an excellent complement of skilled invasive cardiologists, and Hugh, with his new administrative duties, would be unable to meet the "50% rule" that he had promulgated in 1980, in the early days of angioplasty when the increased complexity and pace of change required a greater time commitment. In addition, there were now a number of excellent cardiovascular clinical laboratories (echo, nuclear, pacemaker, vascular, electrophysiology) in addition to the cardiac catheterization laboratory. All were growing in clinical productivity and academic excellence, and all had a compelling need for resources, particularly space, equipment, consultant, and technical staff. A position of relative impartiality would help Hugh in meeting these competing resource requirements.

The cardiac catheterization laboratory continued to perform in an outstanding manner in all three shields under Holmes' leadership, with an acceleration in clinical trial involvement, and exploration of other promising technologies, as outlined below.

Jim Chesebro played a vital role in engaging Mayo Clinic in a series of NHLBI trials under the TIMI family of trials, and the catheterization laboratory staff were active participants in all phases of TIMI's recruitment of patients with acute myocardial infarction for intravenous and intracoronary fibrinolytic therapy. Often these trials also involved nuclear medicine expertise, Ray Gibbons (then working in the catheterization laboratory) and his colleagues, who quantitated the volume of myocardium at risk and, post intervention, the volume of myocardium which had been salvaged.

Lloyd Fisher, at the University of Washington, and Katherine Detre, at the University of Pittsburgh, were principal statisticians on many of these NHLBI trials in the 1970s and 1980s, and they educated many Mayo Clinic investigators on the complexities of trial design and conduct. Both ascribed to the doctrine that, when designed and conducted properly, the statistical conclusions from randomized clinical trials were much more straightforward versus the inherent uncertainties always attached to nonrandomized comparisons. Lloyd Fisher joined the staff and led us to better understand the mysteries of how statisticians think, a daunting prospect in years past, but provided a better understanding of the crucial importance of well-designed studies.

As the field continued to expand, unmet and unexpected opportunities/challenges were recognized. During this time was a proliferation of talks on complications with interesting aphorisms such as "IWIHDT," aka "I wish I hadn't done that" and "larger than God had intended it to be", aka "coronary perforation." Complication management case-based series at local and national and regional meetings were typically completely oversubscribed. Such case-based educational meetings in all areas of medicine have become dominant strategies, maintaining audience attention and participation and having perhaps the best relevance to practice.

Other unmet clinical needs identified included the presence of a chronic total occlusion in native coronary arteries in the absence of acute infarction. The first two studies ever published in that patient group included one from Mayo Clinic involving 24 patients with total occlusion not associated with acute transmural myocardial infarction and documented that, in selected cases, chronic occlusions could be successfully treated percutaneously, leading to the now vibrant field of chronic total occlusion (CTO) intervention (Fig. 3.10) [8]. A subsequent hallmark article from Dr. Mandeep Singh, an advanced fellow at Mayo Clinic, documented the utility of bilateral coronary arterial injections for improving the outcome of CTO by adding the ability to identify the distal vessel, thereby guiding the intervention. This approach, which relied on coronary injections in a contralateral coronary artery which supplied collaterals to the occluded coronary artery allowing assessment of

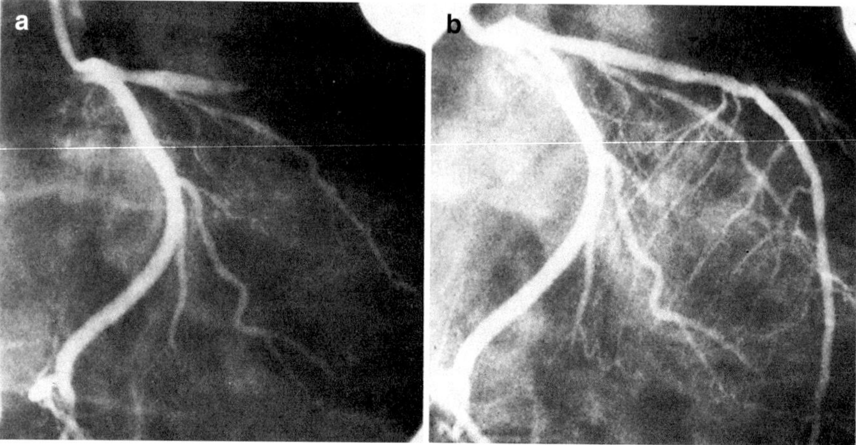

Fig. 3.10 Initial criteria for PTCA included a subtotal stenosis. Very early on, patients presenting for angiography sometimes had a total occlusion even though the patient was not in the throes of an acute myocardial infarction. Two very early publications including that of Holmes documented the efficacy of elective dilatation of a chronic total occlusion in that setting in this case a mid-LAD occlusion. This early report helped set the stage for subsequent interest in the field which continues to grow to this day. (Left panel, baseline; right panel, post-uncomplicated PCI). (**a**) Total occlusion of the middle left anterior descending artery. (**b**) After dilation, there is visualization of the distal left anterior descending artery with minor residual stenosis. (From Holmes et al. [8]; used with permission)

the size and course of the target occlusion, is now the cornerstone in virtually every CTO procedure.

Other unmet needs during coronary intervention were the presence of lesion calcification, large bulky lesions, ostial location, major side branch stenosis, and very severe tortuosity.

Documentation and recognition of the importance of these resulted in the development of what were then novel adjunctive strategies including atherectomy to debulk lesions, rotational atherectomy to treat calcified stenoses, and laser angioplasty for undilatable lesions, and then the initial application of coronary stenting as a bailout procedure for dissections or acute closure after PTCA. These new technologies were all added to the therapeutic armamentarium during this decade. After their initial description in small registry series, they became the subject of randomized clinical trials and registries. Some eventually failed to improve outcomes in randomized clinical trials and registries and became sidelined.

Directional Coronary Atherectomy

At Stanford, the inventive entrepreneur, John Simpson, who had already pioneered the over-the-wire concept for balloon angioplasty catheter, developed a new concept of plaque removal using a cutting tool mounted on a larger catheter, the idea being that, by resecting and removing obstructive tissue, the coronary lumen could be better widened and restenosis might be decreased. He also hypothesized that improving the lumen by plaque removal would lead to a more predictable angiographic result than that achieved by the barotrauma of balloon dilatation and was able to convince the FDA that a select few centers should evaluate his new device. Simpson had had many dealings with Holmes and Vlietstra, and he recruited Mayo Clinic to participate in this very early experience. After gaining approval for the protocol from the CV Practice Committee, Holmes and Vlietstra proceeded with their first case in October 1988, under the watchful guidance of one of Simpson's colleagues, Matt Selmon.

The case went well, and the extracted plaque was sent for pathology review. On this and subsequent cases, there was a high level of success; the major challenge was in obtaining good hemostasis in the femoral artery on withdrawal of the large 11F sheath that was required to accommodate the bulkier catheter delivery system.

In those heady first few weeks, many patients were treated with this new tool; 1 day, we treated five cases. Kirk Garratt, a bright new staff member, quickly joined the team. Bill Edwards, an energetic cardiac pathologist, was able to demonstrate that the cutting tool removed plaque, media, and, in a couple of cases, even extended to the adventitia. No early clinical consequences followed such deep resections. Although with later and sometimes even more aggressive resection, the artery became somewhat bigger than nature had ever intended (aka perforation). In this case, the concept of bigger is better popularized as an approach to prevent restenosis was not always a good idea.

Urs Kauffman, a young cardiologist from Lausanne, Switzerland, was with us at the time, and he oversaw the data collection and follow-up of these patients. This led to a 1989 report on the 50 patients, including 8 with saphenous vein graft stenosis, treated in the first 3 months, [9] and not much later, a comprehensive book on the subject co-edited by Holmes and Garratt (Fig. 3.11) [10].

Other devices, after multiple iterations and transformations with more data and improved technology, became mainstream, essential components for the procedures such as stent implantation. The stent journey has been well described. Endovascular prostheses manufactured with different metals and designs had been tested in animal models in both cardiac and noncardiac vascular beds beginning in the mid-decade years. The first coronary stents were implanted in Europe, in 1986, by Jacques Puel and Ulrich Sigwart. There was much excitement over this new development because it promised to expand the lumen greater than with angioplasty alone and it might rescue those vessels where there was recoil or when acute occlusion had occurred. Restenosis might also be lessened.

Other companies soon introduced stents for evaluation in the USA, including Cook, Inc. in Indiana. Cesare Gianturco, a Mayo Clinic-trained radiologist, worked with the Cook company on several stent designs, possibly applicable in any tubular structures within the body, including, of course, arteries. For his version of a coronary stent, Gianturco worked with Gary Roubin in Birmingham, Alabama, and they came up with the FLEX design, a balloon-expandable stent mounted on a thin coronary catheter.

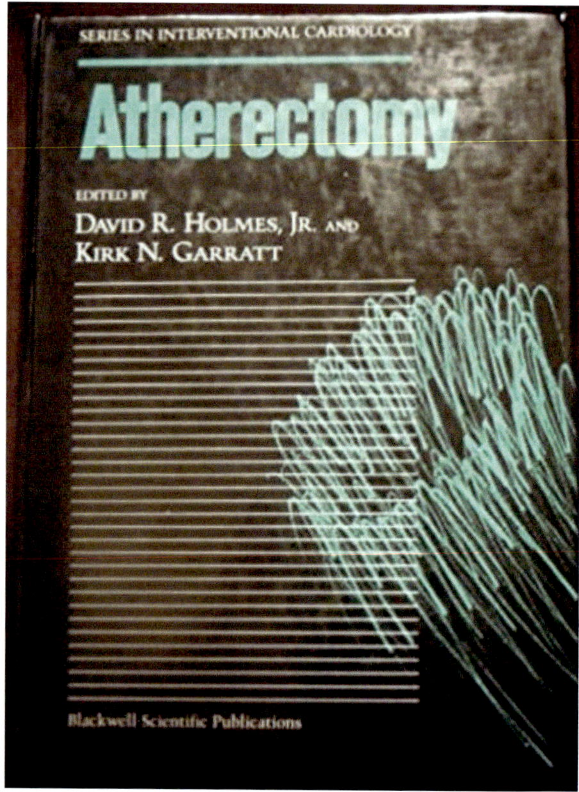

Fig. 3.11 Dissemination of early reports on new technology and strategies of care was an extremely important part of education, practice, and development in the cardiac catheterization laboratory. Such projects which were expected resulted in books as this and formed the underpinnings of the science and practice of interventional cardiology. Of interest the expectation of involvement in publication and presentation of data had been a prerequisite put in place by Frederick Willius when he was the Chief of Cardiology and who many considered to be one of the first "Academic Cardiologists." (Cover image used with permission)

In those early days of interventional cardiology, most of the highly active practitioners knew each other. Grüntzig had introduced his Emory training fellow, Gary Roubin, to Vlietstra in early 1985, and Sigwart was a friend of many of us, even coming to Rochester in 1989. Gianturco stopped by the catheterization laboratory on one of his Mayo Clinic visits. Mayo Clinic was invited to be one of the evaluation sites when the Gianturco-Roubin stent was approved in 1989 for closer investigation.

Early conditions potentially suitable included restenosis, aortocoronary bypass grafts, and acute occlusion following PTCA. However, an early experience of 117 self-expanding stents initiated toward the end of the 1980s [11, 12] documented subsequent complete stent occlusion in 24% of patients, long-term restenosis in 14% of those stents which remained patent, and a 1-year mortality of 7.6%. This

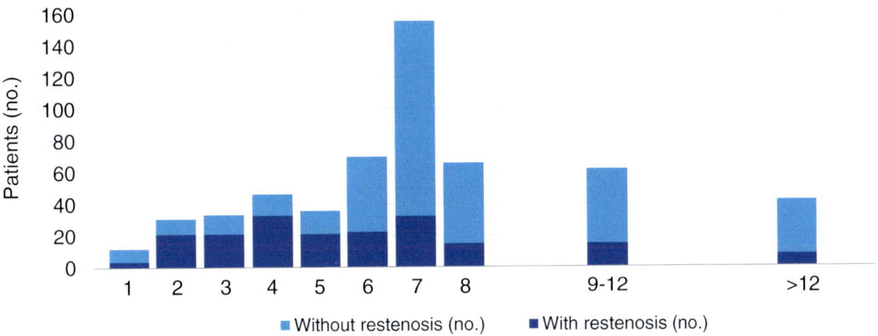

Fig. 3.12 Restenosis post PTCA began to be identified as a cause of recurrent symptoms. The timing of it had remained unclear as had the effect of it on symptoms. In the early days of PTCA, many centers in the NHLBI PTCA Registry had implemented a process of surveillance follow-up angiography. In this initial registry, angiographic restenosis was identified in 33.6% of patients. As seen, restenosis typically occurred early and within the first 7 months. The symptoms were interesting in that not all patients presenting with angina post procedure had restenosis but instead may have had other lesions as the etiology of the clinical presentation. In addition, not all patients with restenosis had symptoms. These data had important implications for subsequent trials that used restenosis as either a clinical or angiographic endpoint for assessment of different approaches. (From Holmes et al. Am J Cardiol 1984;53:77C–81C; used with permission)

specific data cast a pall over the field. Persistence would be needed in the following decade.

As part of this process, the urgent need for data sources was identified. The initial NHLBI PTCA Registry of consecutive patients had been developed [13]. One of the most important early analyses included the description of restenosis (Fig. 3.12). The first publication of this issue coming from Mayo Clinic investigators evaluated the results of follow-up angiography in patients from 27 centers enrolled in the PTCA Registry [4]. In this series, restenosis was documented in 33.6%. Other salient features included the fact that it was documented typically within the first 7 months post procedure with the return of symptoms. Very importantly, however, surveillance in patients undergoing angiography without chest pain revealed 14% had restenosis, and in patients with definite or probable angina, 44% of patients did not have restenosis (Fig. 3.13). This data from 1984 would be identified repeatedly in the field until the introduction of coronary stents. The phenomenon of restenosis has been the focus of a whole field of subsequent new approaches and technology.

In addition, during this time, the need for data led to the development of other local, regional, national, and international sources. Building on the excellent experience with clinical trials that Mayo Clinic had had in the 1970s (CASS and the Chesebro study), catheterization laboratory investigators embraced a national trend for documenting results in national registries and subjecting important questions to randomized trials, both in-house and in collaboration with others around the country. It was a move away from reliance on personal and collective observational experience, and it recognized the statistical power of rigorous patient selection, randomized selection, and large cohort numbers. This Mayo Clinic PTCA database

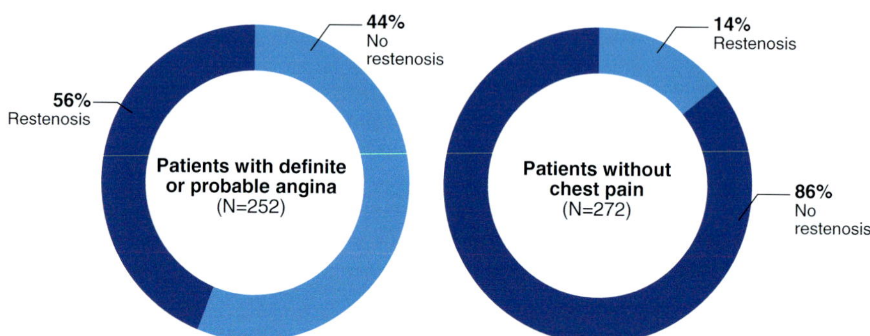

Fig. 3.13 An important consideration related to routine surveillance angiography. In this data from the NHLBI PTCA Registry of surveillance in patients undergoing angiography without chest pain, 14% had restenosis, and in patients with definite or probably angina, 44% of patients did not actually have restenosis. (From Holmes et al: Am J Cardiol 1984;53:77C–81C; used under license)

was designed and implemented by Vlietstra working with Dr. Lila Elveback and Kent Bailey. The Mayo Clinic PTCA Registry enrolled all consecutive patients undergoing percutaneous revascularization at Mayo Clinic and continues to accumulate initial and follow-up data on all patients who have undergone PCI at Mayo Clinic in the past; these data have provided the unique, long-term information available on strategies of care with percutaneous revascularization and have spawned multiple publications and research grants.

The importance of left ventricular function on outcome was increasingly recognized. Ron Vlietstra and Lila Elveback performed an analysis of survival predictors in medically treated patients in Bob Frye's registry of patients who had coronary angiography between 1966 and 1972. The most reliable predictor of 2-year survival was left ventricular ejection fraction (Fig. 3.14a). When medically treated patients were compared with patients who had coronary bypass surgery, 3-year survival was significantly improved ($p < 0.05$) in those who had an ejection fraction between 25% and 50% (Fig. 3.14b), but not if it was <25% or >50% [14].

This survival advantage for those with moderate left ventricular impairment treated surgically was later confirmed in the CASS where 7-year survival was 84% in the surgical group versus 70% in the medical group ($p = 0.01$) of randomized patients with ejection fractions between 35% and 50% [15]. As percutaneous revascularization was more frequently used, this data on baseline left ventricular function became more central.

PTCA and CABG

The role of PCI became more common; its role compared to coronary artery bypass graft surgery (CABG) became an increasing object of discussion and controversy. For patients with multivessel coronary artery disease, CABG had been the standard

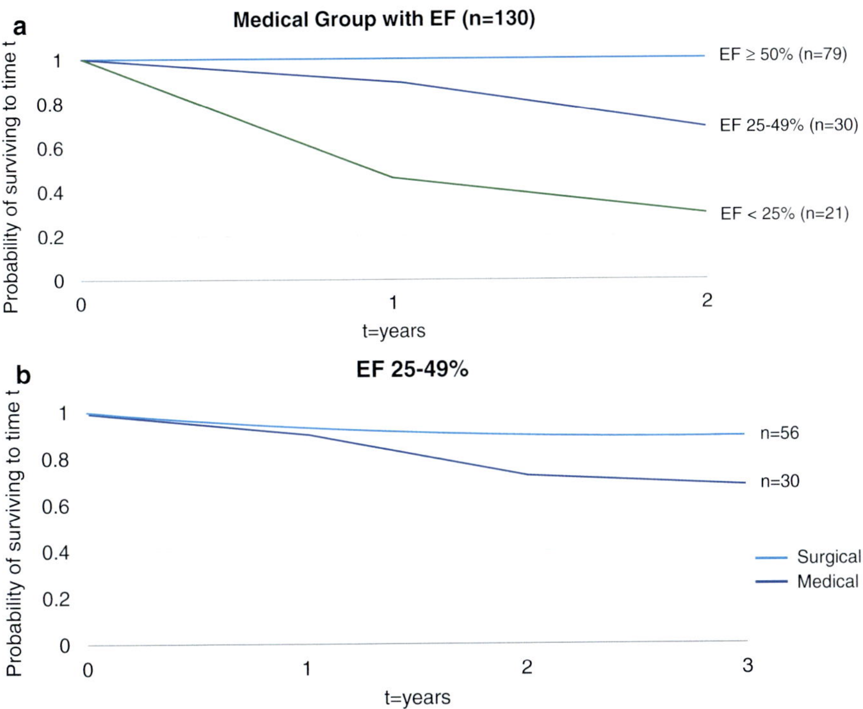

Fig. 3.14 As coronary surgical procedures increased in the late 1960s and early 1970s, Mayo Clinic investigators identified predictors of 2-year survival. Out of a group of 1,879 patients undergoing coronary angiography from 1966 to 1972, they identified 183 patients who would have been candidates for CABG but who were treated medically, and 520 similar patients treated surgically. In the medical group, at 2 years, the single best discriminator of survival was EF (**a**). In the surgical group, EF also had the greatest discrimination. In the patients with moderate decrease in EF (EF 25%–49%), surgery resulted in improved survival at 3 years (**b**). (From Vlietstra RE, et al. Mayo Clin Proc, Feb 1977, Vol 52; used with permission of Mayo Foundation)

of care, particularly for those with LMCA involvement since the initial CASS experience. As PTCA results improved, an increasing number of selected patients with multivessel disease were being treated. This approach was developed and became widely used based on the work of two pioneers in the field, both of whom had trained and worked as staff cardiologists at Mayo Clinic—Drs. Geoff Hartzler and Barry Rutherford. Accordingly, there was great interest at the national level in the development of a randomized clinical trial to compare outcomes of these competitive revascularization strategies. Michael Mock was a Project Leader at the NHLBI during the CASS and was instrumental in starting the first PTCA Registry there. He had a great respect for the Mayo Clinic way of doing things, and he approached Bob Frye to identify opportunities for staff recruitment to the Cardiovascular Division. Support for his transfer to Mayo Clinic was strong and universal, and he proved to be an enormous asset in the planning and conduct of many subsequent trials, especially the BARI study, which was directed by Bob Frye and generously funded by the NHLBI.

Claude Lenfant, Director of the NHLBI, had initially expressed doubt about the willingness of cardiac surgeons to embrace such a trial, comparing bypass surgery with coronary angioplasty, but Michael Mock referred him to John Kirklin, then America's elder statesman of cardiac surgery who strongly supported such a move. The die was cast.

It resulted in the development of a proposed NIH multicenter trial developed by Mayo Clinic with the goal of randomizing patients with multivessel CAD to either PTCA or CABG. The outlines, endpoints, and metrics of that trial formed the basis for the subsequent pivotal trial—Balloon Angioplasty Revascularization Investigation (BARI)—and spawned among others the subsequent international trials of GABI and SYNTAX. These trials form the scientific foundation of professional societal guidelines. During this time, there was intense debate again at all levels of conferences, and in multiple publications. The three co-authors of this chapter debated, published, and refined approaches throughout the decade. Vlietstra

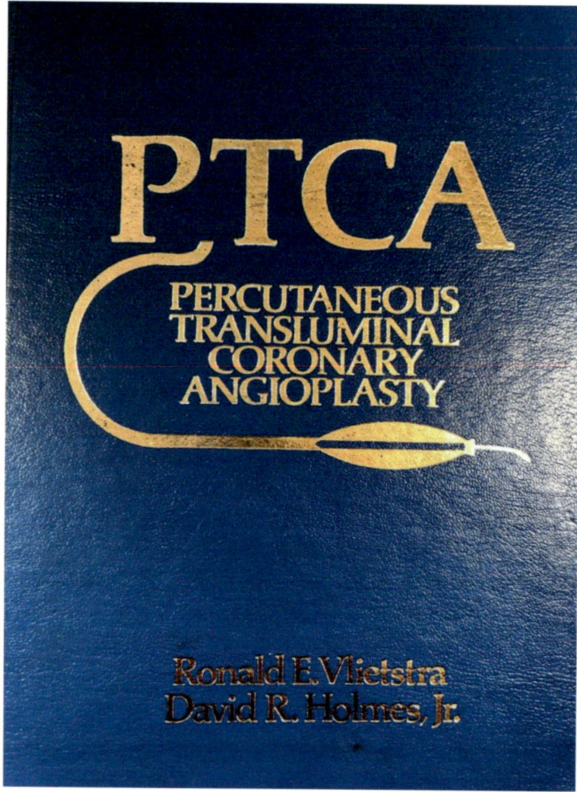

Fig. 3.15 As part of catheterization laboratory participation, the staff was expected to be involved not only in clinical practice but as part of the three shields of Mayo Clinic Philosophy was expected to be involved in research and education. This expectation and the results it achieved were responsible for an exuberant production of important material that affected patient care globally

and Holmes edited their first book together on PTCA in 1984 which showcased the breadth of experience and depth of knowledge accumulated by Mayo Clinic investigators (Fig. 3.15), and other books followed.

During the decade there were improvements in both interventional catheter-based and surgical techniques. In a collaborative grant with CV surgery, Chesebro, working along with Valentin Fuster and cardiac surgeons, designed the seminally important trial of the effect of platelet-inhibitor drugs in the setting of CABG to evaluate their effect on perioperative therapy on early postoperative vein graft patency, the findings of which had long-term effect on the field [16].

The decade of the 1980s led to other increasing interactions with cardiac surgery and anesthesiology, not all of which proceeded smoothly. In the decade of the 1970s, the focus of coronary angiography was to fully delineate the anatomy and facilitate discussions about surgical revascularization. During that period of time, focusing specifically on diagnostic coronary angiography, infrequent patients required urgent surgery either because of identification of severe unstable coronary anatomy, particularly LMCA disease, or the development of a complication from angiography, such as a proximal dissection from coronary intubation. With the advent of PTCA and its introduction into the catheterization laboratory, the need for closer collaboration became even more necessary and sometimes very problematic. Late afternoon or early evening calls, particularly on Friday afternoons, from the cardiac laboratory to the cardiac surgeon on call for emergencies about a patient with acute closure on the cath table which could not be rescued by catheter techniques were sometimes received with less than intense exuberant enthusiasm, although achieving optimal patient care always trumped discussion.

As mentioned, consideration for PTCA involved treatment that included proximal, concentric, nontortuous, noncalcified, subtotal lesions in patients with stable clinical symptoms. Such criteria would also identify patients who would have also been candidates for CABG. As enthusiasm for the procedure increased, however, patient and lesion criteria for PTCA expanded, and there were competing interests between interventional cardiology and cardiovascular surgery.

As originally defined, the Mayo Clinic protocol developed by Vlietstra and implemented under the direction of catheterization laboratory leadership by Smith and subsequent directors involved joint review of patient and lesion selection criteria by clinical cardiology, the interventional cardiologist, and CV surgeon. A common venue for that was the weekly cardiac catheterization meeting which involved multiple participants based on case reviews. It featured "frank and open discussion" by people with strongly held opinions which were often conflicting; a term later used to describe political discussions by people from different sides of the political spectrum. These formed the basis of Heart Team discussions which are now mandated by professional societies and even regulatory agencies. They generated ideas for new alternatives to strategies of care, new scientific studies, and grant submissions. As part of that discussion, initially, a surgical operating theater was held open during each PTCA procedure in case a complication developed which would have involved the need for urgent transport for surgery. Such complications were not uncommon at that time with catheter-induced coronary dissection and acute closure seen in 5%–10% of cases and were associated with increased morbidity for myocardial infarctions and even mortality well documented by Mayo Clinic experience as well as the NHLBI PTCA Registry [4]. While difficult to predict, these complications caused major problems for patient safety and the efficiencies of both the cardiac catheterization laboratory and CV surgery.

As technology became improved as well as improved operator experience, such complications became less frequent although they still caused considerable controversy. The introduction of percutaneous intra-aortic balloon pumps and perfusion balloons during this time was important in this regard; however, it was not until the next decade that the development of more advanced coronary stents and their increasing use dramatically decreased the need for urgent surgery.

These initiatives went hand in hand with advancements in imaging and procedure techniques. There was intense interest in the field regarding contrast material with newer non-ionic contrast agents.

Contrast Nephropathy

The use of contrast media carries a risk for aggravating renal insufficiency in those already with a creatinine of 1.5 mg or greater. In patients who developed this, in-hospital mortality was significantly increased. In the 1980s, we followed practices of good hydration and minimizing the total contrast dose used. Instead of left ventriculography, we would use echocardiography to evaluate left ventricular function, but contrast doses inevitably crept up when faced with more complex multivessel interventions.

Newer contrast agents, with lower osmolality and non-ionicity, promised some reduction in those risks. To test the effects of one of these newer agents on renal impairment, Charlie Taliercio, one of our excellent training fellows, helped set up a randomized trial (with the assistance of Lila Elveback) of a new non-ionic, low osmolar agent and a traditional ionic one in patients with renal impairment.

It was not easy to fund such a study because companies making either the newer or traditional agents were concerned about the negative consequences for their product if it was shown to be inferior. Fortunately, we did identify a company that distributed both types in the USA, and they agreed to support us in comparing their iopamidol (non-ionic and low osmolar) with their diatrizoate (traditional hyperosmolar ionic).

In total, 307 high-risk patients with renal impairment (serum creatinine greater than or equal to 1.5 mg/dL) were randomized in a double-blind manner to either iopamidol or diatrizoate at cardiac angiography with subsequent follow-up study of renal function. Baseline clinical and angiographic variables were similar in the iopamidol ($n = 155$) and diatrizoate ($n = 152$) groups. Change in renal function after angiography was less pronounced with iopamidol compared with diatrizoate as measured by mean (+/− SD) increase in 24-h serum creatinine (0.11 +/− 0.2 versus 0.22 +/− 0.26 mg/dl, $p < 0.001$), mean maximal increase in serum creatinine (0.2

+/− 0.44 versus 0.38 +/− 0.73 mg/dL, p < 0.0001), and percentage of patients with a maximal increase in serum creatinine greater than 0.5 mg/dL (8% versus 19%, p < 0.01). Subsequently published in the 1990s, there was no significant difference between agents in the number of patients (few in either group) developing clinically severe acute renal dysfunction [17].

This study and numerous others around that time helped move catheterization laboratory practice to iso- or hypo-osmolar non-ionic agents and away from traditional hyperosmolar ionic agents. Many studies since that time have failed to show a benefit greater than the old standards of prehydration and minimizing contrast dose.

There were particularly important advances in imaging. Application of video recording had been central to Dr. E.H. Wood's interests. These efforts were continued with the development of high-definition video systems for routine clinical use because of their improved resolution.

Imaging and Radiation Exposure

They found universal application in procedures such as PTCA where high-definition imaging was mandatory to optimize results and identify subtle changes in the vessel architecture which could result in acute or threatened closure. The initial application of these efforts at improving visualization allowed Mayo Clinic to transmit live cases as part of an educational format to both national and international meetings. Digital-based recording techniques were developed in close collaboration by Merrill Wondrow at Mayo Clinic working with General Electric Medical Systems. An

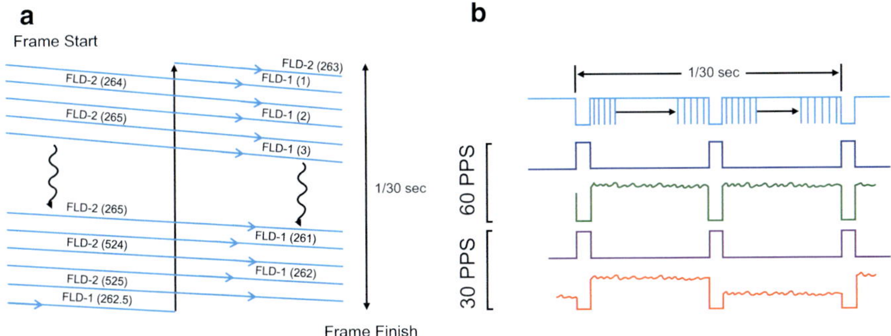

Fig. 3.16 (**a, b**) Radiation exposure and the contrast resolution required for increasingly complex interventional procedures remained an important consideration. The usual approach to conventional video recording consisted of 525-line video frame rate. Each frame was comprised of two fields and then scanned to complete the frame with its requisite radiation pulse. In contrast, interlaced scanning was introduced in the catheterization practice. With this technique (**b**), radiation was decreased by 50%. (From Holmes DR, et al. Mayo Clin Proc 61:3321–326, 1986; used with permission of Mayo Foundation)

important concern as the requirements for superb imaging were understood was the issue of radiation exposure both with cine and video for physicians, paramedical personnel, and patients alike. Regulatory agencies implemented the strategy of ALARA (as low as reasonably achievable) to minimize the impact of radiation exposure. At that time, all video systems were based on interlaced scanning which, by virtue of increasing pulses, resulted in increasing radiation. Working in concert with General Electric, a new progressive scanning system was developed and then implemented for the first time at Mayo Clinic.

The striking advantage was a 50% reduction in radiation to both the patient and the operator without any degradation in image quality (Fig. 3.16a, b) [18]. This type of progressive scan video has become an industry standard. Other imaging enhancements included development and implementation of digital subtraction angiography which became standard for evaluating myocardial perfusion and coronary blood flow as well as enabling a reduction in contrast volume required for left ventricular angiography, the latter a particular concern for patients with abnormal renal function or hemodynamic instability.

Other aspects of imaging continue to change. The advances in echocardiography in the early 1980s now included Doppler technologies that could determine velocities and flows across aortic valves and derive pressure gradients and valve cross-sectional areas noninvasively. Early nonsimultaneous comparison of these derived measures with catheterization data showed promise, but there was enough uncertainty about validity in all cases that most clinicians were reluctant to make the decision about valve surgery based only on these noninvasive findings. Currie [19] reported the results of hemodynamic determination of aortic valve gradients in the catheterization laboratory by simultaneous catheter-based and continuous wave Doppler techniques in a prospective study of 100 consecutive patients ranging in age from 50 to 89 years. The echocardiographer was blinded to the catheter hemodynamic findings, and excellent correlations ($r = 0.91$ to $r = 0.93$) between the various continuous wave Doppler metrics and catheter-based hemodynamics were obtained. Widespread changes in the evaluation and management of aortic valve stenosis occurred following this publication.

The integration of two-dimensional and Doppler techniques became more widely used. Initially used as an adjunct to invasive cardiac procedures, these techniques became mainstream and allowed definitive diagnosis of some cases of complex congenital heart disease. In some patients, the need for cardiac catheterization eliminated the need for invasive studies while, in others, the two procedures were complementary, yielding a definitive diagnosis [20–23]. These techniques were also increasingly used for hemodynamic assessment of complex clinical settings. Appreciation of the issues of restriction versus constriction led to combined echo- and hemodynamic studies. When validated by surgical procedure and pathologic results, new diagnostic criteria were developed, leading to selection of optimal strategies of care with more definitive criteria for constriction which would improve with pericardiectomy (Fig. 3.17).

In routine clinical practice, the left atrium was largely inaccessible up until 1980. Transseptal catheterization had been introduced in 1959 by Ross and later modified

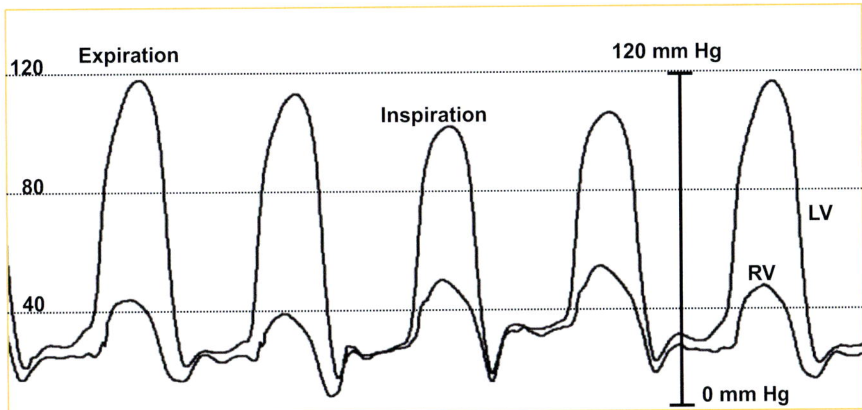

Fig. 3.17 Unmet clinical needs were identified in patients presenting with heart failure often right sided. The clinical issue was to identify constrictive pericarditis from restrictive cardiomyopathy. Distinguishing these was essential as patients with constrictive pericardial disease could be treated with pericardiectomy which would dramatically improve symptoms and outcome. In contrast restrictive cardiomyopathy had no surgical approaches for "cure" or at least marked improvement, while with restriction, medical therapy was all that was possible. Distinguishing between these two options was often difficult. In some patients where the diagnosis could not be made with certainty, they might be recommended to undergo the Chamberlain procedure, with a small thoracic incision to inspect the pericardium; if constriction was found, pericardiectomy would then be performed in contrast in those patients in whom the pericardium was not involved and only medical therapy was used. During this time, new invasive diagnostic criteria for distinguishing constriction versus restriction were developed in the Mayo Clinic Cardiovascular Laboratory by Nishimura working with others. As seen in a patient with constriction, with inspiration there is a decrease in LV filling and LVSP and an increase in RV systole duration pressure. These criteria which have been expanded since that early work have revolutionized the evaluation and care of these patients

by Brockenbrough, but the stiff needle system was hard to maneuver, and the complication rate, in less-experienced hands, was off-putting [24].

The alternative (for the assessment of mitral stenosis) was to obtain pulmonary "wedge pressures" via a right heart end-hole catheter positioned in a very distal small peripheral pulmonary artery. If the blood that leaked back had arterial saturations, then the pressures recorded were believed to represent the pressure in the left atrium. However, obtaining a good "wedge position" was often difficult, and the operator was left frustrated. In addition, there was a shift in pressure recorded from pulmonary wedge to LA pressure.

That all changed when the USCI medical device company released the Mullins sheath. When positioned in the right atrium (via the right femoral vein), this sheath allowed for much easier orientation against the atrial septum and passage of the transseptal needle into the left atrium itself. Once the needle had penetrated through the septum and into the left atrium, the sheath could be advanced, and catheters could be passed through it into the left atrium and left ventricle.

Jim Seward, best known for his pioneering work in echocardiography, began using this sheath in the pediatric lab in 1980, primarily to access the pulmonary veins for retrograde angiography to outline pulmonary artery anatomy in patients with pulmonary atresia. He was quick to see how it would help in the adult lab as well and he taught us in its use.

The biplane imaging systems used in the lab were especially helpful in recognizing landmarks for where the needle could best be advanced through the septum usually at the level of the fossa ovalis. There was a change in pressure recorded via the needle lumen when the left atrium was entered, and confirmation could be made by injecting a small dose of contrast. Should, in rare instances, the needle tip penetrate an atrial wall, this injection would show contrast entering the pericardial space, necessitating prompt two-dimensional echocardiography monitoring for any evidence of cardiac tamponade. In addition, penetration in the ascending aorta would result in obtaining a systemic pressure. In this later case, it was imperative to not advance the sheath into the aorta. In most cases, the tip of the needle could be withdrawn without clinical consequence. In the first 8 years of transseptal catheterization in the Mayo Clinic adult lab, 472 procedures were performed, with 2 deaths (a mortality rate of 0.4%). A detailed account of this approach, and its nuances, is given by Jim O'Keefe et al. in *Interventional Cardiology* [24]. Jim had come to Mayo after training at Rice University in Houston and quickly made his presence felt in the catheterization laboratory and in pacing. An elite middle-distance runner, he soon made many friends inside and outside the clinic.

It quickly became clear that this new access to the left atrium had many additional advantages. Instead of lengthy efforts to cross a heavily diseased aortic valve or a prosthetic valve, left ventricular pressures could be obtained quickly and accurately. The occasional need for direct apical puncture of the left ventricle was reduced, and it opened up the left atrium for electrophysiologic mapping and, later, ablation procedures. It was an essential advance for mitral valvuloplasty, antegrade aortic valvuloplasty, and left atrial appendage occlusion.

Vasodilators

Many patients, mostly young women, were referred to Mayo Clinic for evaluation of primary pulmonary hypertension. In the early 1980s, there was little that could be done for these patients, and the workup was usually limited to excluding alternative causes of the problem, such as an AV fistula, pulmonary embolism, scleroderma, drug toxicity, or lupus. A senior Mayo Clinic cardiologist, Ray Pruitt, first Dean of the Mayo Medical School, challenged us in the lab to explore drug interventions, just as Lou Rubin had just reported in the New England Journal of Medicine [25].

Patients would spend a long time in the lab while we evaluated the effects of hydralazine, verapamil, nifedipine, and a new serotonin receptor blocker, ketanserin, to see if pulmonary pressures would drop and cardiac output increase. Often the calculated pulmonary vascular resistance would fall with one or other drug, but when the patient was tried on that drug little, if any, clinical benefit could be seen. Sometimes their clinical condition even worsened [16].

The only window on the horizon appeared to be heart-lung transplantation, recently introduced by Norm Shumway, at Stanford. During Mayo Clinic's preparation for that surgical step, transplant surgeon John Wallwork visited, and he mentioned that in Cambridge, where he worked, a continuous infusion of prostacyclin was very useful pretransplant, in temporarily improving pulmonary artery dynamics.

Michael McGoon had studied pulmonary vascular reactivity in Paul Vanhoutte's basic vascular physiology lab. He had also performed many of the patient lab studies with vasodilators and had opened a pulmonary hypertension clinic. He worked with Upjohn and the FDA to win approval for trying prostacyclin in selected Mayo patients. This led to a variety of new strategies, some very helpful, to be employed in the 1990s.

There were other opportunities to study vascular reactivity working with Vanhoutte in the coronary arena. Rubanyi et al. evaluated vasoconstrictor activity of coronary sinus plasma in patients with coronary artery disease [23]. For this study focusing on the vasoactive properties of plasma samples were taken from the coronary sinus, a systemic artery, and the superior vena cava in patients with and those with normal coronary arteries at rest and during supine bicycle exercise. Using platelet-rich samples, in a bioassay organ bath preparation of coronary artery rings, the authors found that the coronary sinus blood of patients with CAD exhibited

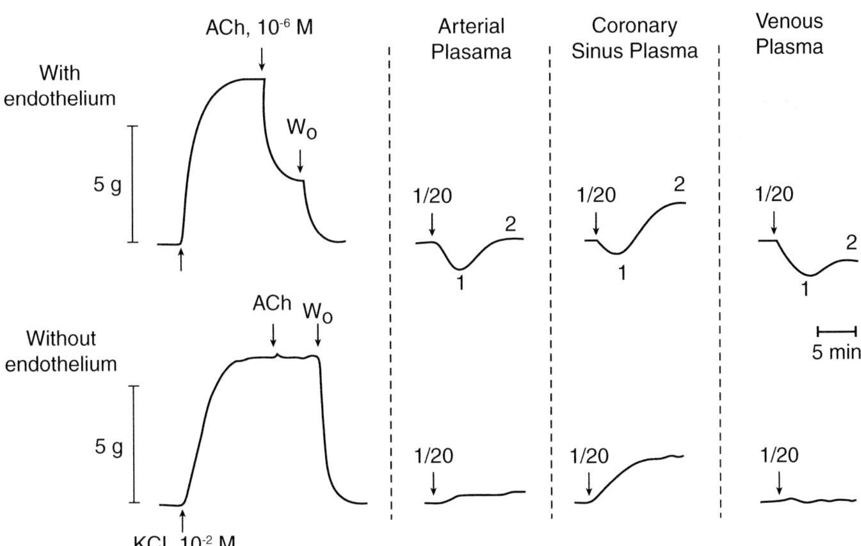

Fig. 3.18 Assessment of vasoactive properties of serum from a patient with coronary artery disease studied in an organ bath in which isolated canine coronary rings were mounted. In rings with endothelium, plasma samples were tested by the response to acetylcholine. In samples from the brachial artery, when the endothelium was intact, there was relaxation of the ring, while in preparations without endothelium, there was no change. In contrast, the pattern of relaxation and contraction was different in the coronary sinus plasma with vasoconstriction. (From Rubanyi et al. JACC 9(6):1243, 1987; used with permission)

vasoconstrictor activity. The impact of the endothelium could also be assessed. These properties were similar irrespective of whether the samples were taken during rest or during supine bicycle exercise (Fig. 3.18). The authors concluded that this vasoconstrictor activity may be associated with 5-hydroxytryptamine. The imbalance favoring vasoconstriction could potentially result in myocardial ischemia [26].

Other "structural" issues were addressed with the involvement of physician extenders which, for the first time, facilitated same-day admission criteria to streamline patient flow and resulted in improved patient satisfaction and convenience.

A final piece of the future looking developed around a GLP animal laboratory in which Mayo Clinic could help develop and test new in-house IP as well as work closely with Industry to evaluate new technologies and address clinical pathophysiologic issues. In 1977, following the groundbreaking innovations by others, the industry was working hard to come up with new designs for coronary stents. Medtronic, located just 80 miles away in Minneapolis, sent two engineers to Mayo Clinic, bringing with them some prospective new stents.

They looked interesting, but for us to realistically work with them, we would need a large budget, enough to fund half of one consultant's time as well as a full-time laboratory assistant. Medtronic would also have to fund a full animal lab, all animal and equipment costs, and Mayo Clinic's overheads, including the legal help needed in setting up a contract. This amounted to a tidy sum, but Medtronic quickly bought into the plan.

After much back-and-forth with Kathy Meyerle in Mayo Clinic's Legal Department, Vlietstra was able to complete such a contract and budget which gave Mayo Clinic total freedom on what studies to perform and no restriction on how and when to report the findings. It was the first time that Mayo Clinic's Cardiovascular Division had established such a close interaction with the industry, and it opened the door for many similar collaborative projects later.

The question now was who would lead the work. Luckily, Rob Schwartz had just joined the staff. He was a dynamic young investigator who thrived on bioengineering projects (he had trained in aeronautical engineering while serving in the US Air Force). He was looking for a research project that combined novel coronary devices with his engineering background. Working with Kathy Meyerle in Mayo Clinic's Legal Department, IACUC, and Medtronic, Dr. Vlietstra was able to come up with funding for staff and laboratory assistants at St. Mary's Hospital. This relationship allowed Mayo Clinic the option of which studies to perform, the questions to be addressed, and the interaction with multiple industry stakeholders. It would prove to be invaluable in the next decade under the leadership of Rob Schwartz who had just joined the staff with a particular interest in bioengineering evaluating novel coronary and vascular devices. Out of that would come extremely valuable information for a practical animal model of restenosis, important information on the pathophysiology of restenosis and approaches for mitigation working with others in the field.

He jumped at the chance.

All these initiatives were carried out in the next decade which was fashioned on the creativeness, networking, hard work, and visioning of those who continued to lay the foundations for the future.

References

1. Gaspard P. History of coronary angioplasty. Europa Digital & Publishing. 2017.
2. Sundt TM Jr, Smith HC, Campbell JK, Vlietstra RE, Cucchiara RF, Stanson AW. Transluminal angioplasty for basilar artery stenosis. Mayo Clin Proc. 1980;55:673–80.
3. Holmes DR Jr, Vlietstra RE, Fisher LD, et al. Follow-up of patients from the coronary artery surgery study (CASS) potentially suitable for percutaneous transluminal coronary angioplasty. Am Heart J. 1983;106:981–8.
4. Holmes DR Jr, Holubkov R, Vlietstra RE, et al. Comparison of complications during percutaneous transluminal coronary angioplasty from 1977 to 1981 and from 1985 to 1986: the National Heart, Lung, and Blood Institute Percutaneous Transluminal Coronary Angioplasty Registry. J Am Coll Cardiol. 1988;12:1149–55.
5. Mabin TA, Holmes DR Jr, Smith HC, et al. Intracoronary thrombus: role in coronary occlusion complicating percutaneous transluminal coronary angioplasty. J Am Coll Cardiol. 1985;5:198–202.
6. Sugrue DD, Holmes DR Jr, Smith HC, et al. Coronary artery thrombus as a risk factor for acute vessel occlusion during percutaneous transluminal coronary angioplasty: improving results. Br Heart J. 1986;56:62–6.
7. Holmes DR Jr, Hartzler GO, Smith HC, Fuster V. Coronary artery thrombosis in patients with unstable angina. Br Heart J. 1981;45:411–6.
8. Holmes DR Jr, Vlietstra RE, Reeder GS, et al. Angioplasty in total coronary artery occlusion. J Am Coll Cardiol. 1984;3:845–9.
9. Kaufmann UP, Garratt KN, Vlietstra RE, Menke KK, Holmes DR Jr. Coronary atherectomy: first 50 patients at the Mayo Clinic. Mayo Clin Proc. 1989;64:747–52.
10. Holmes DR, Garratt KN. Atherectomy. Blackwell Scientific Publications. 1992:256.
11. Sigwart U, Puel J, Mirkovitch V, Joffre F, Kappenberger L. Intravascular stents to prevent occlusion and restenosis after transluminal angioplasty. N Engl J Med. 1987;316:701–6.
12. Serruys PW, Strauss BH, Beatt KJ, et al. Angiographic follow-up after placement of a self-expanding coronary-artery stent. N Engl J Med. 1991;324:13–7.
13. Holmes DR Jr, Vlietstra RE, Smith HC, et al. Restenosis after percutaneous transluminal coronary angioplasty (PTCA): a report from the PTCA Registry of the National Heart, Lung, and Blood Institute. Am J Cardiol. 1984;53:77c–81c.
14. Vlietstra RE, Assad-Morell JL, Frye RL, et al. Survival predictors in coronary artery disease. Medical and surgical comparisons. Mayo Clin Proc. 1977;52:85–90.
15. Passamani E, Davis KB, Gillespie MJ, Killip T. A randomized trial of coronary artery bypass surgery. Survival of patients with a low ejection fraction. N Engl J Med. 1985;312:1665–71.
16. Chesebro JH, Fuster V, Elveback LR, et al. Effect of dipyridamole and aspirin on late vein-graft patency after coronary bypass operations. N Engl J Med. 1984;310:209–14.
17. Taliercio CP, Vlietstra RE, Ilstrup DM, et al. A randomized comparison of the nephrotoxicity of iopamidol and diatrizoate in high risk patients undergoing cardiac angiography. J Am Coll Cardiol. 1991;17:384–90.
18. Holmes DR Jr, Bove AA, Wondrow MA, Gray JE. Video x-ray progressive scanning: new technique for decreasing x-ray exposure without decreasing image quality during cardiac catheterization. Mayo Clin Proc. 1986;61:321–6.
19. Currie PJ, Seward JB, Reeder GS, et al. Continuous-wave Doppler echocardiographic assessment of severity of calcific aortic stenosis: a simultaneous Doppler-catheter correlative study in 100 adult patients. Circulation. 1985;71:1162–9.
20. Sinak LJ, Hoffman EA, Schwartz RS, et al. Three-dimensional cardiac anatomy and function in heart disease in adults: initial results with the dynamic spatial reconstructor. Mayo Clin Proc. 1985;60:383–92.
21. Nishimura RA, Rogers PJ, Holmes DR Jr, Gehring DG, Bove AA. Assessment of myocardial perfusion by videodensitometry in the canine model. J Am Coll Cardiol. 1987;9:891–7.

22. Holmes DR Jr, Bove AA, Nishimura RA, et al. Comparison of monoplane and biplane assessment of regional left ventricular wall motion after thrombolytic therapy for acute myocardial infarction. Am J Cardiol. 1987;59:793–7.
23. Wondrow MA, Bove AA, Holmes DR Jr, Gray JE, Julsrud PR. Technical consideration for a new X-ray video progressive scanning system for cardiac catheterization. Catheter Cardiovasc Diagn. 1988;14:126–34.
24. O'Keefe JH, Jr. The transseptal approach for left heart catheterization. The Practice of Interventional cardiology, FA Davis Publishing. 1989:107–119.
25. Rubin LJ, Peter RH. Oral hydralazine therapy for primary pulmonary hypertension. N Engl J Med. 1980;302:69–73.
26. Rubanyl GM, Frye RL, Holmes DR Jr, Vanhoutte PM. Vasoconstrictor activity of coronary sinus plasma from patients with coronary artery disease. J Am Coll Cardiol. 1987;9:1243–9.

Chapter 4
1990s: Another Move

David R. Holmes Jr., Malcolm Bell, and John F. Bresnahan

The 1990s featured extraordinary growth in the cardiac cath lab with continued acceleration of projects initiated in the 1980s. The practice priorities were expansive. There was continued growth in the number of patients treated, types of devices used, scientific output, involvement of new colleagues and investigators from around the world, new multicenter collaborative networks for investigating studies, a move to new laboratories and equipment, and new unmet clinical needs. We continued to not only move to the future but to define the future and then train for it.

New investigators/colleagues played a large role. Many had come in the past and stayed for the rest of their careers, including Malcolm Bell, John Bresnahan, Guri Sandhu, Andre Lapeyre, and Chet Rihal. In addition to being very talented invasive and interventional cardiologists, they often went on to administrative positions; subsequent catheterization directors (Rihal and Sandhu), Director of the Mayo Clinic Personnel committee (Rihal), Cardiology Department Vice Chair (Bell), Course Director for Mayo Medical Students rotating through cardiology (Bresnahan), and Director of the Mayo Clinic Mobile Catheterization Laboratory (Lapeyre). Many other outstanding interventionalists subsequently moved to other academic institutions, both in the US and abroad, where they have had tremendous careers, including Kirk Garratt, Rob Schwartz, Rob Simari, David Hasdai (Israel), Urs Kaufman (Switzerland), and Peter Berger, among others.

Percutaneous coronary revascularization remained a major focus. Whereas the 1980s had seen the widespread growth of PTCA, the 1990s brought investigations aimed at improving the procedures by either solving complications or by markedly expanding the number of patients and lesions that could be treated. The New

D. R. Holmes Jr. (✉) · M. Bell
Department of Cardiovascular Diseases, Mayo Clinic, Rochester, MN, USA
e-mail: Holmes.david@mayo.edu; Bell.malcolm@mayo.edu

J. F. Bresnahan
Mayo Clinic (retired), Rochester, MN, USA

D. R. Holmes Jr., R. L. Frye (eds.), *The Mayo Clinic Cardiac Catheterization Laboratory*, https://doi.org/10.1007/978-3-030-79329-6_4

Approach to Coronary Intervention (NACI) registry had been brought along to evaluate the new devices; the results of subsequent investigations then led the way to the development of new devices or iterations of older devices and new strategies of care [1]. These devices and strategies were developed by interventional cardiologists working with industry colleagues; interestingly, these interventional cardiologists often had specific and unique catheters with their own respective names attached. Initial published, small registry experiences typically lacked consistent definitions or controlled data entry and also lacked core laboratories. NACI, which had been developed to address these issues, continued to play an increasingly pivotal role. In addition, the 1990s brought to the forefront the use of larger, multicenter randomized clinical trials (RCTs) and registries that have become the hallmark of current cardiovascular science and have provided the standard data set and approaches upon which all professional societal guidelines and clinical practice are based [2].

PTCA had been based on the application of barotrauma delivered at varying pressures to modify and decrease the arterial stenosis responsible for symptoms, ischemia, or both. Although the initial thought was that at inflation pressures of 6–8 atmospheres (available with the devices in use at that time), compression of the atheromatous stenosis might be the mechanism, pathologic studies documented that the resultant improvement was the result of both micro- and macro-disruptions and fractures of the atherosclerotic plaque. However, the disruption produced was not predictable, and subsequently resulted in severe vessel trauma, which then resulted in acute dissection and/or acute vessel closure. Given the unpredictable nature of the result of this vascular trauma, efforts focused on means to render the procedure more predictable.

Directional Coronary Atherectomy

As previously mentioned, in the 1980s directional atherectomy continued to attract the most interest by virtue of its ability to remove tissue with the goal of making the procedure more predictable. Some of the first publications on clinical outcomes were reported in a number of papers from the Mayo Clinic Cath Lab (Kaufman, Garratt, Bell, Holmes, and Vlietstra, among others). Initially developed and applied in the late 1980s, it soon became the focus of two major multicenter randomized clinical trials during the 1990s: first, for the treatment of native coronary arterial disease (CAVEAT) in which we were a participating clinical center, and second, for patients with saphenous vein bypass graft disease (CAVEAT 2) in which Mayo Clinic investigators were the principle investigators [2]. These trials represented the beginning of decades of similarly designed RCTs in coronary interventions, particularly stents. Directional atherectomy had some other important features that resulted in unanticipated consequences, which became important and significantly impacted its application [3–8]; it required larger access sheaths with the potential for increased vascular complications. While "directional," the depth of tissue removal could not always be controlled and, if excessive, could result in coronary perforation or late aneurysm formation, phenomena that had always been

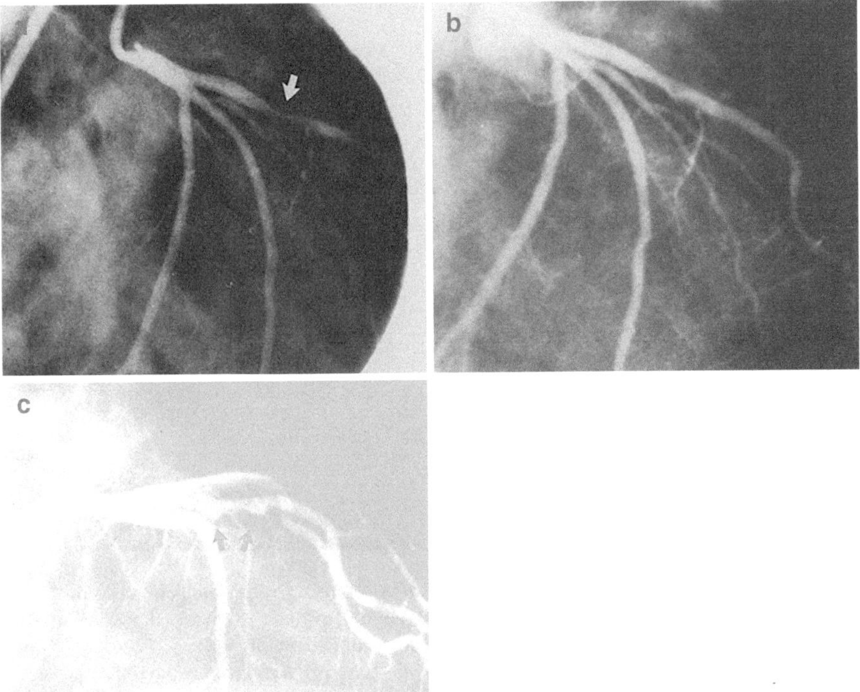

Fig. 4.1 (a) Baseline RAO view of the LAD lesion prior to DCA (*arrow*). (b) Following DCA, the arterial lumen is substantially improved. (c) Follow-up angiography in an anterior oblique cranial view documents fusiform aneurysmal dilation (*arrows*). (From Bell et al. [8]; used with permission)

Fig. 4.2 Photomicrograph of the atherectomy specimen from this patient documents deep wall resection with extensive adventitial tissue. *I* Intima; *M* Media; *A* Adventitia. (From Bell et al. [8]; used with permission)

uncommon with PTCA [5, 8]. Bell et al. evaluated the relationship of deep arterial resection and coronary arterial aneurysms in 64 successful DCA patients undergoing coronary angiography and identified that subsequent aneurysms occurred in 10% (Figs. 4.1a–c) (Fig. 4.2). In this regard, the concept of "bigger is better"

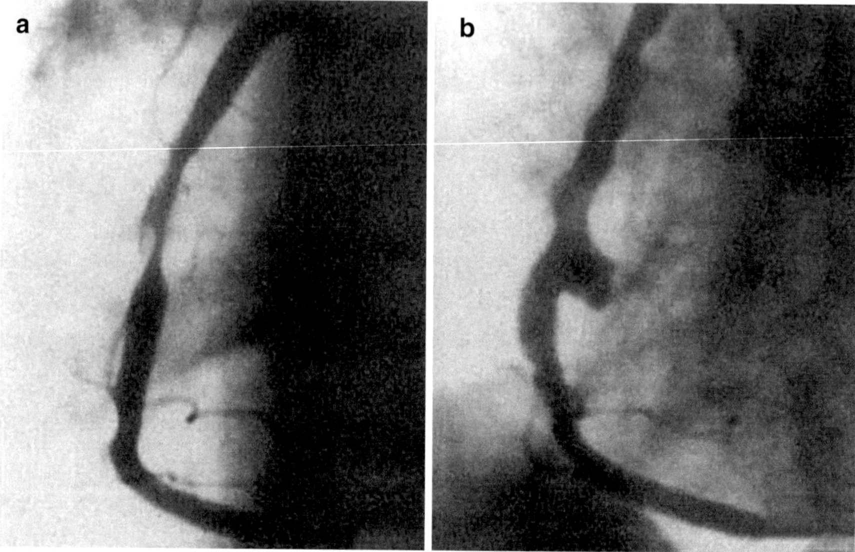

Fig. 4.3 (**a**) DCA of the mid-RCA documenting severe stenosis. (**b**) Immediately following DCA, angiography documented perforation without rupture. (From Holmes DR, Garratt KN, Atherectomy, 1992 Blackwell Scientific Publication; used with permission)

(referring to residual lumen size), which was promulgated at that time in the 1980s as an approach for preventing restenosis, was not always the best strategy, as it might lead to perforation (Fig. 4.3a, b) or aneurysms. Perforation categories and classification schemes were developed and helped to develop strategies. In the setting of perforation, the initial approaches rested on prompt balloon inflation proximal to the perforation to minimize continued leak and stabilize hemodynamics. Perfusion balloon catheters were developed so that even with prolonged inflation, distal flow could be maintained, minimizing the degree of ischemia. Covered stents were developed to seal the perforation, although these devices were typically more bulky and difficult to deliver. Novel strategies were also developed, including the "ping pong" approach (Fig. 4.4), which involved access to another arterial site and placement of an additional guiding catheter. With this approach, the initial perfusion balloon was left inflated across the perforation to prevent continued flow, while a second operator, using the other guiding catheter placed from a second access site, prepared equipment that would be ready to insert for more definitive treatment of the perforation; when that additional equipment was in place, the initial perfusion balloon was deflated, allowing for placement of additional equipment, such as a covered stent, to seal the perforation. This approach minimized perfusion balloon ischemia and avoided free blood flow into the perforation if the perfusion balloon had to be deflated for some time because of severe ischemia.

There were other issues with directional atherectomy that affected its eventual role in PCI. The robust clinical trials documented the issue of vascular access complications because of the large catheter size (11F vs current 5–6F), as well as abrupt vessel closure [3, 4, 6, 7] and distal embolization [3, 4, 6, 7]. Finally, the lack of

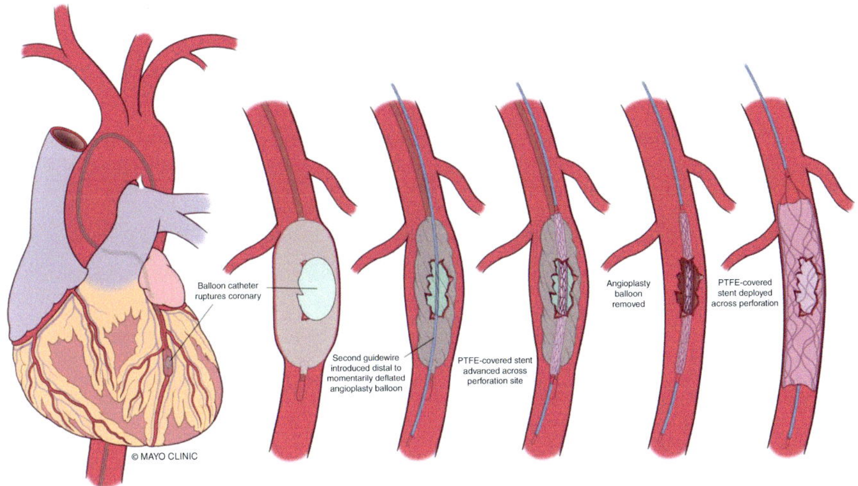

Fig. 4.4 The "ping pong" approach. If perforation is identified, a perfusion balloon is inflated. This allows perfusion distally to the vascular bed to minimize or prevent ischemia while sealing the perforation. A second operator gains access from an alternate arterial site and prepares a second guiding catheter and another device – typically a covered stent. This is positioned in the ascending aorta. Working together, the second operator can then intubate the coronary lesion and deliver a covered stent during the time when the perfusion balloon is being deflated and then removed

clinical improvement compared to other evolving technology, particularly stent implantation, led to the procedure being abandoned in the coronary arena. The technique, however, provided very important and interesting information on differences in the pathophysiology between primary atherosclerotic and restenotic lesions as well as information about the pathology of saphenous vein bypass graft disease [9, 10]. Primary lesions were characterized by foam cells typically seen in atherosclerosis but a predominance of dense intimal fibrosis with necrotic debris. In contrast to this, restenotic lesions had typically looser fibroproliferative tissue found by staining to be primarily smooth muscle cells (Fig. 4.5a–c).

Excimer Laser

Another technology, the excimer laser angioplasty with two different approved laser systems, had also been developed in the 1980s to improve the outcome of percutaneous revascularization and was approved for specific subsets of patients based mainly on lesion characteristics. As this approach became more widely used, it was the focus of development of a large NACI registry experience [12, 13] of 887 patients; although the results were deemed satisfactory, specific complications, such as perforation and long dissections, were problematic (Fig. 4.6a, b) [14, 15]. These long dissections were felt related to intracellular vapor bubble induction during lasing resulting in extensive wall damage or even perforation. For dissections, saline

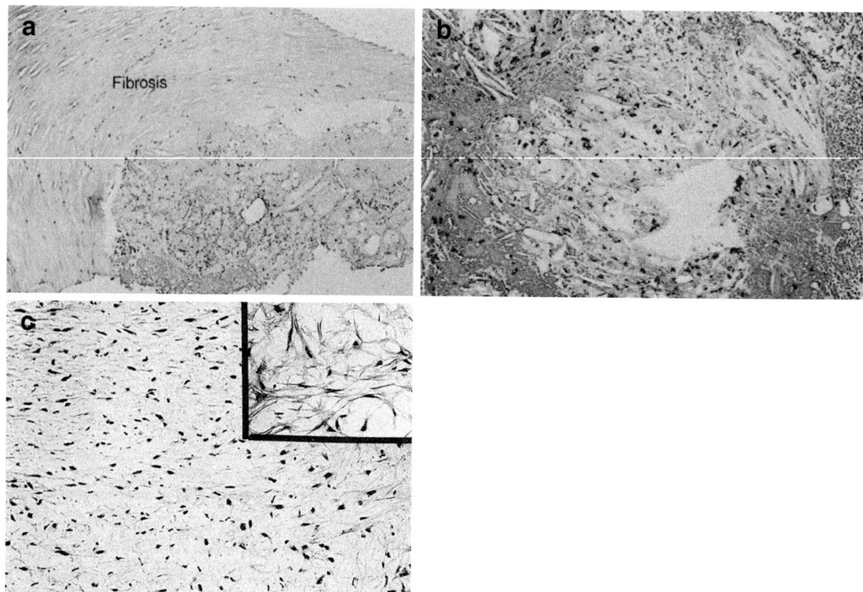

Fig. 4.5 Histopathology of specimens obtained by directional coronary atherectomy. (**a** and **b**) Primary lesions document atherosclerotic plaque with dense fibrosis, foam cells, and cholesterol clefts. They may include necrotic debris. (**c**) In contrast, restenotic lesions are more typically found to include intimal fibrosis and may include loose irregular proliferation of intimal smooth muscle cells. (From Garratt et al. [11]; used with permission)

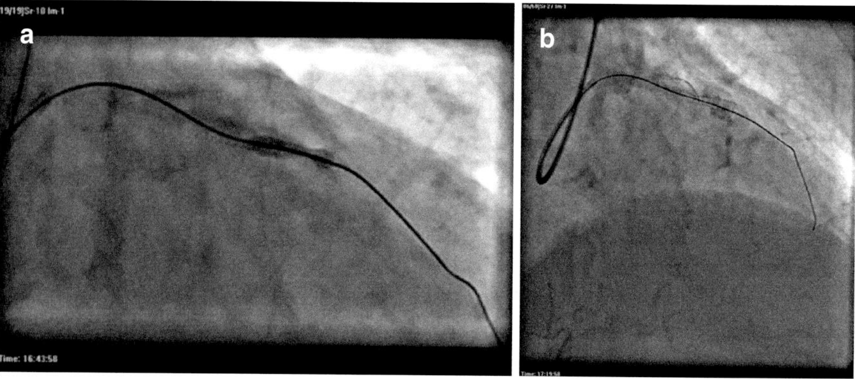

Fig. 4.6 (**a**) ELCA treatment of a long fibrotic lesion in the mid-LAD. Stent implantation was performed, but a residual underployed stent was documented. (**b**) ELCA was performed and resulted in a small perforation tracked into the ventricular myocardium

solution flushing became widely used to mitigate the problem. Other issues related to the fact that an extra stand-alone, relatively large console was needed for every procedure that was not widely used in interventional cardiology for coronary application. In those laboratories that had invested in the console, excimer laser approaches were often not available when needed because the technology and console had been adapted for use in cardiac pacing laboratories, where it had become a standard approach for the removal of older pacing lead systems. These older pacemaker lead systems, which had failed, typically had long, fibrous sheaths enveloping them, making attempts at removal very difficult and, in some cases, very hazardous. For a brief period of time, the application of an excimer laser wire was used for revascularizing chronic total occlusions [13, 16]. This was ultimately abandoned because of coronary perforations and the lack of obvious improvement over other techniques available at that time. Additionally, laser provided no improvement in restenosis rates, had limited catheter sizes, and, during those years, could not ablate calcified lesions.

Rotational Atherectomy

Another promising technology – rotational atherectomy, also developed in the 1980s – was becoming widely used to treat complex calcified coronary lesions that often did not respond favorably with the typical pressures available that were achievable at that time with current PTCA balloons (6–8 atmospheres). The concept was that of differential ablation of calcified/fibrotic tissues, while sparing more normal arterial wall. With that, even a small burr (1.25 mm) in a larger vessel could change the vessel compliance by ablating superficial, calcific fibrotic lesions, thus making it possible to achieve larger final vessel minimal lumen with either conventional PTCA or stent implantation, thus optimizing results. Multiple registries and randomized clinical trials were subsequently performed and documented a specific and significant role for treating calcified lesions, although the technique never became used very widely across the field during that decade due to lack of restenosis reduction, and dissections and perforations in tortuous vessels.

Restenosis

The overriding problematic issue for the interventional cardiology field was restenosis, as documented in the NHLBI Registry in 1984 (Fig. 4.7a–c) [15, 17]. Its impact on the field was increasingly widely recognized [18, 19]. The decade of the 1990s focused intensely on this problem both from the aspect of pathophysiology and its clinical course. Resolution of the problem, or at least its mitigation, would greatly increase the number of patients who might benefit from this less invasive therapy as compared to surgical revascularization. While the clinical consequences of restenosis had become increasingly recognized in the multiple subsets of patients undergoing PTCA and the fact that restenosis or target lesion revascularization (TLR) had been increasingly used as a trial endpoint, the underlying pathophysiology and strategies for prevention and mitigation remained unknown.

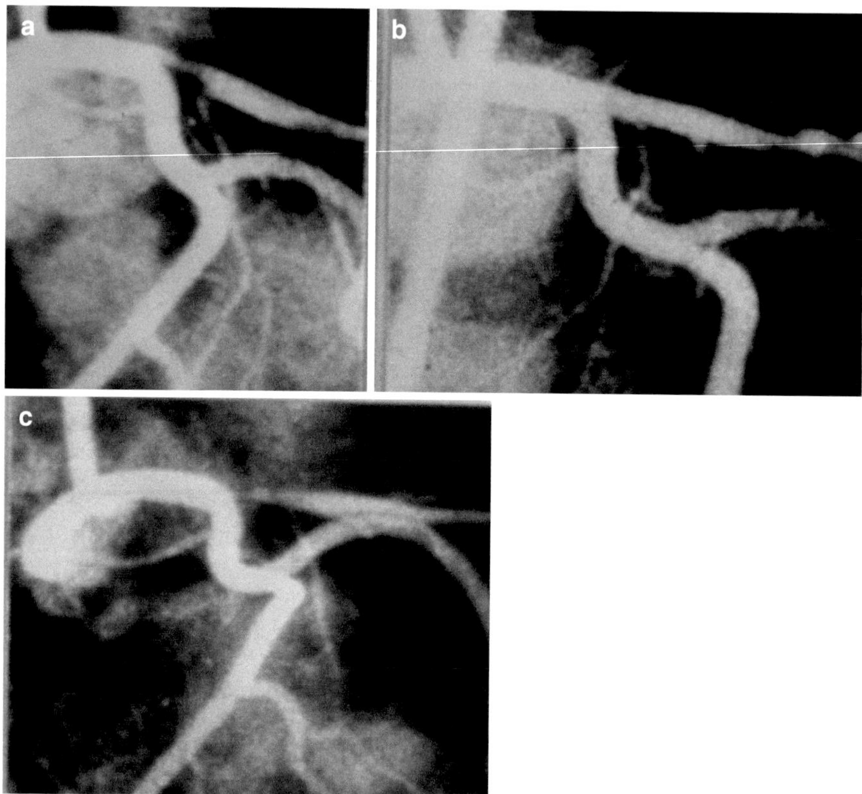

Fig. 4.7 (**a**) Restenosis has remained a problem since the early days of coronary intervention. At baseline, there is a severe ostial stenosis with moderate downstream disease. (**b**) Ostial LAD stenosis treated percutaneously with an excellent result. (**c**) However, 6 months later, symptoms recurred and severe stenosis was documented

Development of Animal Laboratory Practice

To address this, Mayo investigators led by Schwartz, who had joined the staff with one of his unique interests being development and testing of new technology, Chesebro, Fuster, and Bill Edwards in cardiac pathology working alone or in concert with other investigators both nationally and internationally and in the medical industry, collaboratively addressed multiple issues including both device and pharmacologic strategies. The pathology of the phenomenon was assessed in histologic specimens from both primary and restenotic lesions in native and vein graft specimens [9, 10] under the direction of Edwards from Mayo Clinic and Renu Virmani, both prominent cardiac pathologists [20–23]. The Mayo Clinic animal investigational laboratory, put in place to address fundamental issues and evaluate different approaches both pharmacologic and device-based, achieved great prominence. The designation as a Good Laboratory Practices (GLP) facility was of great significance, as the data from experiments conducted according to published standard practice

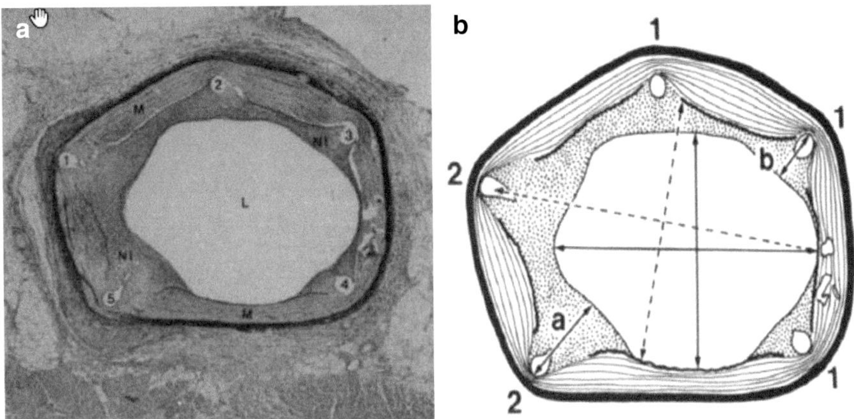

Fig. 4.8 A practical model of restenosis was developed in a porcine model. The resultant tissue had histologic features similar to those seen in human restenosis. This model relied on metallic coils delivered with oversized higher-pressure balloons. (**a**) Photomicrograph at 28 days documenting the relationship with depth of arterial injury by the coils and extent of neointimal hyperplasia. (**b**) Restenosis was proportional to the depth of injury. (From Schwartz et al. [25]; used with permission)

were able to be submitted to US regulatory agencies and formed an important part of presentations used for FDA panel approval meetings. Multiple Mayo Clinic investigators used the facilities for a variety of experiments, which ranged from vascular biology to hemostasis to evaluation of flow parameters in various vascular beds, among others. A unique, practical proliferation model in porcine coronary arteries was developed in the animal laboratory at St. Mary's Hospital by Schwartz and colleagues [22–25]. This model, which used metal coils delivered percutaneously to the coronary arteries along with oversized high-pressure balloon dilatation, resulted in an extensive proliferative response that had histologic features identical to those seen in pathological specimens from patients who had developed clinical coronary arterial restenosis. In this model, light microscopy documented fracture of the internal elastic lamina, which was found to be of central importance and, if damaged, resulted in a cascade of subsequent events [24, 25]. Restenosis due to neointimal hyperplasia restenosis was proportional to the degree of arterial wall injury during therapy (Fig. 4.8a, b); subsequently, an injury score was developed that related the depth of wire penetration and laceration of the internal elastic lamina to the degree of neointimal proliferation. The unique advantages of this model were that it was practical and reliable and closely mimicked the proliferative aspects of human restenosis. This then facilitated testing and screening in the animal laboratory of multiple pharmacologic agents as well as mechanical means, including paclitaxel and heparin coating, local basic fibroblast growth factor, short-wave ultraviolet laser energy, external beam radiation, alpha integrin blockade, C-myc antisense, and angiotensin-converting enzyme inhibition. A unique strategy was developed with a fibrin-coated stent (Fig. 4.9) that was tested in the animal model and then used in an IDE small clinical trial of patients undergoing intervention for severe degenerative vein graft disease [9, 26–28]. While the trial showed no benefit in terms of restenosis and fibrin coating as

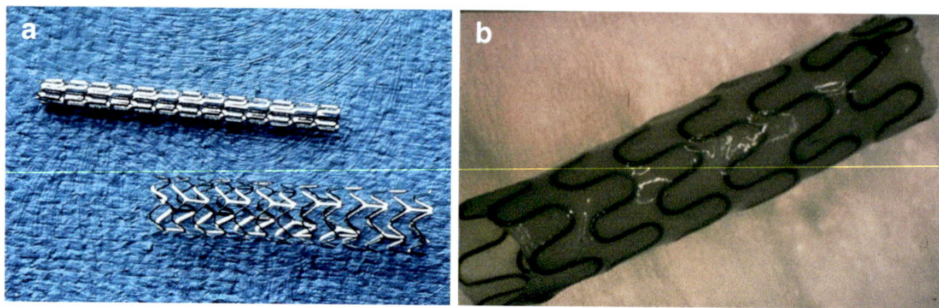

Fig. 4.9 Attempts to find a strategy to facilitate healing of the arterial injury produced by stent implantation resulted in an unique approach where the stent was coated with fibrin (**a** and **b**). The surface with fibrin might facilitate healing. In addition, fibrin coating could allow drugs that could be instilled in the fibrin for local delivery

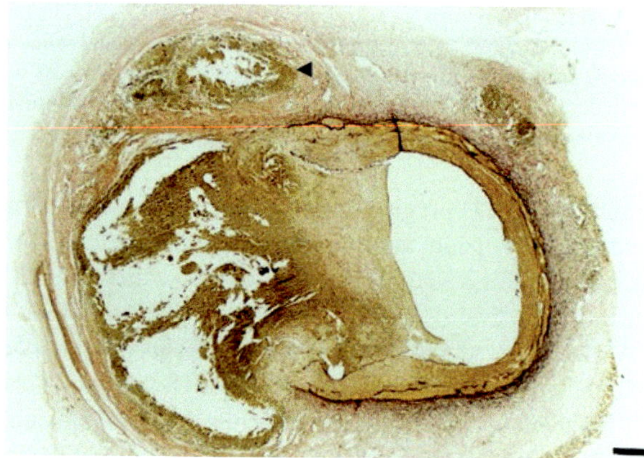

Fig. 4.10 In a porcine coronary artery model, biocompatibility of synthetic polymers was assessed – tested as strips deployed across the circumferential surface of the wire cool stents. As can be seen, at 4 weeks, the biodegradable polymer polyorthoester induced an exuberant inflammation response with destruction of the vessel wall including adventitia. (From van der Giessen et al. [30]; used with permission)

a strategy was discontinued, the concept returned to the field with the development of drug-coated stents for local drug delivery. An important component of the restenosis focus was the development of the "Restenosis Treatment Board." Along with Medtronic, centers from Mayo Clinic, Cleveland Clinic, and the Thoraxcenter in Rotterdam, the Netherlands, worked together to study pathophysiology of restenosis, evaluate new therapeutic and mechanical approaches, and gain important insights into the field. A crucial piece of information identified the marked inflammatory sequelae to implantation of biodegradable and nonbiodegradable polymers in porcine coronary arteries (Fig. 4.10) [29, 30]. This finding focused on the importance of inflammation in these drug/device combinations and issues of whether devices and materials were biocompatible or blood compatible, which varied among different polymers. Such collaborative investigations identified the importance of interactions involving individuals from different backgrounds, including anatomists, biochemists, vascular biologists, and interventionalists, among others.

During the latter part of the 1990s, intense interest remained focused on the neo-intimal hyperplasia and resulted in development of vascular brachytherapy using both gamma and beta emitters. This strategy formed the basis of multicenter investigations and randomized trials that were carried out at the end of the decade and then in the 2000s, identifying the role of both emitters and the practical nature of administration. As mentioned, this strategy had been initially tested by Schwartz in the animal laboratory using the porcine model of restenosis and external beam irradiation.

Given the GLP designation, the animal laboratory, under the direction of Schwartz, helped to develop and test the strategy of local site treatment to prevent stroke in the setting of non-valvular atrial fibrillation. The concept arose from seminal work in Mayo Clinic-Jacksonville by Dr. Joseph Blackshear, which identified in patients with non-valvular atrial fibrillation that stroke and or systemic embolism arose from the thrombus in the left atrial appendage in 90% of cases [31, 32]. Although stroke prevention until that time had focused on oral anticoagulation, many patients were not candidates for such therapy because of bleeding or noncompliance. The limitations of oral anticoagulation and the knowledge of the location of thrombus in 90% of patients led to the concept of mechanical closure of the left atrial appendage, which was investigated and developed. Early development in the animal laboratory in close collaboration with a Mayo Medical Ventures company (Atritech Inc., Plymouth, Minnesota) led to the development of the WATCHMAN device (Fig. 4.11) [33] for left atrial appendage closure. The experiments, performed during development and testing of the early prototypes in the animal laboratory and

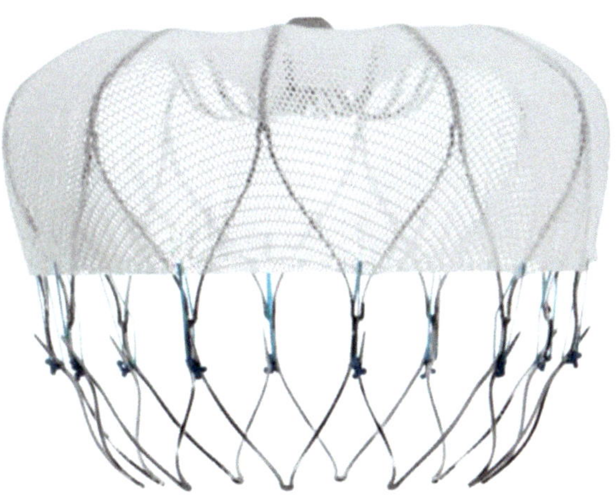

Fig. 4.11 The WATCHMAN device was developed to seal the left atrial appendage and prevent the development of thrombus that could migrate and embolize to result in stroke/systemic embolization

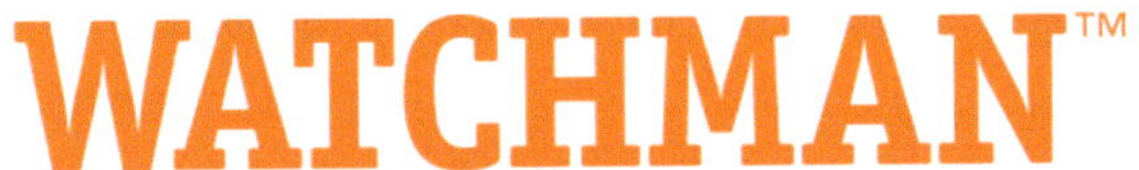

adjunctive therapies used, formed the basis of eventual approval of the WATCHMAN device in the next decades as the only approved device for this indication of stroke prevention. Throughout this decade, the laboratory served as a great repository for interactions with medical device companies as new technology was developed and studied.

Acute Ischemic Syndromes: Pathophysiology

Acute ischemic syndromes remained a focus of interest. The pathways leading to plaque instability in the setting of an otherwise chronic disease remained unclear. Giovanna Liuzzo, who had trained with Attilio Maseri in Italy, came to Mayo Clinic to work with Cornelia Weyand to study, among other things, the role of monocytes that may be active in patients with unstable angina. Such upregulation would result in the production of IL-6 and subsequently acute phase proteins. They studied peripheral blood lymphocytes in patients with unstable and stable angina at the time of hospitalization and after 2 and 12 weeks. The findings were that there were increased frequencies of CD4+CD28null T cells in patients with unstable angina (Fig. 4.12) [34]. The emergence of these cells may result in persistent antigenic stimulation and set the stage for ongoing inflammation. This work led to continued evaluation of T-cell proliferation and plaque instability in acute coronary syndromes

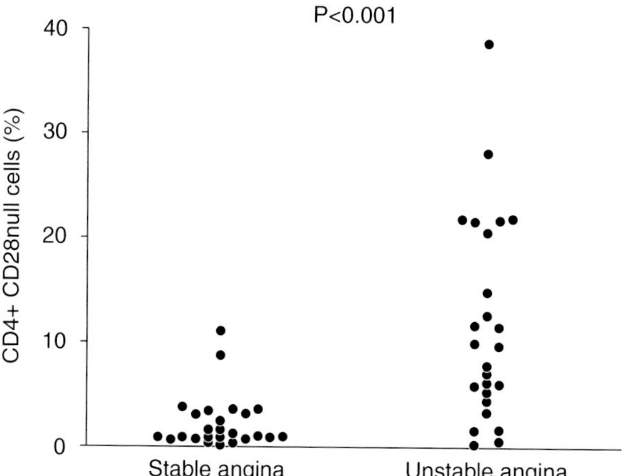

Fig. 4.12 Information on underlying inflammation and its relationship with unstable angina was evaluated using monozytes. In this study, patients with unstable angina had increased frequencies of CD4+ CD28null T cells compared with patients with stable angina. Such T cells may result from persistent antigenic stimulation and may continue to result in the cellular process of inflammation. (From: Liuzzo et al. Circ 100:2135, 1999; used with permission)

[34]. In this work, peripheral blood T cells from patients with and without unstable angina were compared for the distribution of functional blood T cells by flow cytometric analysis. Clonality was identified by spectrotyping and subsequent sequencing. The investigators found that unstable angina was associated with the emergence of monoclonal T-cell populations as compared to patients with stable angina, suggesting that an unstable place may be invaded by clonally expanded T cells and may be involved in plaque disruption. Subsequent studies by Weyand, Holmes, and Frye, among others, identified particular importance to a specialized T-cell subset, "natural killer T cells," which have proinflammatory properties and may contribute to the vascular injury [35]. Basic investigations into the pathophysiology continue in attempts to develop new strategies of care.

Patient Subsets Undergoing Intervention

During the 1990s, the early and subsequent continued application of coronary arterial stents revolutionized the field of restenosis prevention. The first emergency bailout stent at Mayo Clinic was placed by Garratt at the end of a long catheterization laboratory day under the critical eye of the Chief of Cardiovascular surgery. Over the course of their implementation, stents have undergone multiple transformations – from bare metal to drug eluting to biodegradable backbones. Their application spanned the decades from the mid-late 1980s to the present. There was intense focus on issues of acute stent thrombosis with the application of dextran; single, double, and triple antiplatelet therapy; and OAC to prevent the problem (Fig. 4.13).

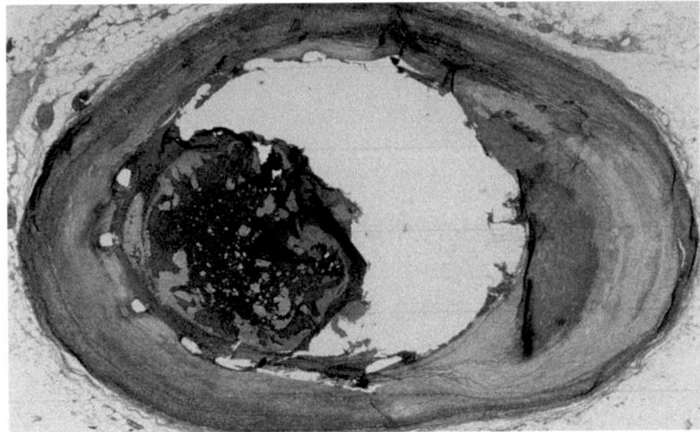

Fig. 4.13 Stent thrombosis in patients post procedure was associated with increased mortality and myocardial infarction, as seen in this specimen from a patient dying following intervention. This phenomena sparked intense interest in pharmacologic and device strategies to eliminate the problem

Vascular complications tended to occur in approximately 15% of patients in the early period post implant because of the intense anticoagulant and antiplatelet therapy. The obligate need for oral anticoagulation disappeared after the introduction of potent antiplatelet therapy and high-pressure balloon inflations, as advocated by Antonio Colombo in Milan, Italy, along with other investigators. These issues were particularly germane in patients with atrial fibrillation who required anticoagulant therapy for stroke prevention but who then required treatment of coronary artery disease with stent implantation. In these patients, triple therapy with the combination of an OAC and dual antiplatelet therapy was associated with a marked increase in bleeding. There was continued discourse about the length of time needed for dual antiplatelet therapy, general European practices tending to favor shorter duration compared with American guidelines. These discussions have continued to be played out beyond the 1990s, as multiple trials and pivotal studies were subsequently performed.

There were other issues in coronary revascularization to be addressed. The implication of renal toxicity with the development of contrast-mediated acute renal failure was well recognized and occurred with increasing frequency related in part to the treatment of more complex lesions and longer procedures guided by contrast angiography. The beginning of multiple studies was initiated by a Mayo Clinic randomized trial comparison of nephrotoxicity of iopamidol and diatrizoate in high-risk patients. Trials such as these focusing on renal toxicity have continued to this day, the majority of which continue to document that the crucial issue has been minimizing contrast dose and maximizing adequate hydration.

Specific patient groups were of special interest, as we studied the wider-spread dissemination of the application of this technology. Bell published one of the early descriptions of gender bias [36] in an assessment of "referral for coronary artery revascularization procedures after diagnostic coronary angiography: Evidence for gender bias?" (Fig. 4.14). Other related evaluations included assessment of in-hospital mortality, specifically in women, after PTCA. Another area of enhanced interest was evaluation of percutaneous revascularization in elderly patients, which was of special importance, as demographics have continued to change.

Since the seminal initial Mayo Clinic description of 16 patients undergoing PTCA for chronic coronary occlusion by Holmes and colleagues in 1984, longer-term follow-up in the entire experience of 365 Mayo Clinic patients became available [16, 21]. Such longer-term follow-up was of extreme importance for the future of this subset of patients in terms of their clinical and functional outcome. As part of this project, Mayo Clinic investigators, led by an interventional fellow (S.S. Srivatsa), performed a detailed histologic analysis [37] of the influence of the duration of coronary occlusion on neovascular channel patterns and intimal plaque composition (Fig. 4.15). This led to the important finding that many "chronic total occlusions" had a very small, persistent lumen that would

1650   JACC Vol. 25, No. 7
                                                                      June 1995:1650-5

SURGERY

Referral for Coronary Artery Revascularization Procedures After Diagnostic Coronary Angiography: Evidence for Gender Bias?

MALCOLM R. BELL, MB, BS, FRACP, FACC, PETER B. BERGER, MD, FACC,
DAVID R. HOLMES, Jr., MD, FACC, CHARLES J. MULLANY, MB, MS, FACC,
KENT R. BAILEY, PhD, BERNARD J. GERSH, MB, ChB, DPhil, FACC

Rochester, Minnesota

Objectives. We sought to determine whether there is a gender bias in the selection of patients for coronary revascularization once the severity of the underlying coronary artery disease has been established with angiography.

Background. It has been suggested that women with coronary artery disease are less likely to be referred for coronary angiography and coronary artery bypass surgery than men. Whether such a referral bias for revascularization procedures, including coronary angioplasty, is present once angiography has been performed is not clear.

Methods. We retrospectively analyzed 22,795 patients with suspected coronary artery disease who underwent coronary angiography between 1981 and 1991 and compared the numbers of women and men who underwent either coronary artery bypass surgery or coronary angioplasty within 30 days of coronary angiography.

Results. Angiography revealed significant (one-vessel or more) disease in 15,455 patients (52% of women, 76% of men). Despite worse symptoms, women had less extensive coronary disease than men as judged by the number of vessels diseased. Women were also more likely to have other co-morbid diseases. An equal proportion of women (54%) and men underwent revascularization procedures. After adjustment for baseline differences and age, differences in the two individual revascularization strategies were very small: More women tended to have coronary angioplasty ([absolute difference ± 1 SD] +3.3 ± 0.7%, p < 0.0001), but fewer had coronary artery bypass surgery than men (−2.5 ± 0.8%, p = 0.003). When the two revascularization strategies were considered together, there was no significant gender difference in overall adjusted use of revascularization (+0.8 ± 0.9%, p = 0.41).

Conclusions. Once diagnostic coronary angiography had been performed, no major differences in the overall utilization of revascularization procedures were noted for women compared with men.

(J Am Coll Cardiol 1995;25:1650–5)

Fig. 4.14 Mayo Clinic focused on specific patient groups. Bell et al. focused on this on an early study on gender bias. (From Bell et al. J Am Coll Cardiol 1995;25:1650–5; used with permission)

not be identified during angiography; however, that could be crossed with specially designed guide wires to access the distal vessel and facilitate successful treatment.

Chronic Total Occlusion

As the field of percutaneous coronary intervention expanded and matured, Mayo Clinic was heavily involved and worked with the American Board of Internal Medicine, focusing on guidelines for training, credentialing, and maintenance of competence for the performance of both angiography and interventions [22, 26, 29]. These initiatives were spearheaded by the Society of Cardiac Angiography and Intervention. An early group participated fully in these agendas, including Holmes in his role as President of that organization. Subsequent to this, Garrett occupied

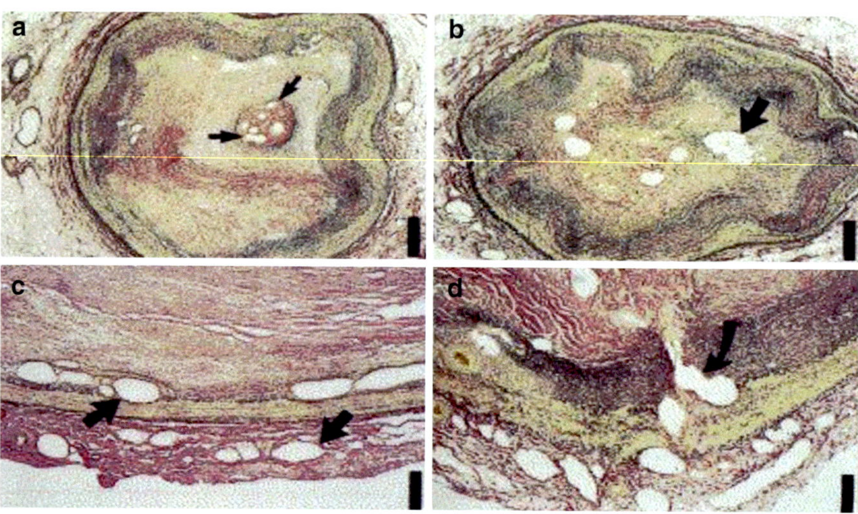

Fig. 4.15 Chronic total occlusion of coronary arteries has been one of the most common reasons to refer patients for CABG rather than PCI. An early Mayo Clinic study evaluated pathologic specimens of patients who were found to have a chronic total occlusion at autopsy. Srivatsa et al. found that even though the angiography performed previously in these patients had been felt to be complete occlusion of the specific vessel, that microchannels were often present. Subsequent advances in CTO procedures had come to be facilitated by the presence of these microchannels. (**a**) Low-power view (elastic van Gieson stain) of an advanced chronic total occlusion (CTO) lesion demonstrating lumen recannalization with small and medium neovascular channels (NCs) (arrows). (**b**) Low-power view (elastic van Gieson stain) of a CTO, demonstrating several large intimal plaque (IP) NCs (arrow) within the IP. (**c** and **d**) High-power views (elastic van Gieson stain) demonstrating several large NCs within the adventitia and also traversing the media between the adventitia and the IP (curved arrow) (From Srivatsa et al. [37]; used with permission)

that same role with great impact on invasive and interventional cardiology and worked closely with regulatory agencies and multiple professional societies on reimbursement and coding.

As part of these processes, there was interest in the development of certification standards for interventional cardiology. Working with the Board of American Internal Medicine, under the leadership of Dr. Spencer King, a group developed an examination for added qualifications in interventional cardiology. An early group including Holmes met frequently with the American Board of Internal Medicine, learning about optimal test question writing, development of standardized tests, and grading strategies. This important project resulted in national testing and certification for individuals working in the field. Importantly, it set in place the development of other sub-specialties such as pacing and electrophysiology, which followed along the same pathway for certification and credentialing.

Treatment of Multivessel CAD

The relationship between interventional cardiology and cardiovascular surgery remained central to the field. Important differences between the two strategies were emphasized and debated, including several factors: (1) an invasive versus less invasive procedure; (2) the fact that restenosis only pertained to PTCA; (3) the presence of chronic total occlusions that could be bypassed by surgery but only successfully treated in very carefully selected patients with PTCA; (4) the importance of completeness of revascularization on outcome. These issues had major importance that continue to the current day as the frequency of achieving complete revascularization is substantially better as a whole with CABG compared with PCI; and (5) the role of PTCA for more complex LMCA and 3VD patients. These formed the basis for multiple subsequent registries and trials that have formed the fundamental professional societal guidelines.

Evaluation of the new therapeutic procedures that had been implemented was pursued vigorously. An early study of PTCA versus CABG in patients with MVD had been championed by Dr. Michael Mock in the 1980s. After the development of the protocol and case report forms, submission for an NIH grant was not funded. Subsequently, it was transitioned to the BARI (Bypass Angioplasty Revascularization Investigation) Trial, comparing CABG with PCI funded by the NIH. This study, headed by Frye, was toward its final endpoint at 5 years. It had enrolled 1829 patients with multivessel coronary artery disease suitable for either CABG or PCTA and found at an average of 5.4 years that survival with coronary surgery was not statistically different compared to PTCA (89.3% vs 86.3% ns). The authors, however, found that diabetic patients, who made up 19% of the total enrollment in the BARI Trial, had enhanced survival at 5 years with CABG – 80.6% for CABG vs 65.5% for PTCA group ($p = 0.003$) (Fig. 4.16a, b) [32]. In contrast, in nondiabetic patients at 5 years, there was no significant difference in death and myocardial infarction (80.5% for CABG vs 78.7% with PTCA). Repeat revascularization, however, was increased in the PTCA group, which again led to increased interest in approaches for prevention or mitigation of restenosis. This trial, particularly with the finding in diabetics, affected the entire field of coronary intervention, influencing the care of patients (Fig. 4.17); the subsequent development of new devices as well as later scientific investigations, including both large single and multicenter registries, and RCT, including BARI 2D, continued to focus on diabetic patients.

The original NHLBI PTCA Registry, in which Mayo Clinic had been the 16th center, had been closed to new patient enrollment, though follow-up continued. It was transitioned to a new NIH Registry (NACI – New Approaches to Coronary Intervention); Mayo Clinic was the third highest enroller studying these new strategies of care. During this time, Mayo Clinic participated in five industry protocols, which led to FDA product approval for TEC atherectomy, directional

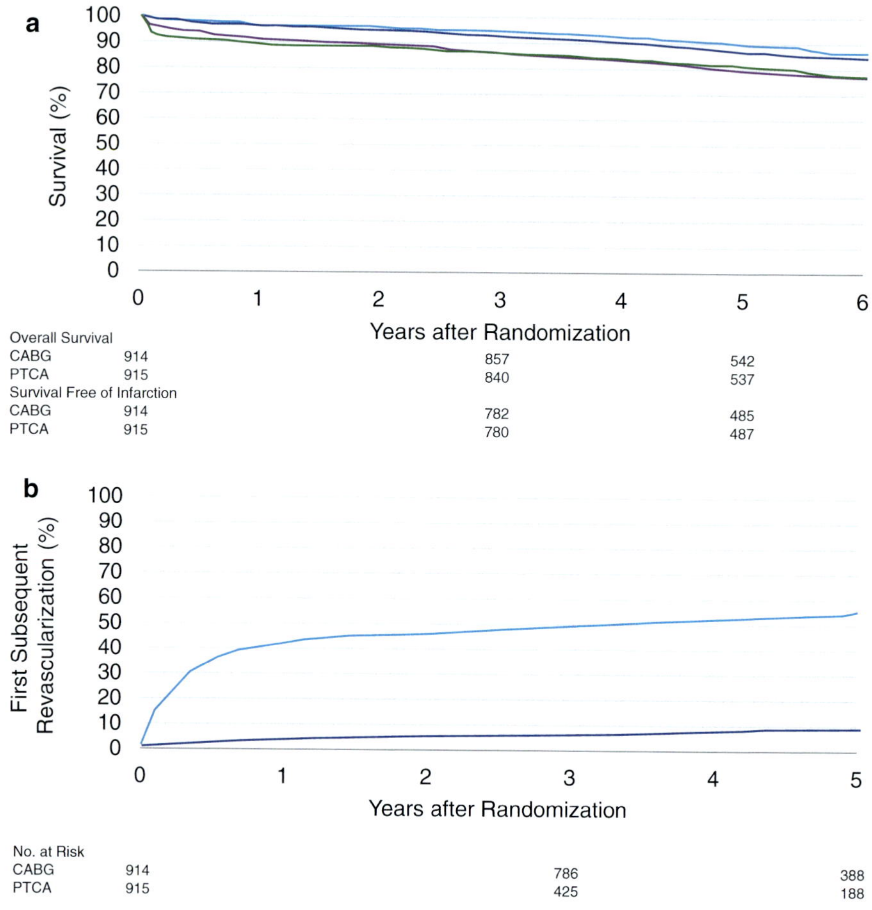

Fig. 4.16 (a) Kaplan-Meier plots of survival in BARI Trail with no difference between CABG and PTCA. (b) In BARI Trial, the results of subsequent revascularizations were strikingly different with increased rates with PTCA. (From NEJM 1996;335(4);217–225; used with permission)

coronary atherectomy, the Gianturco-Roubin stent for coronary bail out, and both aortic and mitral balloon valvuloplasty. In the latter case, Mayo Clinic presented on behalf of the company (Mansfield Inc.) to the FDA panel for which approval for mitral balloon valvuloplasty was granted. This approval opened the way for initiation of percutaneous mitral procedures, which subsequently became standard of care for selected patients with rheumatic mitral stenosis [5, 14]. Mayo investigators during that time published papers on the long-term follow-up of patients undergoing closed transventicular mitral commisurotomy as a surrogate for percutaneous balloon mitral valvuloplasty and served as the basis for a

Fig. 4.17 An important, although not pre-specified, BARI analysis evaluated outcome in diabetes and found as per USA today that…

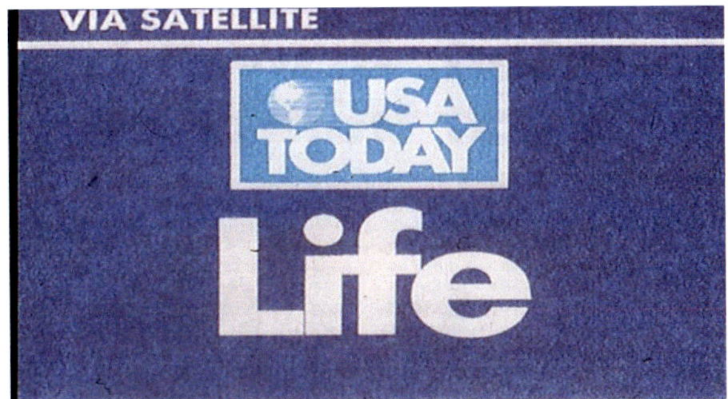

Angioplasty not best option for diabetics

By Doug Levy
USA TODAY

Diabetics with heart disease are better off with bypass surgery than angioplasty, the National Heart, Lung and Blood Institute said Thursday.

A study of 1,829 people with blockages in two or more heart

Dr. George Sopko, an NHLBI cardiologist. However, the recommendation only applies to patients with both severe diabetes and two or more blocked coronary arteries.

Such patients who already have had angioplasty should be monitored carefully, he says, "but there's no need to panic."

subsequent randomized trial in the field, which led the way to the acceptance of mitral balloon valvuloplasty as the treatment of choice for selected patients with mitral stenosis. We also published information on the optimal specific technology to be used [12]. Although that disease has become less prevalent in "Western countries," it remains a significant global problem affecting younger patients and has been particularly difficult in the setting of young women during pregnancy with resultant morbidity and even mortality for both mother and fetus. In addition, Mayo Clinic was an enrolling center, and multicenter trials evaluating IVUS which had been found to play an important role in evaluating coronary arterial lesions specifically left main coronary artery stenosis and planning optimal interventional strategies and documenting results [12]. Despite excellent scientific data on the clinical importance of IVUS, it remained underutilized in the US, a pattern which continued in subsequent decades.

An important milestone was reached in 1993. In the late 1980s, the cath lab had shifted the practice, becoming more eager to explore the relative merits of PTCA versus thrombolytic therapy for acute myocardial infarction. As part of this interest, Ray Gibbons, an early invasive cardiologist by training and working in the cath lab at Mayo Clinic, had designed a randomized clinical trial of immediate angioplasty versus tissue plasminogen activator. Enrollment started in April 1989 and finished in June 1991. The primary endpoint was the change in and size of the perfusion defect assessed by matched admission and discharge tomographic imaging using technetium-99 m sestamibi (Fig. 4.18) [38]. In the 108 patients enrolled, there was

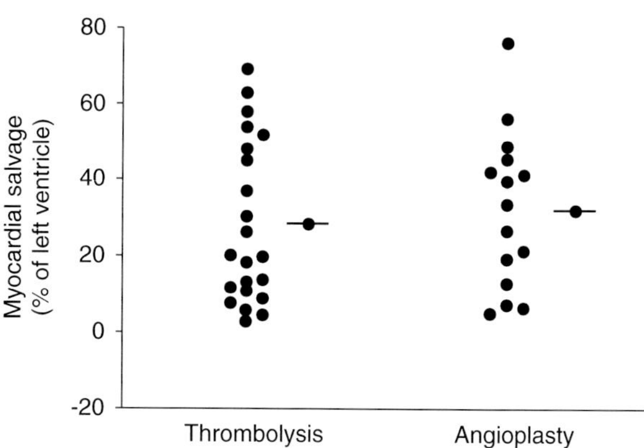

Fig. 4.18 Using myocardial salvage (the percentage of left ventricle) assessed with sestamibi in patients with anterior infarction, there was no difference between thrombolytic therapy and PTCA. Such analyses have become standard endpoints. (From NEJM 1993;328:685–91; used with permission)

no significant difference in myocardial salvage between the two approaches. There were several limitations of this small study, which affected Mayo Clinic's subsequent work:

(a) Data on the primary endpoint was missing from five patients because of technical reasons.
(b) The confidence intervals chosen for comparison in the study.
(c) The fact that many patients underwent revascularization for recurrent ischemia.

These issues and limitations were addressed in subsequent studies using the endpoint of myocardial salvage, initially identified and chosen by Gibbons working along with other Mayo Clinic investigators and which became widely used in the field of studies on reperfusion therapy in acute infarction.

Other work in the field of acute myocardial infarction involved the use of adjunctive therapeutic agents aimed at further improving myocardial salvage. Mayo authors, led by Garratt, designed a study administering a combination of adenosine and lidocaine as a bolus delivered to the infarct-related artery in patients with STEMI prior to immediate angioplasty. This small study included 45 patients. Compared with historical controls, late perfusion defects were improved with the combination of adenosine and lidocaine. Although the authors recommended that randomized clinical trials were justified, they were not carried out for lack of industry funding in part because both adenosine and lidocaine were widely available generic drugs. Such issues of funding may have a large impact on eventual practice patterns. In the field of acute myocardial infarction, these trials and results of catheter-based reperfusion were part of the information that resulted in primary PCI being identified as the treatment of choice for acute myocardial infarction, provided that resources and experienced personnel were available. In regions where those resources were not available, strategies for lytic therapy and then urgent transfer to an experienced infarction center (so-called "drip and ship") were put in place. During that time, Mayo Clinic, working throughout the area of referral, identified processes to facilitate urgent transfer.

An important component of the treatment of STEMI and non-STEMI involved patients who presented with or who developed cardiogenic shock [3, 39, 40]. This group of patients had been the focus of great interest because of the rates of 60% of mortality and morbidity associated with that complication. Mayo Clinic investigators, including Hasdai from Israel, identified information on frequency and characteristics, basic pathophysiology, timing, outcome, and the need for optimization of strategies of care in patients with both STEMI and non-STEMI. Investigations of these patients formed the basis of multiple randomized clinical studies that have followed since that time.

In addition to the trials and procedures, there were other major changes in the cath lab. As mentioned, the animal laboratory became a central resource for the development and testing of new devices and understanding basic mechanisms of disease. During this decade, a new approach to vascular molecular biology was initiated. Dr. Rob Simari, who had entered the Mayo Clinic program as an advanced fellow in interventional cardiology, became interested in basic underlying principles of cardiovascular diseases. After discussion, Simari modified his career plans. He selected a different track and was given the opportunity to obtain advanced training in vascular molecular biology as a Mayo Foundation scholar working under the direction of Dr. Elizabeth Nabel at the University of Michigan. Upon return to Mayo Clinic, he became a national leader and well-established investigator, interacting closely with the NIH and study sections on regenerative medicine before leaving to eventually become the Chancellor of the University of Kansas.

A central component of the mission of the laboratory required superb cardiac imaging, which was fundamental for diagnosis and treatment. At that time, cine films formed the platform for archival storage [41]. Such coronary angiographic data were the basis upon which strategies of care were based – namely, medical therapy, PTCA, or CABG. Unfortunately, each vendor of angiographic equipment had their own unique format, such that images from one vendor were not always able to be read by other systems. This resulted in the application of the term "Tower of Babel"; the worst-case scenario was a patient coming for evaluation of coronary artery disease, who had recently undergone diagnostic coronary angiography at another institution, which provided images on a CD that could not be reviewed and analyzed on our system, and which occasionally necessitated recommending that the patient have a repeat angiographic study. Working under a collaborative agreement with General Electric (GE), a prototype archival system was developed for cine film replacement by Merrill Wondrow, Jack Cusma, and others. Such systems became the focus of national committees with input from Mayo Clinic aimed at identifying a preferred system for image transfer. The standards for this became the DICOM 3 initiative which was successfully adopted as standard industry formats and allowed angiographic images from different systems to be read by all institutions. As part of this, Mayo Clinic investigators, particularly Merrill Wondrow, were involved with a proposal for high-speed data image transmission. Government funding for this project linked Mayo Clinic Rochester with sister facilities in Eau Claire, Wisconsin, and Scottsdale, Arizona, and allowed transfer of images during catheterization procedures to facilitate patient management. Other imaging projects included the validation of a new UNIX-based quantitative coronary angiographic system, three-dimensional reconstruction of the coronary arterial tree, and the use of image reconstruction for better assessment of complex congenital cardiac lesions to optimize subsequent procedural performance, either transcatheter or surgical.

Other imaging modalities were also being tested, including intravascular ultrasound and angioscopy. Under the direction of Dr. Amir Lerman, a full program evaluating endothelial function in coronary anatomy was implemented for the evaluation of patients with microvascular disease utilizing intracoronary Doppler, allowing the study of flow and resistance and identifying patients in whom coronary vasospasm or microvascular disease was the pathophysiology of clinical presentation. These studies formed the basis for incorporation of the use of L-arginine in practice today for patients with coronary microvascular disease in combination with calcium channel antagonists [24].

There were other major changes. During the period from 1989 to 1993, there had been an increase in full-time equivalent staff consultants with a significant growth in major laboratory procedures and a dramatic growth in stent-based approaches. Projected growth of 5% per year was estimated for the rest of the decade. A particularly important program of outreach was developed and administered by Dr. Byron Olney. Mayo Clinic had placed outreach cardiologists in Mankato, Eau Claire, La Crosse, and Austin to provide cardiac care closer to patient homes. These practices continued to grow, and the concept of more advanced outreach strategies was initiated.

Mobile Cardiac Cath Lab

Early discussions in the literature had identified a potential role for mobile cardiac catheterization facilities, which had initially been used beginning in 1989. As part of these conversations, Mayo Clinic developed their own program. Multiple issues and scenarios were considered. These included facilities at the sites for mobile laboratory equipment, close proximity to the regional site, trained nursing care and bed capacity, video communications, facility and processes for urgent transport back to St. Mary's Hospital via helicopter or urgent ground transport, close relationships with the regional center internists and cardiologists, Mayo Clinic staffing for the procedure both for the angiographic equipment and procedural nursing staff, and patient selection, among other important issues. For each of these potential issues, specific protocols were developed and vigorously discussed. Concerns, in part, related to focusing all cases only on diagnostic angiograms. Specific questions raised included what to do if, while at the regional site, a patient arrived with cardiogenic shock related to an acute myocardial infarction. In that circumstance, would emergent angiography and dilatation be able to be offered? After a long discussion, the decision was made that only diagnostic studies would be performed. Other important issues included other patient demographics. In a report from a registry of 1001 patients being seen in a mobile cath lab setting [42], the indications included angina CCA II–IV in 46.4%, atypical chest pain in 36.9%, and a positive exercise stress test in 25.6%. These criteria mirrored those used in the Mayo Clinic mobile

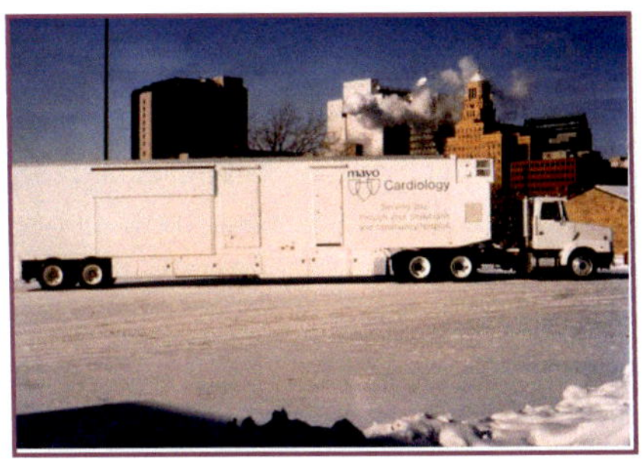

Mobile Cath Lab
Hospitals Currently Signed-Up
(February 1991)

Austin MN – Wednesday
Winona MN – Tuesday
Mankato MN – Thursday

First patient procedure – February 20, 1991

Fig. 4.19 The mobile cath lab – 1991

Fig. 4.20 Only one casualty
was identified one early
morning on the way to
Austin, Minnesota

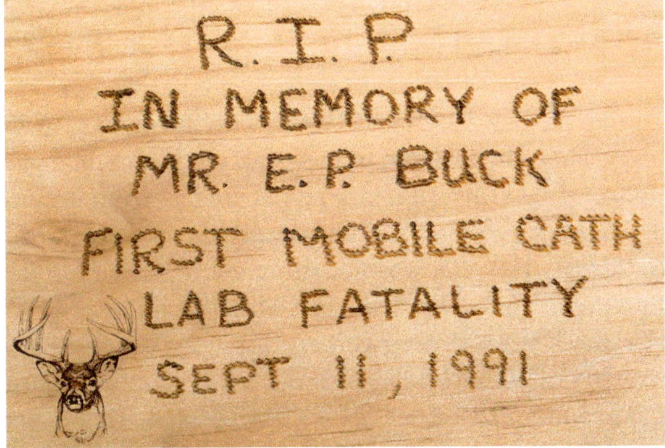

cath lab throughout the time it was administered under the supervision of Dr. Andre Lapeyre (Fig. 4.19). In our experience, there were no significant patient complications, and no patient required urgent transfer. The response of the communities was very positive, both the hospitals and the patients, and the presence of these mobile laboratories helped to foster growth of cardiology in their respective hospitals. In one of the locations, it was eventually added as a permanent placement when the radiology suite there was upgraded (La Crosse, Wisconsin). The only casualty of the laboratory was a deer that was hit during the early morning hours as the mobile laboratory was being transported to Austin, Minnesota (Fig. 4.20). Of the three mobile sites, two of them were converted to fixed facilities. Accordingly, the mobile cath lab was no longer needed.

The Mankato fixed cath lab construction was completed in late 1998. To become operational, nurses and techs went to Rochester for training and then worked through having the T3 lines in place to support real-time bidirectional video during a case, if needed, with images and hemodynamic data with backup systems in place if anything failed. Several transportation dry runs were done in the event of complications to make sure patients could get to the OR in Rochester in as short a time as possible. For the first several cases, the Mayo-1 helicopter was flown to Mankato to stand by in case of complications. All that work to get ready to safely do the first cases took several months of preparation. At that time, ACC guidelines said this should not be done. This was another great example of the capacity of the CV department to develop the best treatment options for patients because, although there were great "door to needle times" for thrombolytics, there were more patients that were untreated for MIs because they were past the time window. At that time, the 2-hour ground transport time to Rochester or Minneapolis was costly in terms of muscle and outcomes. Even when patients could be flown, it was a 25-minute flight time from Rochester to Mankato, 10–15 minutes onsite in Mankato and another 25 minutes in the air back to Rochester to get the patient in the cath lab from the Mankato ER or hospital.

Facility Expansion

During the late 1980s and 1990s, with the rapid growth in the numbers and type of procedures, the addition of new staff physicians and paramedical personnel, and the influx of new investigators and scientists from around the world, it had become apparent that the initial clinical cath lab on the sixth floor of the Alfred building at St. Mary's Hospital was not sufficient in size (19,000 square feet) and shape, configuration, and equipment. The Mayo Clinic overall Chair of the Clinical Practice (Dr. Mark Warner) reviewed and approved a request in 1993 that the cath lab executive committee, working with our administrative assistant, Alice Flood, had developed to move to a new area – Mary Brigh 4. That expanded facility would increase to 43,000 square feet with 12 new laboratories, 10 of which would be ready for immediate use and dedicated to invasive and interventional cardiology, pacing, and electrophysiology. The request included 37.0 full-time equivalent (FTE) allied health personnel. The total cost was projected to be $19,633,500 (to be realized by 1995). There were also structural changes. The design included three pods of four procedure rooms, each of which surrounded and was connected with the central core for equipment for that pod of rooms. This eliminated the need for staff to leave the pod to find equipment in other areas of the cath lab during procedural performance. Accordingly, this radial strategy improved efficiency. There was also a developmental procedure room for new equipment; this room had a dedicated closed and secured gallery for physician and industry observers from around the world who had been involved in the development of more advanced equipment. This was essential, as new flat-panel imaging systems were brought into Mayo Clinic for first US evaluation. These new systems had been developed to meet the increasing need for visualization of the fine guide wires in use and to facilitate identification of very-fine arterial structures such as small micro-dissections as part of optimizing procedural performance. Physicians from around the world came to evaluate the images. Of interest, the individual operators from different countries sometimes had specific differences in their desired image format concerning contrast and pixilation and display of the entire image set. During this time, there was a GE "Edison" engineer assigned full time at Mayo Clinic who worked very closely with Merrill Wondrow and Jack Cusma on optimizing image quality and for continued development and testing of new equipment. An important application was the transfer of images from the procedure rooms to the outpatient Mayo Building several blocks away and to satellite facilities. This process allowed the catheterization personnel to immediately transfer images during the diagnostic procedure to the referring physician or surgeon to discuss and then implement therapeutic strategies such as coronary intervention and to review the procedure while it was being performed. Intense interest on radiation safety for both patients and staff also became a priority at this time, with reports published on the amount of radiation exposure in complex procedures such as treatment of CTOs. Cusma, who had come from Duke, was a central figure in the balancing of excellent images in complex clinical settings, with the need for minimizing radiation. Other changes in the new cath lab included an extended prep and recovery room that had specific capabilities for pediatric patients and other spaces for family consultation, as well as rooms that were used for cardioversions.

Disappointments

One final enhancement was never realized, to our disappointment. During the decade there was increased interest in other imaging modalities, including MRI and CT, that would add important information for patient care. These other modalities had specific structural requirements, particularly for shielding of MRI units. The potential to combine either of these imaging modalities with cardiac angiography offered tremendous possibilities not available at any other institution. For example, an MRI study combined with coronary angiography would allow documentation of the extent of left ventricular necrosis and enable more focused dilatation; or with CT, the rotational aspect could help to define areas in the pulmonary arteries that would benefit from stent implantation. When we planned the new cath lab on the fourth floor of St. Mary's Hospital, a room was specifically designed and built facing out on the outdoor wall of the hospital. It had the shielding required for MRI and had external windows that could be removed for new equipment installation, which could be lifted up outside and installed without the need to disrupt the rest of the cath lab function. This room was large enough and positioned so that it would include MRI, coronary angiography, and CT that could be used as clinical protocols mandated. High-level discussions were made with GE for installation of a research MRI unit in that room, and tacit agreement by GE was obtained by the head of the cath lab. However, navigating such an arrangement with Mayo Clinic competing vested interests in radiology intent on maintaining complete control of that modality proved too much of a challenge to overcome, and the whole concept of combining imaging modalities in the same procedure room to optimize patient care and provide a platform for scientific investigation was shelved. This would have been an amazing opportunity for science and development that would have benefited patient care and helped to shape the future but, at that time, with competing interests, was not to be consummated but hopefully to be resurrected at some time in the future as part of more collaborative practices.

The decade was one of the amazing growths in the breadth of patient care, the advancement of science, the development of brilliant careers at Mayo Clinic and globally, and the excitement of networking with many stakeholders to create and envision the future that would continue into the next decade to come.

References

1. Holmes D Jr, Myler R, Kent K, et al. National Heart, Lung, and Blood Institute Percutaneous Transluminal Coronary Angioplasty Registry as a standard for comparison of new devices. When should we use it, and what should we compare? Circulation. 1991;84:1828–30.
2. Holmes DR Jr, Topol EJ, Califf RM, et al. A multicenter, randomized trial of coronary angioplasty versus directional atherectomy for patients with saphenous vein bypass graft lesions. CAVEAT-II investigators. Circulation. 1995;91:1966–74.
3. Hibbard MD, Holmes DR Jr, Bailey KR, Reeder GS, Bresnahan JF, Gersh BJ. Percutaneous transluminal coronary angioplasty in patients with cardiogenic shock. J Am Coll Cardiol. 1992;19:639–46.
4. Holmes DR Jr. The mobile catheterization laboratory: should we pick it up and move it? The trustees of the Society for Cardiac Angiography and Interventions. Catheter Cardiovasc Diagn. 1992;26:69–70.
5. Rihal CS, Schaff HV, Frye RL, Bailey KR, Hammes LN, Holmes DR Jr. Long-term follow-up of patients undergoing closed transventricular mitral commissurotomy: a useful surrogate for percutaneous balloon mitral valvuloplasty? J Am Coll Cardiol. 1992;20:781–6.
6. Popma JJ, Topol EJ, Hinohara T, et al. Abrupt vessel closure after directional coronary atherectomy. The U.S. Directional Atherectomy Investigator Group. J Am Coll Cardiol. 1992;19:1372–9.
7. Holmes DR Jr, Simpson JB, Berdan LG, et al. Abrupt closure: the CAVEAT I experience. Coronary angioplasty versus excisional atherectomy trial. J Am Coll Cardiol. 1995;26:1494–500.
8. Bell MR, Garratt KN, Bresnahan JF, Edwards WD, Holmes DR Jr. Relation of deep arterial resection and coronary artery aneurysms after directional coronary atherectomy. J Am Coll Cardiol. 1992;20:1474–81.
9. Murphy JG, Schwartz RS, Edwards WD, Camrud AR, Vlietstra RE, Holmes DR Jr. Percutaneous polymeric stents in porcine coronary arteries. Initial experience with polyethylene terephthalate stents. Circulation. 1992;86:1596–604.
10. Garratt KN, Holmes DR Jr, Bell MR, et al. Restenosis after directional coronary atherectomy: differences between primary atheromatous and restenosis lesions and influence of subintimal tissue resection. J Am Coll Cardiol. 1990;16:1665–71.
11. Garratt K, et al. Differential histopathology of primary atherosclerotic and restenotic lesions in coronary arteries and saphenous vein bypass grafts: Analysis of tissue obtained from 73 patients by directional atherectomy. J Am Coll Cardiol. 1991;17:442–8.
12. Nishimura RA, Higano ST, Holmes DR Jr. Use of intracoronary ultrasound imaging for assessing left main coronary artery disease. Mayo Clin Proc. 1993;68:134–40.
13. Litvack F, Eigler N, Margolis J, et al. Percutaneous excimer laser coronary angioplasty: results in the first consecutive 3,000 patients. The ELCA investigators. J Am Coll Cardiol. 1994;23:323–9.

14. Rihal CS, Nishimura RA, Reeder GS, Holmes DR Jr. Percutaneous balloon mitral valvuloplasty: comparison of double and single (Inoue) balloon techniques. Catheter Cardiovasc Diagn. 1993;29:183–90.

15. Holmes DR Jr, Reeder GS, Ghazzal ZM, et al. Coronary perforation after excimer laser coronary angioplasty: The Excimer Laser Coronary Angioplasty Registry experience. J Am Coll Cardiol. 1994;23:330–5.

16. Holmes DR Jr, Forrester JS, Litvack F, et al. Chronic total obstruction and short-term outcome: the Excimer Laser Coronary Angioplasty Registry experience. Mayo Clin Proc. 1993;68:5–10.

17. Reeder GS, Lapeyre AC, Edwards WD, Holmes DR Jr. Aspiration thrombectomy for removal of coronary thrombus. Am J Cardiol. 1992;70:107–10.

18. Jeong MH, Owen WG, Staab ME, et al. Porcine model of stent thrombosis: platelets are the primary component of acute stent closure. Catheter Cardiovasc Diagn. 1996;38:38–43.

19. Vlietstra RE, Holmes DR Jr, Rodeheffer RJ, Bailey KR. Consequences of restenosis after coronary angioplasty. Int J Cardiol. 1991;31:143–7.

20. Schwartz RS, Holder DJ, Holmes DR, et al. Neointimal thickening after severe coronary artery injury is limited by a short-term administration of a factor Xa inhibitor. Results in a porcine model. Circulation. 1996;93:1542–8.

21. Schwartz RS, Edwards WD, Bailey KR, Camrud AR, Jorgenson MA, Holmes DR Jr. Differential neointimal response to coronary artery injury in pigs and dogs. Implications for restenosis models. Arterioscler Thromb. 1994;14:395–400.

22. Forrester JS, Topol EJ, Abele JE, Holmes D, Skorton DJ. Proceedings of the 28th Bethesda conference. Practice guidelines and the quality of care. Bethesda, Maryland, October 21-22, 1996. J Am Coll Cardiol. 1997;29:1125–79.

23. Schwartz RS, Murphy JG, Edwards WD, Camrud AR, Vliestra RE, Holmes DR. Restenosis after balloon angioplasty. A practical proliferative model in porcine coronary arteries. Circulation. 1990;82:2190–200.

24. Lerman A, Burnett JC Jr, Higano ST, McKinley LJ, Holmes DR Jr. Long-term L-arginine supplementation improves small-vessel coronary endothelial function in humans. Circulation. 1998;97:2123–8.

25. Schwartz RS, Huber KC, Murphy JG, et al. Restenosis and the proportional neointimal response to coronary artery injury: results in a porcine model. J Am Coll Cardiol. 1992;19:267–74.

26. Holmes DR Jr, Hirshfeld J Jr, Faxon D, Vlietstra RE, Jacobs A, King SB 3rd. ACC Expert Consensus document on coronary artery stents. Document of the American College of Cardiology. J Am Coll Cardiol. 1998;32:1471–82.

27. Holmes DR Jr, Berger PB, Hochman JS, et al. Cardiogenic shock in patients with acute ischemic syndromes with and without ST-segment elevation. Circulation. 1999;100:2067–73.

28. McKenna CJ, Camrud AR, Sangiorgi G, et al. Fibrin-film stenting in a porcine coronary injury model: efficacy and safety compared with uncoated stents. J Am Coll Cardiol. 1998;31:1434–8.

29. Hirshfeld JW Jr, Banas JS Jr, Brundage BH, et al. American College of Cardiology training statement on recommendations for the structure of an optimal adult interventional cardiology training program: a report of the American College of Cardiology task force on clinical expert consensus documents. J Am Coll Cardiol. 1999;34:2141–7.

30. van der Giessen WJ, Lincoff AM, Schwartz RS, et al. Marked inflammatory sequelae to implantation of biodegradable and nonbiodegradable polymers in porcine coronary arteries. Circulation. 1996;94:1690–7.

31. Blackshear JL, Odell JA. Appendage obliteration to reduce stroke in cardiac surgical patients with atrial fibrillation. Ann Thorac Surg. 1996;61:755–9.

32. Holmes DR Jr, Nishimura RA, Reeder GS. In-hospital mortality after balloon aortic valvuloplasty: frequency and associated factors. J Am Coll Cardiol. 1991;17:189–92.

33. Fountain R, Holmes DR Jr, Hodgson PK, Chandrasekaran K, Van Tassel R, Sick P. Potential applicability and utilization of left atrial appendage occlusion devices in patients with atrial fibrillation. Am Heart J. 2006;152:720–3.

34. Liuzzo G, Goronzy JJ, Yang H, et al. Monoclonal T-cell proliferation and plaque instability in acute coronary syndromes. Circulation. 2000;101:2883–8.
35. Weyand CM, Goronzy JJ, Liuzzo G, Kopecky SL, Holmes DR Jr, Frye RL. T-cell immunity in acute coronary syndromes. Mayo Clin Proc. 2001;76:1011–20.
36. Bell MR, Berger PB, Holmes DR Jr, Mullany CJ, Bailey KR, Gersh BJ. Referral for coronary artery revascularization procedures after diagnostic coronary angiography: evidence for gender bias? J Am Coll Cardiol. 1995;25:1650–5.
37. Srivatsa SS, Edwards WD, Boos CM, et al. Histologic correlates of angiographic chronic total coronary artery occlusions: influence of occlusion duration on neovascular channel patterns and intimal plaque composition. J Am Coll Cardiol. 1997;29:955–63.
38. Gibbons RJ, Holmes DR, Reeder GS, Bailey KR, Hopfenspirger MR, Gersh BJ. Immediate angioplasty compared with the administration of a thrombolytic agent followed by conservative treatment for myocardial infarction. The Mayo Coronary Care Unit and Catheterization Laboratory Groups. N Engl J Med. 1993;328:685–91.
39. Hasdai D, Holmes DR Jr, Califf RM, et al. Cardiogenic shock complicating acute myocardial infarction: predictors of death. GUSTO investigators. Global utilization of streptokinase and tissue-plasminogen activator for occluded coronary arteries. Am Heart J. 1999;138:21–31.
40. Hasdai D, Holmes DR Jr, Topol EJ, et al. Frequency and clinical outcome of cardiogenic shock during acute myocardial infarction among patients receiving reteplase or alteplase. Results from GUSTO-III. Global use of strategies to open occluded coronary arteries. Eur Heart J. 1999;20:128–35.
41. Holmes DR Jr, Wondrow MA, Bell MR, Nissen SE, Cusma JT. Cine film replacement: digital archival requirements and remaining obstacles. Catheter Cardiovasc Diagn. 1998;44:346–56. discussion 357
42. Bersin RM, Elliott CM, Elliott AV, et al. Mobile cardiac catheterization registry: report of the first 1,001 patients. Catheter Cardiovasc Diagn. 1994;31:1–7.

Chapter 5
1980–1990: Structural Heart Interventions

Guy S. Reeder and David R. Holmes Jr.

Catheter-based structural heart interventions in adult patients naturally evolved from coronary artery intervention techniques. Since the main interventional tool initially available during this decade was the balloon catheter, it is no surprise that dilatation of stenotic cardiac valves became the main target of interest. The basic techniques, such as antegrade, retrograde, and transseptal approaches, evolved along with refinements in catheter technology and coexistent developments in imaging technology to yield a wide variety of catheter-based interventional procedures currently available (Table 5.1). A timeline of these events is shown in Fig. 5.1.

Table 5.1 Structural heart disease interventions have become an increasingly large component of the adult catheterization laboratory practice

Current adult structural interventions
TAVR
Aortic valvuloplasty
TMVR, mitral valve in valve, mitral valve in ring
MitraClip
Mitral balloon valvuloplasty
Alcohol septal ablation for HCM
Peri-leak closure
PFO closure
Coronary fistula closure
LV false aneurysm closure
PFO, ASD, VSD closure

G. S. Reeder (✉) · D. R. Holmes Jr.
Department of Cardiovascular Diseases, Mayo Clinic, Rochester, MN, USA
e-mail: reeder.guy@mayo.edu; Holmes.david@mayo.edu

© Mayo Foundation for Medical Education and Research,
under exclusive license to Springer Nature Switzerland AG 2021
D. R. Holmes Jr., R. L. Frye (eds.), *The Mayo Clinic Cardiac Catheterization Laboratory*, https://doi.org/10.1007/978-3-030-79329-6_5

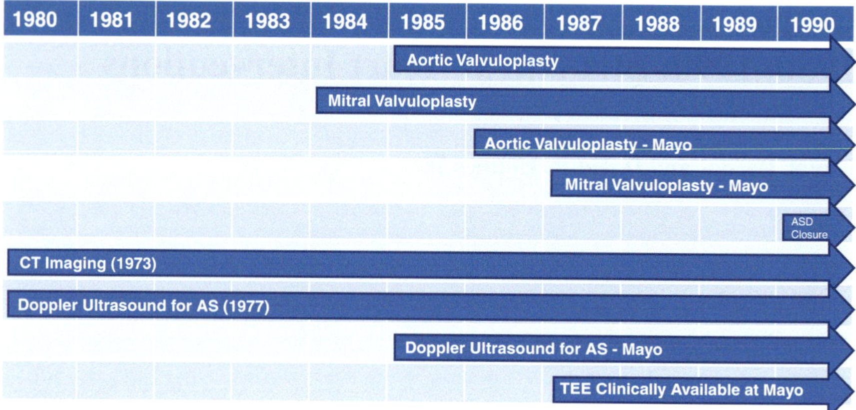

Fig. 5.1 The timeline of the adult interventional cardiology practice documents that while PTCA was increasingly used as an integral part of the practice beginning in the late 1970s to early 1980, treatment and evaluation of valvular heart disease followed 3–4 years later and then followed a similar dramatic growth in procedural performance

Aortic Balloon Valvuloplasty

In 1986, Cribier described three patients with valvular aortic stenosis treated by aortic balloon valvuloplasty [1]. A brachial cutdown with retrograde approach to the aortic valve was utilized, and stepwise inflation was performed with 8-, 10-, and 12-mm-diameter, 4-cm-long balloons of a type then available for dilatation of pulmonary valve stenosis. A reduction in symptoms and valve gradient was noted. An additional 11 patients were treated in the interval between manuscript submission and publication. That same year, the first aortic valvuloplasty at Mayo Clinic was performed by Drs. David Holmes Jr and Rick Nishimura [2]. Other interventional cardiologists performing valvuloplasty in this timeframe included Drs. John Bresnahan and Guy Reeder.

Later that year, the French registry experience of 443 patients undergoing aortic balloon valvuloplasty for severe aortic stenosis was presented [3]. The patients undergoing these procedures were older and typically had tricuspid aortic stenosis pathophysiology, the result of senile calcific changes that restricted normal leaflet function. The procedure was considered successful if the mean transvalvular aortic gradient was reduced by 50% or more, and the aortic valve area increased by 25% or greater. The procedure was complicated by a 2% incidence of stroke and a 4% periprocedural mortality. The mechanism of valvuloplasty was determined to the fracture of calcific plates within the valve leaflets and stretching of the valve tissue, and possibly relief of commissural fusion, though the majority of patients did not have rheumatic valve disease. Although patients did have a positive clinical response, it was only temporary, due to restenosis of the valve within 3–6 months. Even in cases considered successful, patients were often left with moderate or even severe residual valve obstruction. There was, however, continued great enthusiasm, as the patients being treated were not felt to have other options related to either advanced age or multiple comorbidities. An NHLBI Registry was initiated with the coordinating center in Seattle, Washington, and it enrolled approximately 1000 patients. Multiple publications from the registry confirmed the initial findings of modest improvement in gradient and nearly ubiquitous restenosis. By the end of the decade, it was becoming clear that valvuloplasty alone was not a long-term solution to the clinical problem. Balloon valvuloplasty in older patients with senile calcific degenerative aortic stenosis is rarely used alone today, but has been often incorporated into the TAVR procedure along with rapid ventricular pacing to stabilize balloon position during inflation. The basic methods of retrograde crossing of the aortic valve and positioning of a stiff guide wire in the LV learned during aortic valvuloplasty are virtually the same as those used in TAVR today. Alternatively, early in the experience, a transseptal approach was used with antegrade passage of a guide wire through the mitral apparatus to cross the aortic valve. This wire was then advanced to the descending thoracic aorta and used as a rail to position the balloon dilatation catheter. This process was cumbersome and could have led to damage of the mitral apparatus. Subsequently, it never became standard of care and was abandoned.

Mayo Clinic's contribution to the knowledge base regarding aortic balloon valvuloplasty was severalfold. The mechanism of gradient reduction by percutaneous valvuloplasty was documented in a detailed analysis of five cases and a literature review (Fig. 5.2) [4]. Appreciation of fracture of intravalvular calcium led to evaluation of the potential for lithotripsy to fragment the aortic cusp nodules and thereby increase their flexibility (Fig. 5.3). Large valvuloplasty balloons were modified such that a lithotripsy catheter could be designed within the balloon. The concept was

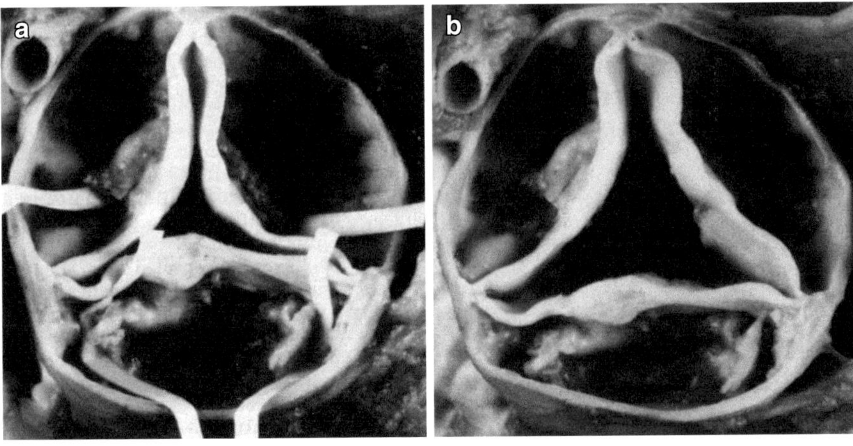

Fig. 5.2 Aortic valve, viewed from above, from a 93-year-old with degenerative (senile) calcific aortic stenosis. (**a**) Four ribbons of white paper demonstrate sites of fracture of archlike calcific excrescences. No commissural fusion is present. (**b**) Photograph of valve in simulated systolic opened position indicates appreciable cuspid mobility and correlates well with clinical reduction in transvalvular gradient from 77 mm Hg to 38 mm Hg. (From Kennedy et al. [4]; used with permission)

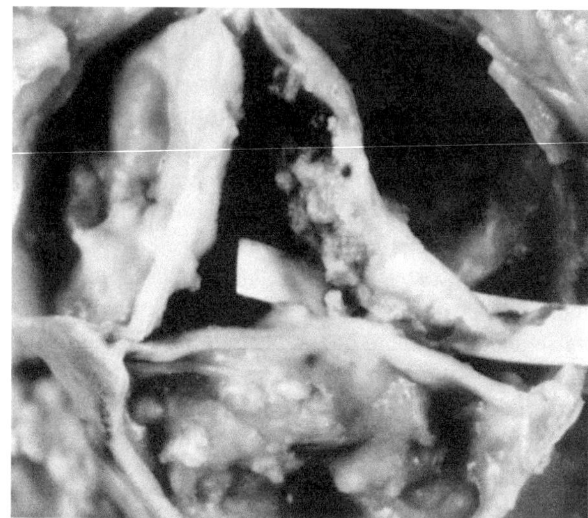

Fig. 5.3 Aortic valve, viewed from above, from an 82-year-old woman with degenerative (senile) calcific aortic stenosis. Ribbon of white paper demonstrates site of tear in the right aortic cusp. In addition, there was fracture of nodular calcium on ventricular aspect of cusp. Calcium in left and posterior cusps was not fractured. (From Kennedy et al. [4]; used with permission)

that such a balloon could be placed across the valve and, during inflation, lithotripsy performed. This led to a postmortem study using electrohydraulic shock-wave decalcification, and a small surgical study led by Dr. Mike King tested whether this mechanism might be beneficial in gradient reduction [5]. Ultimately, it proved to not be helpful, as direct lithotripsy damaged the valve leaflets leading to aortic regurgitation and the need for aortic valve replacement. Follow-up studies of the clinical outcomes of patients undergoing aortic balloon valvuloplasty at Mayo Clinic were also published, demonstrating gradual return of stenosis [6]. The concept of using the temporary improvement in aortic gradient and valve area obtained by valvuloplasty led to the use of this technique as a bridge to aortic valve replacement in select patients with severe reduction of left ventricular function, as a diagnostic test when the cause of left ventricular dysfunction was uncertain or as a bridge to noncardiac surgery in the setting of severe aortic stenosis.

During this time, there was close collaboration between the Mayo Clinic Cardiac Cath Lab and the Mayo Clinic Echocardiographic Laboratory. This close collaboration resulted in significant improvements in patients with congenital heart disease, adult congenital heart disease, or structural heart disease. These improvements included confirmation that echocardiographic assessments could be used to reliably document abnormalities of cardiac valves and function noninvasively, and they were found to be important for implementing and guiding interventional procedures. Continuous-wave Doppler methods had been shown to predict gradients across valvular stenosis lesions using the Bernoulli equation. Simultaneous correlation studies were performed in the cath lab to document the reliability of Doppler methods to accurately measure aortic transvalvular gradients in a population of

Fig. 5.4 Example
demonstrating changes in
subvalvular velocity and
aortic valve velocity
tracings at the three time
periods. Note an
immediate decrease in
aortic valve velocity after
the procedure. This results
in an immediate increase in
aortic valve area (AVA).
Additionally, 1 day after
the procedure
(24–36 hours), there is a
continued increase in
subvalvular velocity with
little change in aortic valve
velocity, resulting in a
further increase in aortic
valve area. (From
Nishimura et al. [9]; used
with permission)

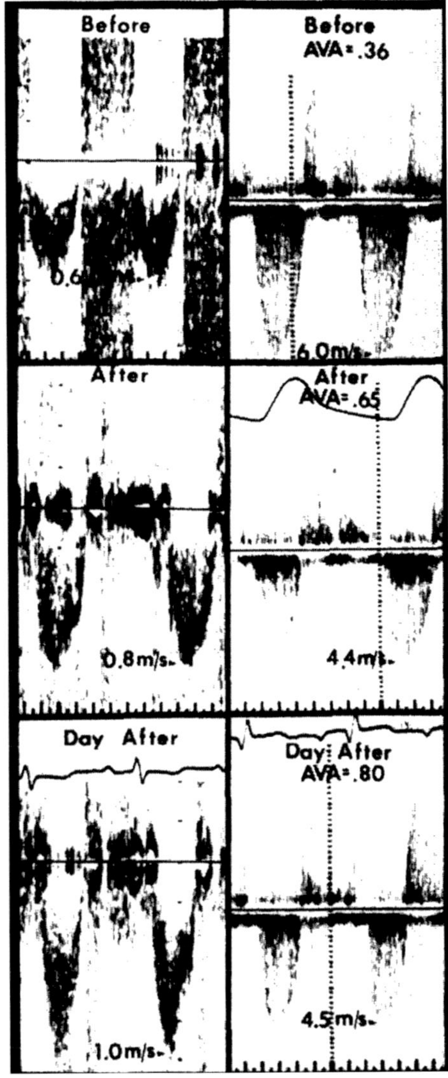

patients undergoing diagnostic catheterization for aortic stenosis, and later in determination of gradients pre- and post-aortic balloon valvuloplasty (Fig. 5.4) [7–9]. Similar studies were performed for the prediction of RV systolic pressure in patients with varying degrees of pulmonary hypertension. These studies ultimately led to the reduced use of diagnostic invasive pressure measurements in favor of the simpler and less costly Doppler echo methodology.

Mitral Balloon Valvuloplasty

Surgical mitral commissurotomy was performed as early as the 1940s with a closed type of procedure, giving way to open commissurotomy in the 1960s with the advent of the heart-lung bypass machine. In 1984, Inue published the results of six patients treated with balloon mitral valvuloplasty using a novel 3-stage balloon [10]. This was followed by other reports using single- and double-balloon approaches to perform commissurotomy, with results similar to surgical open commissurotomy. In 1987, the first mitral balloon valvuloplasty at Mayo Clinic was performed by Drs. David Holmes and Guy Reeder [2]. The mechanism of mitral valvuloplasty is primarily separation of fused commissures. The best results are obtained in patients with pliable, noncalcified leaflets, mild, or no preexisting mitral regurgitation, and the absence of significant calcification in one or both commissures. Unlike aortic valvuloplasty, results are relatively long lived. In a randomized trial of 60 patients undergoing mitral balloon valvuloplasty versus open surgical commissurotomy, the initial increase in mitral valve area was similar in both groups, but after 3 years of follow-up, patients with the percutaneous procedure had a higher average valve area and lower New York Heart Association functional classification compared with the surgical group [11]. Mitral balloon valvuloplasty remains an important technique for patients with appropriate valve anatomy. Although rheumatic mitral stenosis is uncommon in many more well-developed "Western countries," it is still a major problem worldwide. It often is seen in younger patients and causes significant problems, for example, during pregnancy. In those countries with a high continuing prevalence of rheumatic heart disease, percutaneous mitral procedures are widespread. In contrast, the population of patients referred to Mayo Clinic often have characteristics unsuitable for balloon valvuloplasty, and other techniques, such as more recently transvalvular mitral replacement (TMVR), are an active area of investigation.

Mayo Clinic's contribution to the development of mitral valvuloplasty included confirming the important observation that the mechanism was that of commissural splitting and that calcification located in the commissural location identified a population with a worse outcome, since these areas were less likely to yield to the dilating balloon, resulting in trauma to the body of the leaflets, inadequate dilation, or both, any of which may result in procedural-related severe mitral regurgitation requiring urgent and sometimes emergency surgery (Fig. 5.5) [12]. Additionally, Mayo Clinic interventionalists confirmed the practice of transthoracic echo monitoring of mitral balloon positioning during inflation and immediately post inflation. This allowed immediate determination of procedural success, as well as prompt detection of complications such as increase in mitral regurgitation. The gradual and stepwise balloon inflation procedure is widely accepted.

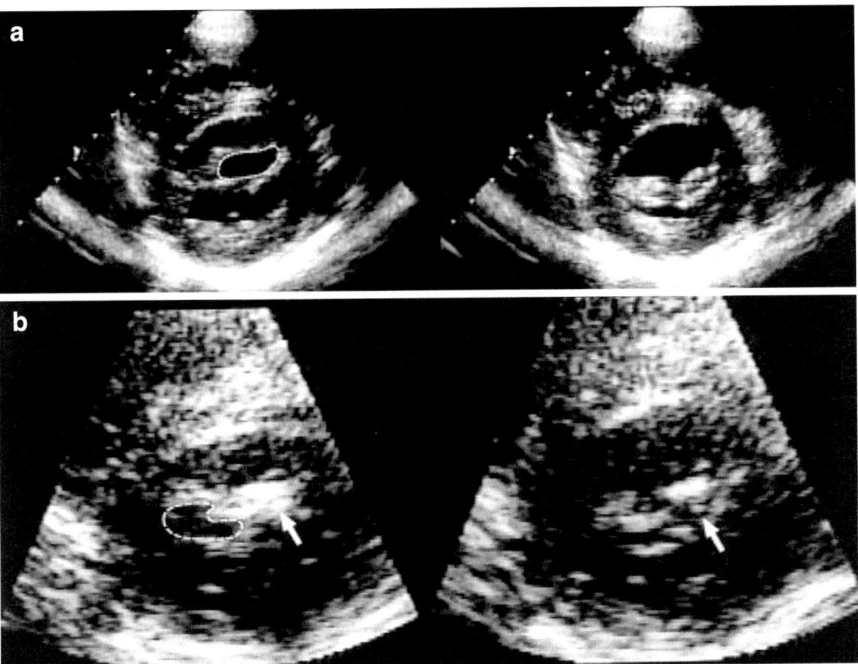

Fig. 5.5 (**a**) Parasternal short-axis view of the mitral valve during diastole (*left*) and systole (*right*) in a 32-year-old woman with severe mitral stenosis. Although thickening of the valve is present, there is no calcification in either the lateral or medial commissures. (**b**) Parasternal short-axis view of the mitral valve during diastole (*left*) and systole (*right*) in a 38-year-old man with severe mitral stenosis. Calcification and fusion are present in the lateral commissure as marked by the *white arrows*. (From Cannan et al. [12]; used with permission)

Atrial Septal Defects

Surgical closure of atrial septal defects utilizing cardiopulmonary bypass was successfully performed in the 1950s. Transcatheter devices were used in animal studies in the 1970s, and in 1975, a 2.5-cm ASD was successfully closed using a catheter-based umbrella-type device [13]. In 1987, a clamshell-type device was developed by Lock and others and ultimately utilized in about 1000 patients before being withdrawn due to device malfunctions [14]. In 1995, the Amplatzer septal occluder became available for investigational use, initiating the modern era of catheter-based atrial septal defect closure [15]. Mayo Clinic's involvement with this practice also occurred in the mid-1990s, primarily by the pediatric cardiac laboratory group, but subsequently included adult structural interventionalists and extended to the practice of closing the patent foramen ovale in patients with suspected paradoxic embolization. During this time period, multiple RCTs of PFO closure were performed. The results were relatively concordant that in broad groups of patients with poorly documented neurologic symptoms, PFO closure was not better than medical therapy. These findings led to a lack of adoption of PFO closure, until the more recent decade when newer results have documented that PFO closure in carefully selected patients was significantly superior to antiplatelet therapy.

Atrial Septostomy

Balloon atrial septostomy was developed in 1966 by Rashkind and Miller [16] for the creation of an atrial septal defect in infants with transposition of the great vessels. This procedure involved insertion of a 5 French balloon catheter across a patent foramen ovale and then quickly pulling the inflated catheter back, resulting in deliberate tearing of the septum.

In the early 1980s, it was observed that among patients with primary pulmonary hypertension, those with an atrial septal defect or a sizable patent foramen ovale, allowing right-to-left atrial shunting, had better survival than those with no atrial communication [17]. This led to the concept of performing atrial septostomy in patients with primary pulmonary hypertension and low output states [18–20]. Initially, transseptal puncture was performed using only fluoroscopic guidance, but this quickly evolved to transesophageal, and currently intracardiac echocardiography for positioning of the transseptal puncture site, and balloon dilatation of the septum with balloon diameters of sufficient size to yield a final resulting atrial septal defect of 8–10 mm in diameter. While many patients improved symptomatically, results were of variable duration due to subsequent healing and closure of the atrial septal defect or the creation of too large a defect and worsening of arterial desaturation. With the advent of an increasing number of effective drugs for the treatment of primary pulmonary hypertension, the need for atrial septostomy in this condition has diminished greatly. On the other hand, the increasing number of patients seen with left atrial hypertension due to heart failure with preserved ejection fraction, or stiff noncompliant left atrial syndromes following multiple ablation procedures, has produced a new cohort of patients who may benefit from atrial septostomy and creation of a left-to-right shunt with unloading of elevated left atrial pressures (Figs. 5.6 and 5.7) [21]. In the modern era, devices for regulating the amount of shunting are in the final testing phases and will soon be ready for more widespread application.

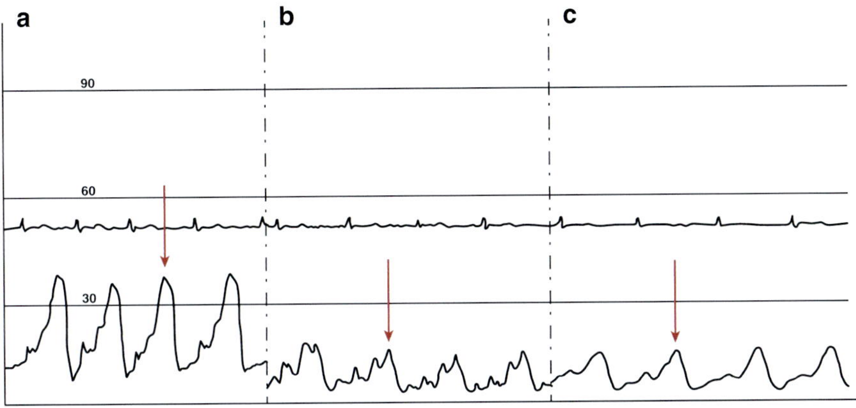

Fig. 5.6 Direct left atrial hemodynamic pressure tracings obtained after transseptal puncture. (**a**) Prior to septostomy, demonstrating giant V waves to 39 mm Hg (*red arrow*). (**b**) Immediately after septostomy, demonstrating significantly decreased V wave to 20 mm Hg (*red arrow*). (**c**) One year post-procedure tracing, showing sustained decrease in V wave pressure (*red arrow*). (Reprinted with permission; from Chandrashekar et al. [21])

Education and Teaching

During this decade and following, Mayo Clinic cardiologists in both the cath lab and echocardiography laboratory had a strong educational relationship with the American College of Cardiology and regularly presented courses at national meetings as well as at the Heart House Learning Center in Bethesda, Maryland. This resulted in the dissemination and sharing of concepts and techniques regarding these new interventions at a national level.

Cardiac Imaging

Most of the current structural interventions rely on two- or three-dimensional imaging for patient selection and procedural guidance. Multidetector-gated CT cardiac imaging is essential for TAVR, aortic prosthetic paravalvular leak closure, transcatheter mitral valve replacement, valve-in-valve and valve-in-ring, and false aneurysm closure procedures. Two- and three-dimensional echocardiography are necessary for procedure guidance with TAVR, peri-leak, and closure of ASD and a patent foramen ovale. Transesophageal echocardiography was available clinically in the mid-1980s, when it was used both on an outpatient basis and in the operating room for intraoperative evaluation of valvular repair and replacement procedures. Continued improvements in both of these X-ray and echo modalities have culminated in their absolute necessity for patient selection and procedural guidance.

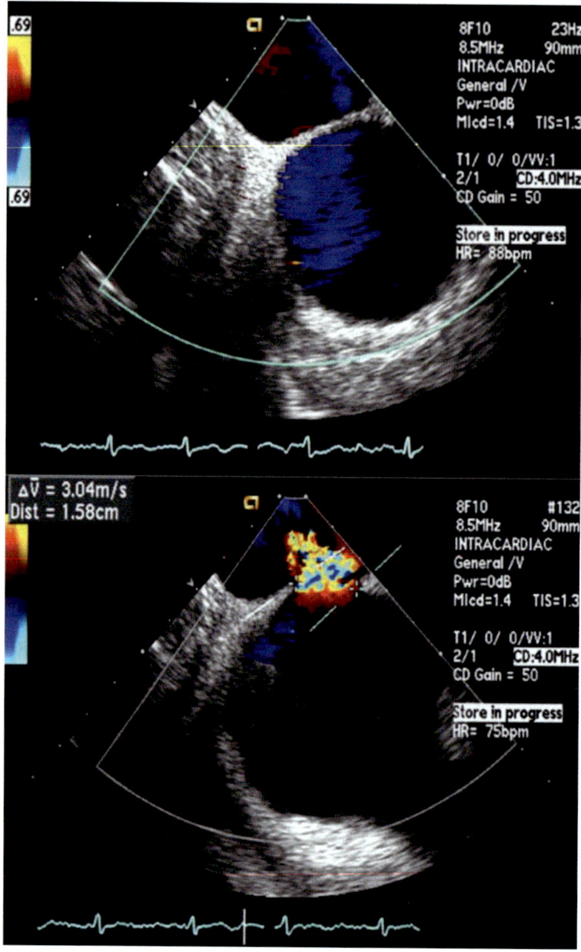

Fig. 5.7 Post-septostomy transthoracic echocardiogram demonstrates an interatrial shunt with blood flow from left to right. (Reprinted with permission; from Chandrashekar et al. [21])

Summary

The field of structural heart interventions, as will be seen in subsequent decades, has been robust and greatly expanded options for unmet clinical needs. This area is increasingly integrated with collaboration between imaging (both cardiology and radiology), cardiovascular surgery, interventional cardiology, and adult congenital heart disease, working closely with industry colleagues and regulatory agencies to form the transformational approaches that have become standard.

References

1. Cribier A, Savin T, Saoudi N, Rocha P, Berland J, Letac B. Percutaneous transluminal valvuloplasty of acquired aortic stenosis in elderly patients: an alternative to valve replacement? Lancet. 1986;1(8472):63–7.
2. Fye W. Caring for the heart, vol. 672. New York: Oxford University Press; 2015.
3. Cribier A, Letac B, Lancelin B. Percutaneous balloon valvuloplasty (PBV) for acquired aortic stenosis: preliminary immediate results of the French registry. Circulation. 1986;74:208.
4. Kennedy KD, Hauck AJ, Edwards WD, Holmes DR Jr, Reeder GS, Nishimura RA. Mechanism of reduction of aortic valvular stenosis by percutaneous transluminal balloon valvuloplasty: report of five cases and review of literature. Mayo Clin Proc. 1988;63(8):769–76.
5. Worley SJ, King RM, Edwards WD, Holmes DR Jr. Electrohydraulic shock wave decalcification of stenotic aortic valves: postmortem and intraoperative studies. J Am Coll Cardiol. 1988;12(2):458–62.
6. Holmes DR Jr, Nishimura RA, Reeder GS, Wagner PJ, Ilstrup DM. Clinical follow-up after percutaneous aortic balloon valvuloplasty. Arch Intern Med. 1989;149(6):1405–9.
7. Oh JK, Taliercio CP, Holmes DR Jr, Reeder GS, Bailey KR, Seward JB, et al. Prediction of the severity of aortic stenosis by Doppler aortic valve area determination: prospective Doppler-catheterization correlation in 100 patients. J Am Coll Cardiol. 1988;11(6):1227–34.
8. Nishimura RA, Holmes DR Jr, Reeder GS, Tajik AJ, Hatle LK. Doppler echocardiographic observations during percutaneous aortic balloon valvuloplasty. J Am Coll Cardiol. 1988;11(6):1219–26.
9. Nishimura RA, Holmes DR Jr, Reeder GS, Ilstrup DM, Small RS, Tajik AJ. Hemodynamic results of percutaneous aortic balloon valvuloplasty as assessed by sequential Doppler echocardiographic studies. Int J Cardiol. 1988;20(3):317–26.
10. Inoue K, Owaki T, Nakamura T, Kitamura F, Miyamoto N. Clinical application of transvenous mitral commissurotomy by a new balloon catheter. J Thorac Cardiovasc Surg. 1984;87(3):394–402.
11. Reyes VP, Raju BS, Wynne J, Stephenson LW, Raju R, Fromm BS, et al. Percutaneous balloon valvuloplasty compared with open surgical commissurotomy for mitral stenosis. N Engl J Med. 1994;331(15):961–7.
12. Cannan CR, Nishimura RA, Reeder GS, Ilstrup DR, Larson DR, Holmes DR, et al. Echocardiographic assessment of commissural calcium: a simple predictor of outcome after percutaneous mitral balloon valvotomy. J Am Coll Cardiol. 1997;29(1):175–80.
13. King TD, Thompson SL, Steiner C, Mills NL. Secundum atrial septal defect. Nonoperative closure during cardiac catheterization. JAMA. 1976;235(23):2506–9.
14. King TD, Mills NL. Transcatheter closure of ASDs and PFOs: a comprehensive assessment. Minneapolis: Cardiotext; 2010. p. 37–63.
15. Masura J, Gavora P, Formanek A, Hijazi ZM. Transcatheter closure of secundum atrial septal defects using the new self-centering amplatzer septal occluder: initial human experience. Catheter Cardiovasc Diagn. 1997;42(4):388–93.
16. Rashkind WJ, Miller WW. Creation of an atrial septal defect without thoracotomy. A palliative approach to complete transposition of the great arteries. JAMA. 1966;196(11):991–2.
17. Montanes P, Rozkovec A, Oakley CM. The natural history of primary pulmonary hypertension (abstract). Bull Eur Physiopath Respir. 1982;18:87.
18. Rich S, Lam W. Atrial septostomy as palliative therapy for refractory primary pulmonary hypertension. Am J Cardiol. 1983;51(9):1560–1.
19. Sandoval J, Gaspar J, Pulido T, Bautista E, Martínez-Guerra ML, Zeballos M, et al. Graded balloon dilation atrial septostomy in severe primary pulmonary hypertension. A therapeutic alternative for patients nonresponsive to vasodilator treatment. J Am Coll Cardiol. 1998;32(2):297–304.

20. Sandoval J, Gaspar J, Peña H, Santos LE, Córdova J, del Valle K, et al. Effect of atrial septostomy on the survival of patients with severe pulmonary arterial hypertension. Eur Respir J. 2011;38(6):1343–8.
21. Chandrashekar P, Park JY, Al-Hijji MA, Reddy YNV, Zack CJ, Reeder GS, et al. Atrial septostomy to treat stiff left atrium syndrome. Circ Heart Fail. 2017;10(7):e004160.

Chapter 6
2000s: New Field of Focus

David R. Holmes Jr. and Charanjit S. Rihal

The turn of the century brought continued change and evolution in the cardiac cath lab as well as its share of controversy. The foundations remained the same, built on the principles of science, education, and practice. New physicians, both fellows and staff from the United States and abroad, joined and added immeasurably. They included Jassim Al Suwaidi (UAE), David Hasdai (Israel), Max Sangiorgi (Italy), Brendan Doyle (Ireland), Aaron Grantham, Verg Mathew, Peter Berger, Patti Best, Joerg Herrmann, Abhi Prasad, and Sam Asirvatham, among others. As had been the approach dating back to Fredrick Willius when he had been head of cardiology in the early twentieth century, staff were expected to be involved in academic projects as well as being expert in full-time clinical practice. Involvement in such projects was important for both staff and fellows as it increased their intellectual scientific investigative skills, gave them a chance to add to the scientific literature as well as their own academic record, and offered the opportunity to present data at local, regional, and national/international meetings. During the 2000s, there were multiple areas of substantial clinical interest which afforded excellent opportunities for such individual and group projects. Mentorship during that decade ranged from informal to more structured sessions and interactions. These relationships and the academic rigor from them resulted in improvements in the entire process of education and research and also enhanced processes to optimize patient care.

The 1980s and 1990s had seen the implementation of multicenter randomized clinical trials (RCTs) with well-outlined scientific methods which were embraced by interventional cardiology. An important advantage of being an active enrolling institution in these trials was that Mayo Clinic investigators could submit requests for proposals to obtain data on specific subsets of patients for analysis and subsequent publications. In many trials, then as now, high-enrolling sites were given

D. R. Holmes Jr. (✉) · C. S. Rihal
Department of Cardiovascular Diseases, Mayo Clinic, Rochester, MN, USA
e-mail: Holmes.david@mayo.edu; rihal@mayo.edu

preference by the sponsor for data requests. During the 2000s, that strategy was used repeatedly which resulted in multiple important manuscripts by both staff and fellows. A review of these topics and the resulting manuscripts allows identification of the important issues in the field that were the focus of intense study and formed the continued basis of training fellows in designing protocols and analyzing data.

Acute Ischemic Syndromes

Patients with acute ischemic syndromes (AIS) were the focus of multiple studies at Mayo Clinic, in part, related to the fact that the population of patients was very large with high rates of morbidity and mortality. There was increasing information about the pathophysiology, and new technology was being utilized to optimize care. Emphasizing the importance of this topic, professional societies embraced initiatives based on the scientific studies and focused on "door-to-balloon" (Fig. 6.1) and "Get with the Guidelines" among others that were widely promulgated and eventually made their way into professional guidelines, becoming quality indicators of care.

Randomized clinical trials in interventional and urgent cardiovascular care focused on STEMI as well as non-STEMI and unstable angina which dominated the landscape. The family of three GUSTO trials by Topol and Califf had been designed and implemented in 1990 to address issues of acute myocardial infarction, which had remained unanswered despite careful studies that had involved >100,000 patients.

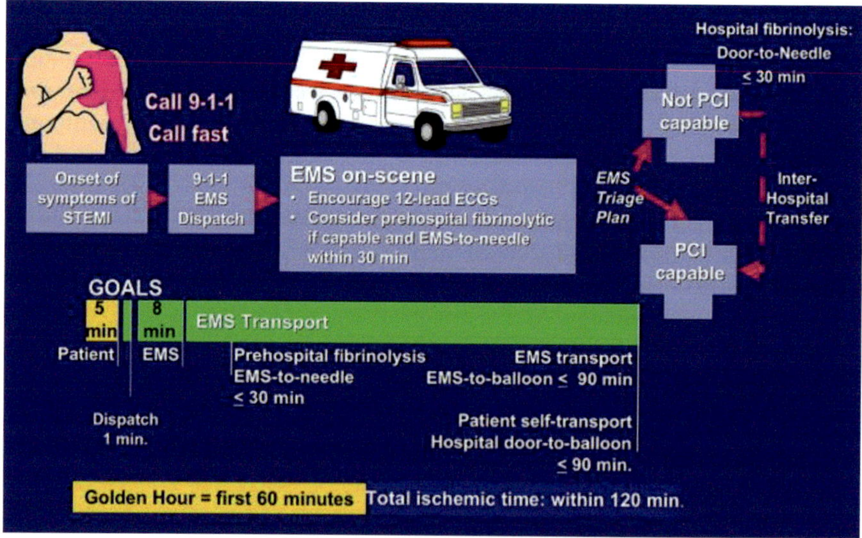

Fig. 6.1 Intense interest in processes of care for STEMI patients focused on the golden hour of reperfusion and mobilizing healthcare systems to achieve earliest access

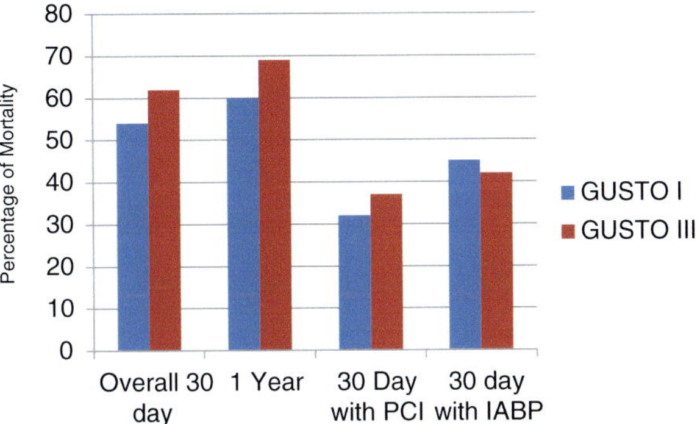

Fig. 6.2 Despite focus on cardiogenic shock in the 1990s, the GUSTO-III trial documented an increase in 30-day and 1-year mortality. (From V. Menon JS et al. Eur Heart J 2000;21:1928–1936; used under license)

The initial GUSTO-I study, that had involved 41,021 patients randomized to either tissue-type plasminogen activator (TPA) or streptokinase for STEMI, was unequivocally positive with TPA associated with a 15% reduction in mortality. It had, however, not answered all of the questions for all of the subsets of patients as well as the critical issue of lytic therapy compared with PCI [1]. An important component in the field was cardiogenic shock. Hasdai was part of an international group which published on the lack of progress in these patients in lessons from GUSTO-I and GUSTO-III (Fig. 6.2). In GUSTO-I, carried out from 1990–1993, shock had been identified in 2,814 patients (7.2%); in GUSTO-III, carried out from 1995–1997, 695 patients with cardiogenic shock (5.5%) were identified. The mortality in GUSTO-III was 62% and actually higher than that seen in GUSTO-I (54%) ($p = 0.001$). In addition, reinfarction and recurrent ischemia rates were also both higher in GUSTO-III (14% vs 11% and 35% vs 27%, respectively). These findings led to increased emphasis on the development of newer strategies of care for these high-risk patients who account for the majority of mortality in patients hospitalized with acute myocardial infarction. As part of this work, Hasdai also evaluated the use of platelet glycoprotein IIB/IIIA blockade in patients with cardiogenic shock complicating acute coronary syndromes including unstable angina or non-STEMI but without STEMI [2, 3]. He also documented the fact that cardiogenic shock may occur on presentation or develop after hospitalization in patients with either non-STEMI or unstable angina and developed algorithms for predicting its occurrence and mortality [2–4]. The development of shock in non-STEMI patients was still relatively unexpected as "non-Q wave infarctions" were felt to have better prognosis. Accordingly, new information reflected outcome more accurately. He also studied a variety of other issues including cigarette smoking and the outcome of mild to moderate congestive heart failure as a complication of STEMI. Out of this work, while in training, Hasdai edited a book on the field (Fig. 6.3). Projects such as these expanded our understanding of shock which, as mentioned, is the most common lethal event in acute coronary syndromes. He also fulfilled one of the objectives of cardiac cath lab training of enhancing the experience in the study of data and science.

Out of these and other efforts for patients with acute ischemic syndromes, multiple changes were implemented at Mayo Clinic. A specific 24/7 STEMI protocol

Fig. 6.3 Hasdai et al. developed a large scientific dataset on cardiogenic shock and was the background for the Contemporary Cardiology book on the field which has continued implications for practice (cover image used with permission)

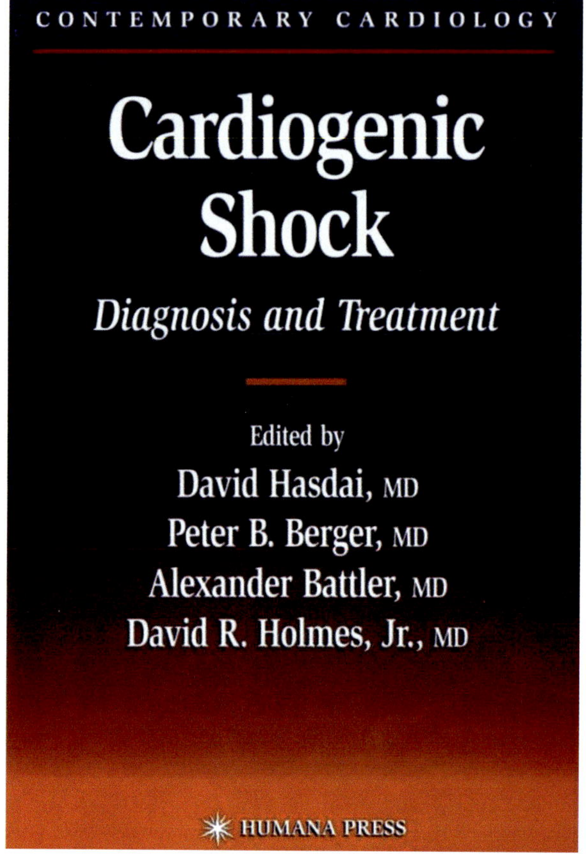

was developed and put in place. This involved a central phone system triage center where STEMI calls where sent and an initial review of a faxed ECG was performed. That central phone system activated a dedicated STEMI pager. The cath lab consultant on call as well as the cardiology trainee, the CCU consultant, and the cath lab technical people were paged simultaneously, and the time of arrival for procedural performance was identified. By protocol, personnel were expected to be in the cath lab within 30 minutes of the call and ready to proceed. For some of the cath lab staff who lived a longer distance from the hospital, they would stay overnight in town. The next day, a "report card" would come out about the response times and the outcome. Such information was used as a continued quality of care initiative. One of the authors (DRH) remembers being somewhat late because he was exercising at the Rochester Athletic Club and had missed the initial call. That tardiness was noted as part of the morning report the next day.

Given the documented poor outcome of higher risk patients including those with cardiogenic shock and the lack of significant improvement with conventional IABP, more advanced strategies for hemodynamic support were incorporated. TandemHeart, a concept and product that had been developed by a colleague, Dr. Howard Cohen, was implemented. This technique provided excellent circulatory support but was more complex. It involved transseptal catheterization and placement of a large bore catheter into the left atrium as well as large arterial sheaths for creating a circuit to unload the left ventricle, thus resting it to optimize the chance for ventricular salvage. Given our large experience with transseptal catheterizations for mitral valve interventions, left atrial appendage occlusion, and electrophysiologic ablations, Mayo Clinic was well suited to provide this treatment, even in patients during cardiogenic shock. The concept for this had arisen from the finding in an early reperfusion trial – TAMI – that patients with STEMI who had failed reperfusion but who had undergone emergent CABG had the best improvement in LV function, potentially related to the fact that during CABG with the LV vented and complete unloading, salvage could be maximized. During TandemHeart procedures, TEE was often performed; during the procedure, the aortic valve leaflets could be visualized as immobile even though aortic pressure was maintained. This technology was also used during high-risk left ventricular electrophysiologic ablation procedures. Subsequently other left ventricular unloading support procedures such as Impella and ECMO were used in selected STEMI and other high-risk clinical situations.

Other aspects of acute coronary syndromes were also studied, particularly the role of inflammation. During the 2000s decade, new agents were being tested to address this unmet clinical need and included enrollment in the APEX trial of pexelizumab, a bioengineered single-chain variable fragment of a monoclonal antibody designed to target component 5 of the complement system. These trials were focused on decreasing inflammatory pathways in patients with acute STEMI undergoing primary PCI. Such efforts would also be applied in patients receiving thrombolytic therapy or for the treatment of other cardiovascular diseases. While the results of this specific trial were negative, efforts continued as inflammation had been identified as an important component in the pathophysiology of AIS and remained an unmet need. We participated in other trials including a trial of nitric oxide inhibition in patients with persistent cardiogenic shock complicating acute myocardial infarction [5]. The cath lab also enrolled in trials evaluating the merits of invasive strategies for patients with unstable angina and non-STEMI which were important for developing pathways of care. Such trials continue to be performed up to the current era.

Stent Implantation

Not all efforts in the cath lab included the study of AIS. There was a virtual explosion in the development and testing of new stent designs and application of these designs to improve outcomes for patients with a variety of anatomic subsets of disease. In addition, new problems with unintended consequences of stent implantation included stent thrombosis and restenosis. All of these strategies with new equipment presented opportunities for study by the staff and fellows in training as well as the paramedical technical staff.

Particularly vexing and anxiety provoking was the problem of stent thrombosis following implantation of drug-eluting stents. It had been known for some time that the mechanism of action of the drugs initially used—paclitaxel and sirolimus—involved interrupting and delaying healing of balloon- and stent-induced vascular injury. In most cases, this injury subsequently healed with a layer of endothelial cells, but in some patients this did not occur. A series of cases with angiographically confirmed late stent thrombosis presented from Rotterdam unleashed a maelstrom of controversy regarding drug-eluting stents and tempered the community's enthusiasm for them [6]. Numerous media reports sensationalized these observations ("ticking little time bombs") and impacted worried patients who sometimes refused stents during the throes of an acute myocardial infarction, or demanded that their previously implanted stents be removed. The solution to the problem came from careful pathologic analysis of an autopsy series demonstrating delayed, or sometimes a complete lack of endothelialization in patients dying of stent thrombosis, or intense inflammation with disruption of the normal arterial wall. The original Rotterdam cases [6] all developed acute stent thrombosis following holding of anti-platelet therapy for elective noncardiac procedures, emphasizing the need for careful attention to antiplatelet therapy following PCI. Spearheaded by Peter Burger, Mayo Clinic contributed to the development of the field initially using the combination of aspirin plus ticlopidine and subsequently aspirin plus clopidogrel. These studies were part of the foundation for the modern recommendation of 1 year of dual anti-platelet therapy following drug-eluting stent implantation. These recommendations continue to evolve with more robust data, clinical trials, and as experience accrues.

Also important was learning how to implant drug-eluting stents at the time of the initial procedure. Dr. Antonio Columbia of Rafael Hospital, Milan, documented the utility of intravascular ultrasound following stent implantation and the use of high-pressure post-dilatation to optimize stent expansion, apposition to the vessel wall, and to exclude local trauma such as proximal or distal dissections and localized thrombosis. These innovations were to change the face of interventional cardiology and arguably rescued coronary stent deployment from the abyss that had loomed after the initial NEJM publication of the results of 24 patients [7].

At Mayo Clinic, Drs. Amir Lerman, Stuart Higano, and Rick Nishimura led the development of a comprehensive coronary imaging program that is now recommended as a routine part of stent implantation. It has been repeatedly shown that intracoronary imaging with ultrasound allows for detection of problems and subsequent optimization with better outcomes for patients. Wide uptake is still lagging, however, and remains a challenge. Utilizing these technologies, the cardiac catheterization lab in collaboration with cardiac transplantation had implemented a protocol of the use of annual intravascular ultrasound examinations for the assessment of transplant vasculopathy, the leading cause of lead death following cardiac transplantation. These anatomic studies have led directly to the use of sirolimus as the preferred post-allograft immunosuppressive therapy in many patients. Ironically and fittingly, this, of course, is the same drug used in one of the two initial first-generation drug-eluting stents (Cypher; Johnson and Johnson).

Particularly fruitful areas for study included stent versus stent trials, localized intracoronary gamma-radiation therapy to inhibit restenosis, evaluation of sirolimus-eluting stents versus bare metal stents in native coronary lesions, and placement of sirolimus-eluting stents for the treatment of coronary bifurcation lesions.

Randomized Clinical Trials and Multicenter Registries

In the 1980s and 1990s, in addition to RCTs, interventional cardiology had also embraced the design and implementation of multicenter registries. These registries involved a more "real-world" experience of cases being treated but without randomization. There were continued robust conversations about the scientific validity of the data obtained from registries because of the presence of confounders which could not be completely adjusted for despite the application of multiple statistical approaches such as propensity matching. Despite this concern, these registry experiences, which did not have multiple careful and rigid inclusion and exclusion criteria, more fully represented what is conventionally called "real-world" experience. When properly carried out with common standard data forms which could be reviewed, adjudicated, and which included comprehensive and complete datasets, information from such registries can provide important data which can be used in professional societal guidelines such as has been seen in Scandinavian registries which include all patients countrywide with specific conditions and therapeutic strategies.

The New York State model under the mandate of the New York State Board of Health is a classic representative of an excellent approach for registries. Statewide enrollment for all patients undergoing the treatment being studied was required with standard forms and data which were adjudicated and then reviewed by a committee that included statisticians, epidemiologists, clinical cardiologists, and interventional cardiologists under the careful direction of Ed Hannan [8]. As part of this registry, New York State appointed two experts from outside of the state to an official position on the committee which included review of the statewide data, setting up standards (e.g., those related to the development of cardiac catheterization laboratories and PCI without surgical backup) as well as criteria for stroke centers within the state. These efforts provided guidance for subsequent professional society guidelines. Holmes was one of those two individuals selected, as well as Spencer King from Emory, and participated in multiple important analyses. This registry provided information on the relationships between procedural volume and outcome of PCI (Fig. 6.4), the development of a risk score for PCI which Mayo Clinic studied [9], the effect of strategies for treating multivessel disease during acute myocardial

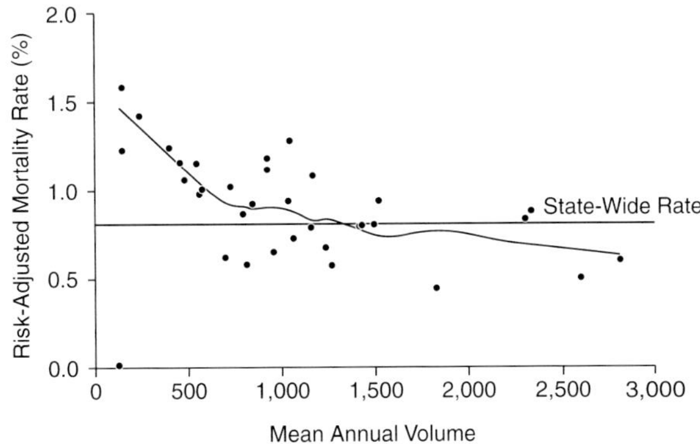

Fig. 6.4 Data from the New York State model documented the relationship between risk-adjusted mortality rate on mean annual volume of PCI procedures. (From Hannan EL et al. Circulation. 2005;112:1171–1179; used with permission)

infarction (i.e., culprit only), treatment of other vessels during the index hospital stay or delayed staged procedures, and finally the effect of completeness of revascularization on outcomes. One of the first papers comparing mortality, myocardial infarction, and repeated revascularization rates of sirolimus and paclitaxel-eluting stents was published from this New York State Registry [10] as well as a comparison of coronary artery stenting outcomes before and after the introduction of drug-eluting stents [11]. Another important study related to point-of-care measurements of platelet inhibition and outcome of PCI in the GOLD Multicenter trial [12]. Although not randomized, these registries inform us about care patterns and can be used for policy decisions at local, state, and even national levels.

Mayo Clinic was also involved in other registries. The new approaches in coronary interventions provided information on a national level focusing on race, baseline characteristics, and clinical outcomes of patients [13]. Such registries allowed evaluation of changes in the field over the life of the specific registry, outcomes of specific disease subsets available for study including left main coronary artery disease, and outcomes in women [14]. Such longitudinal "looks" are essential as the field is evaluated in the context of how devices, patient groups changes, and outcomes evolve. These registries by virtue of broad inclusion were helpful in designing and testing risk prediction models [15]. They also enabled evaluation of subsets of diseases such as diabetes mellitus, those with mild or moderate coronary artery disease, patients with peripheral arterial disease, small coronary arteries treated with stents, race, and outcome in patients with acute coronary syndromes, lesion length and the effect of lesion length on fractional flow reserve (FFR) in intermediate coronary lesions, and the outcome of patients with chronic renal disease. These focused analyses among others were the subject of individual or multiple papers by Mayo Clinic authors during that time, which again fulfilled the reason for including this as part of fellowship to encourage developing experience with the scientific method, providing data to improve care not only at Mayo but working with professional societies for the country as a whole. The results then could be used to design larger prospective or even multicenter RCTs.

Mayo Clinic PTCA Registry

Data from the Mayo Clinic PTCA Registry, designed and implemented by Drs. Ron Vlietstra and Kent Bailey in the early 1980s on different strategies of care or specific disease subsets, was of great importance given the complete enrollment of all patients undergoing treatment at Mayo Clinic and the superb data entry by Lavonne Hammes and her colleagues with statistical support from Ryan Lennon. The importance of prompt statistical input was identified early on. At Mayo Clinic, requests for data analysis were traditionally put into an institutional queue that included all investigators in the institution. This procedure led to some delays. To mitigate this, the cath lab received permission from Mayo Clinic to hire a dedicated analyst, Ryan

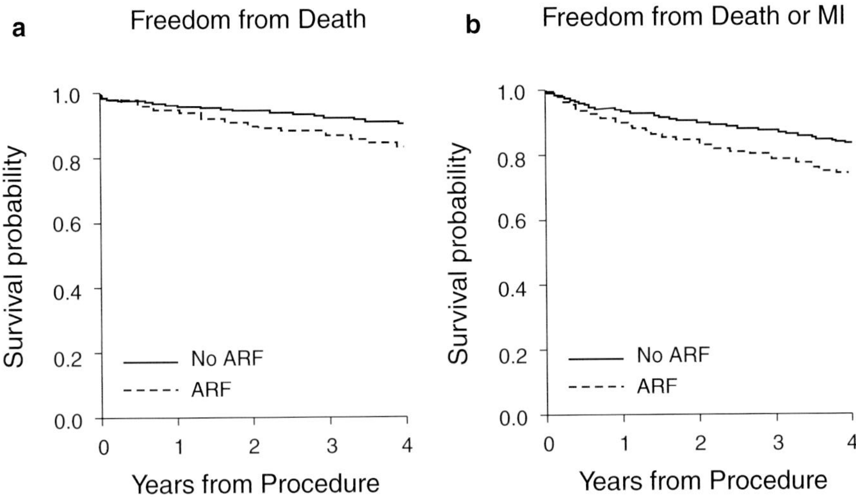

Fig. 6.5 The importance of the development of acute failure as a complication of PCI was documented with worsening of freedom from death as well as freedom from death or myocardial infarction out to 4 years. (From Rihal CS et al. Circulation. 2002;105:2259–2264; used with permission)

Lennon, who became fundamentally important for accessing data used for quality initiatives and publications and presentations in a very timely manner. Some of these focused on specific strategies of care such as Mayo Clinic experience with "true bifurcation lesions," direct stent implantation of vein graft disease, mild coronary disease and endothelial dysfunction, glycemic control and outcome of diabetic patients after successful PCI, long-term survival after successful PCI in patients with chronic renal failure, and the result of abciximab for reducing thrombus burden in vein graft disease, among other topics. Of particular importance was Rihal's evaluation of the incidence and prognostic importance of acute renal failure after PCI (Fig. 6.5); this helped in the development of RCTs aimed at mitigating this important complication which when it occurred resulted in markedly increased inhospital mortality [16]. Early work in the field by Prasad studied the issues of isolated troponin T post procedural in 383 patients undergoing nonemergent PCI and found that elevation was associated with worsened mortality and worsened survival free to MI out to 3 years later (Fig. 6.6a, b) [17]. This early study focused its interest on the issues of biomarkers as indicators of disease such as NSTEMI as well as being indicators of procedural complications. In addition, Mayo Clinic published more extensive and comprehensive articles on coronary artery stents which helped to put the field in perspective. An important component of these studies included the long-term follow-up based on the Mayo Clinic PTCA Registry, for example, the 20-year data on diabetics and their outcome after PCI [18] and the long experience on preexistent coronary artery thrombus on outcome of PCI by early and subsequent decades of treatment as well as the longer-term outcome of PCI in octogenarians. Along those same lines, Mathew evaluated changes in patient

Fig. 6.6 Measurement of biomarkers for myocardial necrosis became increasingly common. As such, they were used to define and assess complications of PCI. As seen, isolated troponin elevates >0.03 postprocedure in nonemergent patients was associated with excess mortality (**a**) and mortality and MI at 3 years (**b**). (From Prasad A et al. J Am Coll Cardiol 2006;48:1765–70; used with permission)

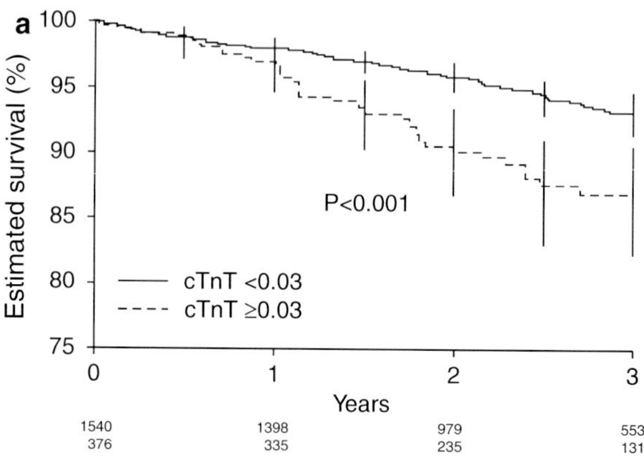

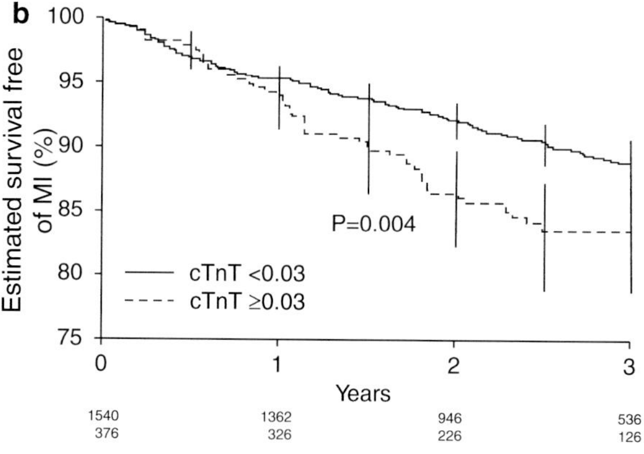

characteristics and outcome over two consecutive decades in PCI in patients with prior coronary artery bypass graft surgery [19] as well as the decreasing mortality in primary PCI during acute myocardial infarction. Given the large number of patients and complete follow-up, important information could be gathered; Doyle evaluated the effect of major femoral bleeding on long-term survival on 17,901 patients treated at Mayo Clinic from 1994 to 2005 (Fig. 6.7) [20]. Such long-term experiences in a single-center experience were not available from any other institution; the observations gained from these unique datasets were used to develop RCTs and NIH grants.

Other important information available in the Mayo Clinic PTCA Registry included processes of care. Ting et al. evaluated the 2-year Mayo Clinic experience of low-risk PCI without on-site cardiac surgery [21] and documented that it was not only feasible but safe and effective [Table 6.1]. This had important implications for other centers embarking on a strategy to facilitate incorporation of PCI in smaller medical centers and resulted in continued paradigm shifts in cardiovascular medicine [22]. Related issues included assessment of pharmacologic facilitation of primary PCI for acute infarction by Gersh [23] which has formed a standard

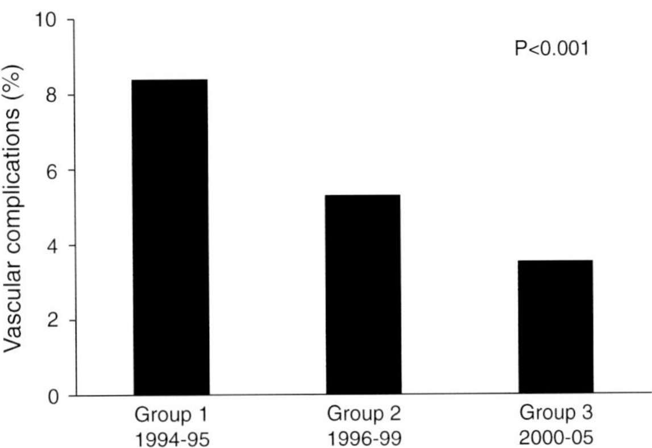

Fig. 6.7 The Mayo Clinic PTCA Registry facilitated the study of complications such as procedural vascular complications over the course of time. As can be seen, changes in practice from 1994 resulted in a significant reduction in this complication. (From Doyle et al. J Am Coll Cardiol Intv 1(12):202,2008; used with permission)

Table 6.1 Clinical outcomes for elective PCI patients

Outcome	Elective PCI (n = 196)	95%CI
Procedural success* (%)	195 (99.5)	97.2–99.9
Inhospital death (%)	1 (0.5)	0.01–2.8
Inhospital myocardial infarction	0	
Inhospital emergent coronary bypass surgery	0	
Inhospital elective coronary bypass surgery	0	
Inhospital repeat PCI	0	
Inhospital stroke or transient ischemic attack (%)	1 (0.5)	
Inhospital vascular complication (%)	2 (1.0)	
Mean follow-up (months), mean ± SD	8.2 ± 6.5	
Follow-up cardiac death	0	
Follow-up noncardiac death (%)	2 (1.0)	
Follow-up myocardial infarction (%)	7 (3.6)	
Follow-up target vessel revascularization (%)	15 (7.7)	
Composite end point of any death, myocardial infarction, or target vessel revascularization (%)	20 (10.2)	

* Procedural success defined as <50% residual stenosis and without in-hospital death, myocardial infarction, coronary bypass surgery, or repeat PCI.
From Ting HH et al. Am Heart J 2003;145:278–84; used with permission

of care for design and implementation of new approaches (Fig. 6.8). This classic conceptual slide of the issues of salvage, open artery, and time has been used repeatedly in publications and forms the background on strategies of reperfusion. This was further explored in developing the Mayo Clinic STEMI protocol for regional systems of optimizing timeliness of reperfusion in peripheral stroke hospitals [24]. This was the focus of further work by Singh with documentation of the outcomes of a system-wide Mayo Clinic protocol for elective and non elective coronary angioplasty at sites without on-site surgery [25] which has influenced the field as it continues to evolve at other centers.

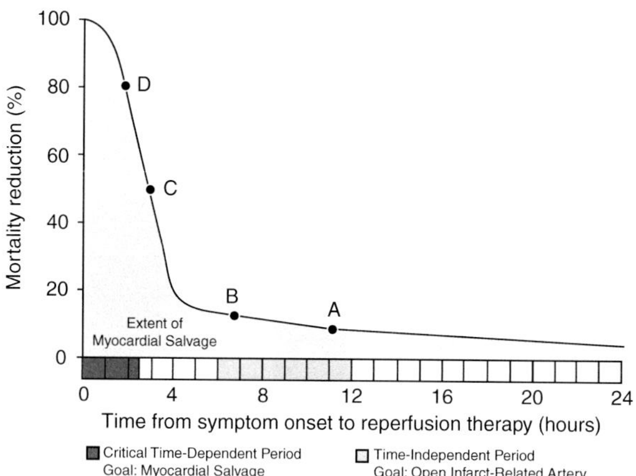

Fig. 6.8 Graph of relationship between mortality reduction and myocardial salvage as a function of time from symptom onset to reperfusion therapy. The extent of myocardial salvage is time dependent. Strategies to decrease mortality depend on time to reperfusion. Strategies to move the curve from point B to C may improve mortality reduction, but may not have a large effect on myocardial salvage. (From Gersh BJ et al. JAMA 2005;293:979–986; used with permission)

Carotid Stenting

Not all interest was focused on the coronary arena, with the development of initiatives to expand the field of interest of cardiologists to renal and iliac artery stenting and carotid and intracranial disease [26]. The latter was of particular importance to consider at that time and continues to resonate today. The more recent data on the use of catheter-based skills and approaches to dramatically improve outcome of some patients presenting with ischemic stroke has presented an opportunity for interventional cardiology to participate in the treatment of these patients with this most feared disease. Working with neurosurgery (Dr. N. Hopkins) in early and very controversial topics, we decried the issue of turf wars and their impact on patient care and outcome [26]. This and other input resulted in the development and implementation of the multicenter CREST trial which randomized patients with carotid arterial disease to either carotid stenting or carotid endarterectomy. Mayo Clinic had arranged for Holmes to develop expertise in carotid stenting. This was contracted by working with the pioneer, experienced, and visionary neurosurgeon, Nick Hopkins in Buffalo who had been involved in developing distal protection and who was an advocate for carotid stenting. During that experience, Holmes had also brought IVUS to that center, where early experience was obtained visualizing intracerebral vessels superior to the siphon. In addition, Holmes also spent time with a Mayo Clinic-trained cardiovascular physician Dr. Michael Bacharach in Sioux Falls, South Dakota, who had extensive experience with carotid arterial stenting. As part of this training, three Mayo Clinic physicians (Holmes, Bresnahan, and Gulati), working collaboratively and sometimes competitively with neurology and neuroradiology, developed expertise in carotid stenting with excellent early results. These procedures were all performed with embolic protection devices, which we had extensive experience with by virtue of their routine use in the treatment of saphenous bypass graft interventions to prevent distal embolization. These new procedures where performed in the cardiac catheterization lab after the training of the staff in terms of equipment, imaging, and pharmacologic adjunctive therapy. We also performed carotid arterial stenting in the Mayo Clinic Health System in La Crosse, Wisconsin, working with general surgery colleagues already performing carotid endarterectomy at that site. Despite early pushback from neurosurgery at both the local and national levels, carotid arterial stenting with embolic protection has become the standard of care. The interactions during that time between cardiology and neuroradiology presage the current dialog around acute stroke interventions which continues to play out with major implications for delivery of care in these high-risk patients.

Restenosis

Restenosis remained the target of increased study as it was felt to represent the Achilles heel of PCI (Fig. 6.9). Mayo Clinic had a unique presence in this field. One specific drug, tranilast, had received great attention after it had been studied in two small Japanese studies and looked very promising for the prevention of restenosis. It had several important properties; it inhibited release or upstream production of chemical mediators, cytokines, and active oxygen transport by inflammatory cells and macrophages. It had also been found to interfere with the proliferation and migration of vascular smooth muscle cells induced by platelet-derived growth factor. These properties, taken together, appeared to provide an excellent potential treatment for the prevention of restenosis. Accordingly, it formed the basis for the PRESTO trial which, at that time, was the largest trial evaluating restenosis [27]. Mayo Clinic (Holmes) was the PI of this international 11,500 patient trial supported by Smith Kline Beecham Pharmaceuticals. Patients with successful PCI of at least one lesion dilated to <50% residual stenosis without a periprocedural complication were randomized to one of the five treatment groups. The primary composite clinical end point included death, MI, or the need for ischemia-driven TVR. The trial was developed and then implemented with the input from basic scientists, pharmacologists, interventional cardiologists, clinical cardiology, statisticians, and clinical trialists. It included a core angiographic and echocardiographic analysis, both of which would be important for assessing important parameters of function of this drug. Important considerations in planning the trial included determination of a sample size to adequately power test the hypothesis. The design of the PRESTO trial was based on the assumption of a 9-month placebo composite end point of 18% and a 30% relative reduction in any of the four treatment groups receiving the different dosing strategies of tranilast.

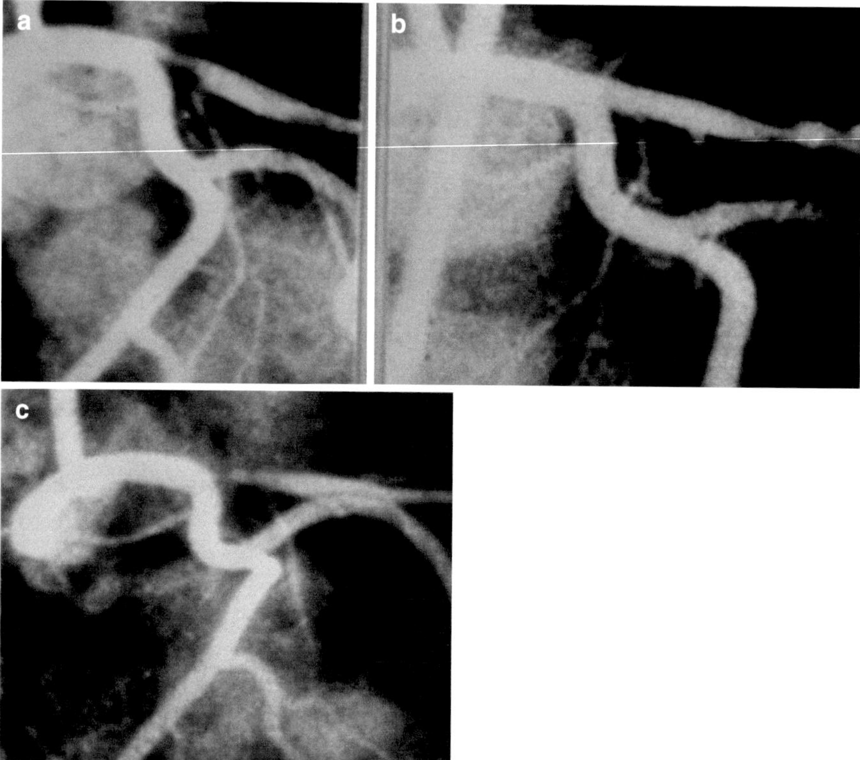

Fig. 6.9 (**a**) Restenosis has remained a problem since the early days of coronary intervention. At baseline, there is a severe ostial stenosis with moderate downstream disease. (**b**) Ostial LAD stenosis treated percutaneously with an excellent result. (**c**) However, 6 months later, symptoms recurred and severe stenosis was documented

Enrollment was rapid and interest very high because the issue of restenosis had become increasingly important as more subsets of patients were being treated with PCI. At the end of trial recruitment and data lock at follow-up, the sponsor had decided to have a meeting in Paris of all the sites and principle investigators. This satellite meeting was held in conjunction with another European meeting to unveil trial results. This strategy of a meeting of sites and investigators to present data before it was released to the cardiovascular community at large has been standard practice for large multicenter, multinational trials.

In a magnificent ballroom setting, in this large trial, the 9-month placebo MACE rate was presented to a large group of very interested audience members, press, and industry leaders. The data and the take-home messages were different than what had been expected; the composite end point in the control group was 15.7% and in the four tranilast dose groups was virtually identical – 15.4–16.0% (Fig. 6.10) [27]. After the presentation of the results, there was profound silence in that same ballroom which moments before had been quite engaged. The very next day, when the

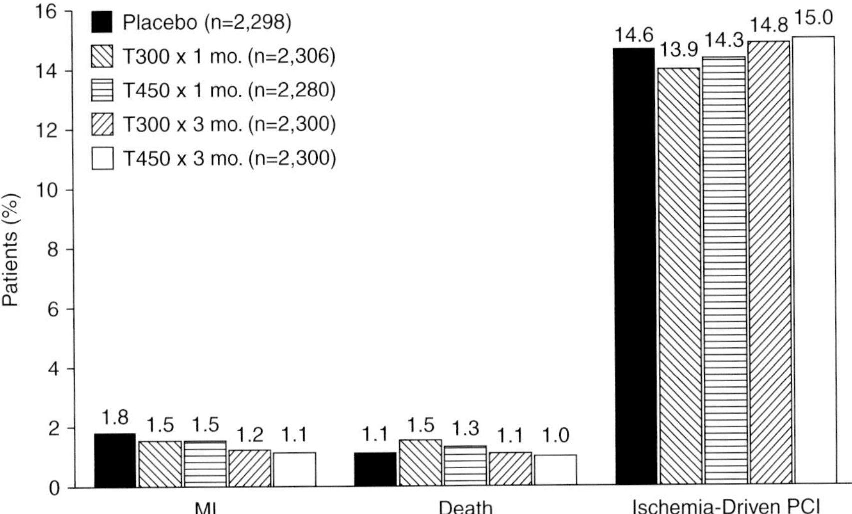

Fig. 6.10 The large PRESTO trial randomized four dosing strategies of tranilast to control in patients undergoing PCI. As can been seen, there was no difference in restenosis rate at follow-up angiography. (From Holmes DR et al. Circulation. 2002;106:1243–1250; used with permission)

PI (Holmes) called the phone number of the sponsor contact, the response was that sponsor contact and the whole team on this project had been reassigned to another project. The fate of a well-conducted but negative trial, lessons learned in a business world.

A positive side to the trial was the possibility of analysis of subsets of enrolled patients. For these, all five groups of patients were included. Subsequent Mayo Clinic analyses included assessment of predictive factors for ischemic TVR, as well as information on the frequency of unstable angina as the presenting symptom of restenosis, both of which were important to more fully understand the phenomenon [28]. In addition, the outcomes of diabetics in the trial as a subset were also analyzed. During this decade, other drugs were also tested including cilostazol which also did not prove to be beneficial, illustrating the multifaceted clinical issues of restenosis.

Stents, Restenosis, and Vascular Brachytherapy

Although native vessel PTCA restenosis had been extremely resistant to a pharmacologic approach, bare metal stents had been developed and had found wide acceptance. The stents acted to minimize acute closure and were responsible for the dramatic decrease in need for urgent CABG related to acute or threatened closure during PTCA, as well as reducing restenosis again compared with conventional PTCA. During the last decade, stents had become so widely used that the term percutaneous transluminal coronary angioplasty had been changed to percutaneous coronary intervention (PCI). Patients had been treated with stent implantation initially with bare metal stents and then drug-eluting stents to prevent the restenosis rates seen with conventional PTCA. However, relatively rapidly, the issues of stent restenosis appeared. Several different forms were identified that had variable clinical consequences. In particular, diffuse in-stent restenosis was characterized by a marked increase in recurrent restenosis. The etiology had been found to be diffuse neointimal hyperplasia. Out of this information came the approach of vascular brachytherapy initially using gamma radiation. Harnessing an ancient and fundamental physical process, gamma rays have ultrashort wavelengths and hence have incredibly high energies and are difficult to stop and shield against. Indeed some of the highest energy processes in the universe such as supernovas are associated with the so-called gamma-ray bursts which, if they were to encounter the earth, would basically cook us like a microwave (actually far more energetically). Although Mayo Clinic had been an investigative site in the original multicenter randomized trials, there were many issues to be addressed from a clinical practice standpoint in bringing this therapy forward. Centers had to develop close working relationships with radiation therapy, develop strategies to shield the patient and the staff performing the procedure, as well as making sure that the cath lab room itself was adequately shielded. Specific details resolved around calculating the dose required, the distance from the source to the surrounding catheterization laboratory and details about transfer, procurement of the source, and then follow-up removal and storing of the radiation source. Elaborate protocols were put into place involving all the stakeholders particularly because of the intensity, strength, and penetration of gamma irradiation. In particular, collaboration with James Martenson, MD, and his colleagues from radiation oncology was critical in establishing the brachytherapy program. Specific issues related to the danger of penetrating radiation from the iridium source had to be thought through. For example, once the source was placed in the coronary artery, all operators had to leave the room, leaving the patient strangely isolated and able to communicate only by audio connections. People whose offices and workplaces were in close proximity including one of the authors (CSR) had to vacate their space while the source was in the patient. Strange words such as bremsstrahlung (braking radiation) became part of the interventional vocabulary. In a strange twist of physics, wearing a protective lead apron could paradoxically be harmful to operators as gamma rays encountered lead atoms, induced dangerous secondary forms of radiation. Counterintuitively, not wearing a lead apron and simply allowing gamma rays to pass through one's body was the safest approach; however, no one to our recollection felt comfortable with that approach. Needless to say, we all breathed a sigh of relief when gamma coronary brachytherapy passed into the annals of medical history and "scatter" came to mean what it had always meant.

Another catheter-based system was developed and tested using beta irradiation, which had significant advantages in terms of radiation protection. Beta radiation, which essentially was electrons, was of much lower energy with limited penetrative power and relatively simple to shield against. Mayo Clinic was involved in both gamma and beta approaches. Based upon the data, vascular brachytherapy using beta irradiation became the only approved therapy for restenosis following bare metal stent implantation.

During this time, however, the interventional cardiology community had the opportunity to begin widespread evaluation of drug-eluting stents. Early efforts using sirolimus-eluting stents were extremely positive for the prevention of restenosis in native coronary arterial stenoses. These devices were complex with a metal frame, a polymer, and a drug within the polymer. Multiple issues had to be addressed including identification of the specific polymer and the specific drug, the elution time kinetics of the drug, and the subsequent stability or lack of stability of the polymer. Early work from the Restenosis Treatment Board comprised of Mayo Clinic, Cleveland Clinic, and the Thoraxcenter in Rotterdam with the funding of Medtronic, had identified that some polymers that had been found to be biocompatible by testing the material in the subcutaneous space were not blood-compatible when delivered in the coronary vasculature, and during healing, severe inflammation and vessel occlusion occurred in animal models, a finding which gave pause for concern by industry and investigators (Fig. 6.11) [29]. However, the field advanced and two drug-eluting stents were brought to market; sirolimus and paclitaxel. The former became more widely used. The strategy of DES was to prevent restenosis, not to treat it. However, because of the success of DES in preventing restenosis, many investigators adopted application of these stents to actually treat in-stent restenosis occurring with bare metal stents.

Accordingly, the field was primed for another multicenter RCT of DES versus vascular brachytherapy for the treatment of in-stent restenosis within bare metal stents. The SISR randomized trial was developed with Mayo Clinic as the PI (Holmes) [30]. The SISR randomized 384 patients with in-stent restenosis between February 2003 and July 2004 to either vascular brachytherapy using gamma

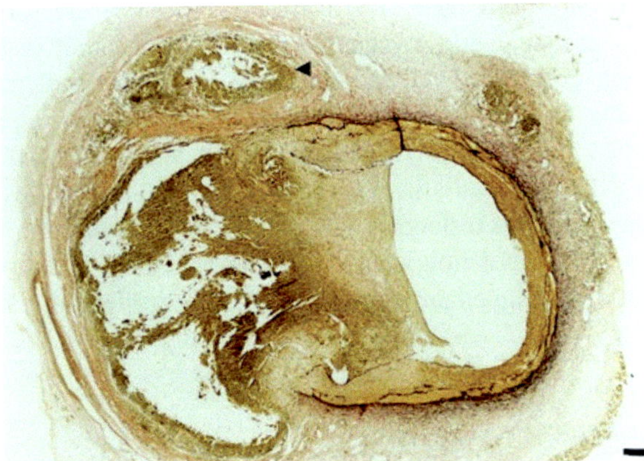

Fig. 6.11 In a porcine coronary artery model, biocompatibility of synthetic polymers was assessed – tested as strips deployed across the circumferential surface of the wire cool stents. As can be seen, at 4 weeks, the biodegradable polymer polyorthoester induced an exuberant inflammation response with destruction of the vessel wall including adventitia. (From van der Giessen WJ et al. Circulation 94;7, 1 October 1996:1690–1697; used with permission)

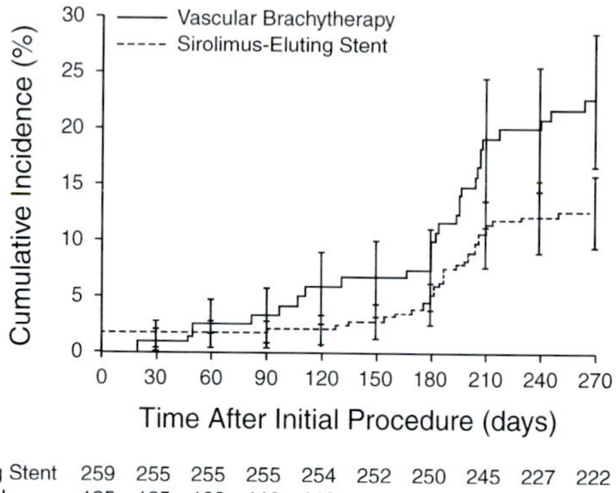

Fig. 6.12 The SISR trial randomized patients with in-stent restenosis of bare metal stents to either gamma vascular brachytherapy or a sirolimus-eluting stent. The cumulative incidence of target vessel failure was worse with brachytherapy. (From Holmes DR et al. JAMA 2006;295: 1264–1273; used with permission)

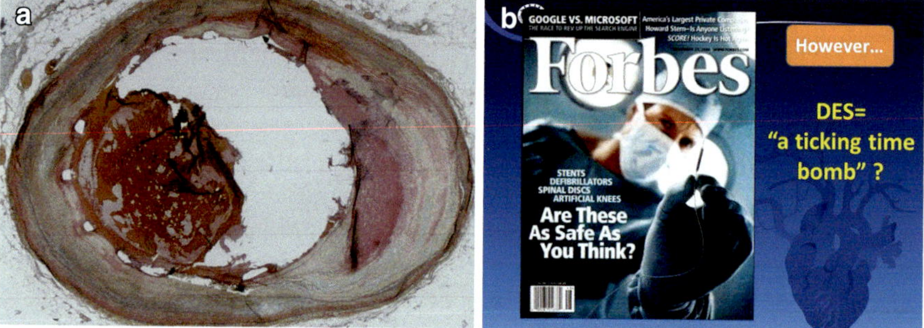

Fig. 6.13 Pathologic section from a patient who died from stent thrombosis (**a**). Such iconic slides were used by some to refer to drug eluting stents as "ticking time bombs" (**b**)

radiation or to the sirolimus DES. The main outcome measure was target vessel failure defined as cardiac death, myocardial infarction, or target vessel revascularization at 9 months postprocedure. Procedural success was excellent at 99.2% and 97.3%, respectively, for VBT and SES. The rate of target vessel failure was 21.6% for VBT versus 12.5% for SES (RR 1.7, 95%CI 1.1–2.8, $p = 0.02$) (Fig. 6.12). Compared with VBT, SES had a larger minimal lumen diameter, less target lesion revascularization, and more restenosis [30]. This trial and other information in the field relegated VBT to a position where it was only offered in a small number of centers and never again played any important role in treatment of restenosis.

Stent Thrombosis

During this time, the phenomenon of stent thrombosis was also identified with its profound implications for both morbidity and mortality (Fig. 6.13a, b). This was found to be more frequent than had been seen with bare metal stents [31, 32]. Sandhu reviewed the Mayo Clinic experience during 1 year of follow-up [33].

Multiple etiologies were discussed, ranging from inflammation related to polymer degradation to immune reactions to the drug, among others. As previously mentioned, it received great press, and in one well-documented incidence (Fig. 6.13a, b), it was said that DES were a "time bomb" ticking in the patient's chest. This was seized upon as argument for and against their use by both cardiologists and cardiovascular surgeons. Initially given the pathology of a thrombus, anticoagulation was used typically along with dual antiplatelet therapy with resultant increased rates of bleeding [34, 35]. This led to strategies relying on dual antiplatelet therapy and the eventual design of the multicenter DAPT trial of which Mayo Clinic was a member of the steering committee [36]. Given early safety data concerns using ticlopidine with ASA, there was increased incorporation of clopidogrel which had fewer significant side effects; however, this led to concern about the issue of nonresponders, namely, patients given the prodrug did not convert it to the effective drug and then would be at increased risk for adverse outcomes as they would be on ASA alone. This resulted in a "Boxed Warning" from the FDA which was circulated on the eve of the American College of Cardiology national meeting which typically had up to 20,000 participants both physicians and industry. This caused great angst for cardiologists and patients alike and resulted in rapid development of an ACC to review the information and publish an official professional societal response aimed at clarifying the issues and focusing on strategies of care [37]. It was was the first of many discussions about that subject which have continued over the next two decades.

The information on underlying pathophysiology continued to accrue the result of international collaborations on monoclonal T-cell proliferation in unstable angina [38] and the role hyperfibrinogenemia on the histocytological composition of atherosclerotic carotid plaques in patients with transient ischemic attacks, as well as the relationship between extracranial thrombotically active carotid plaque as a risk factor for ischemic stroke (Fig. 6.14a–d). Other studies evaluated the stimulation of endothelin B receptor in experimental hypercholesterolemia [39] and the effect of simvastatin on preserving coronary endothelial function in hypercholesterolemia independent of changes in lipids. As part of the evaluation of the effects of hypercholesterolemia on vascular biology, imaging of the coronary vasa vasorum in animal models was performed [40]. Cholesterol lowering was also found to be associated with improvement in coronary vascular remodeling and endothelial function in patients with normal or only mildly diseased coronary arteries [41]. New markers were also studied, particularly pregnancy-associated plasma protein, which was found to be a marker of acute coronary syndromes [42].

Procedural Risk and Strategies of Care

During this timeframe the interventional community became interested in the systematic assessment of procedure risk [43–45]. Coronary angioplasty had always been associated with procedural risk, and while standby operating rooms were no longer necessary, accurate and quantitative assessment of risk became increasingly

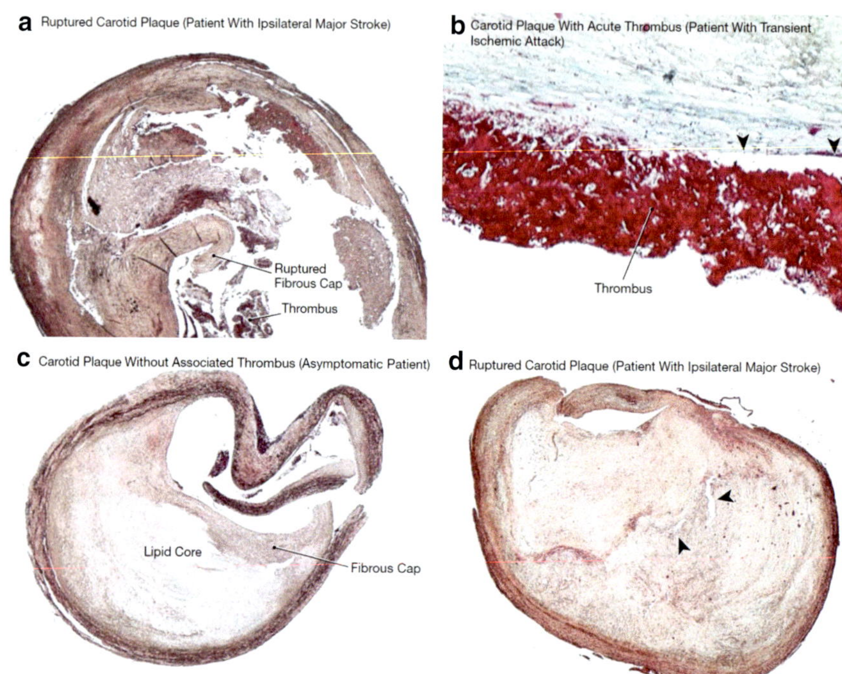

Fig. 6.14 Representative histopathology micrograph from patients undergoing carotid endarterectomy. (**a**) Ruptured fibrous cap and thrombus in a patient with an ipsilateral major stroke. (**b**) Acute thrombus identified in a carotid plaque (arrowheads) with thrombus in the setting of a transient ischemic attack. (**c**) Plaque in an asymptomatic patient undergoing elective endarterectomy. There is no evidence of thrombus. (**d**) Ruptured plaque (arrowheads) in a patient with a major stroke. No apparent thrombus. (From Spagnoli LG et al. JAMA 2004;292:1845–1852; used with permission)

important for patient counseling and risk adjustment in scientific reports. Mandeep Singh developed the Mayo Clinic Risk Score which built upon the work from the New York State Registry and other observations demonstrating the importance of noncardiac comorbidities and determining both acute and long-term outcomes [46–48]. Collaborating with biostatisticians, and using the Mayo Clinic PCI Registry as a data source, we analyzed all procedural complications and developed a standard multivariable model of predictors of complications. The coefficients from this model were subsequently turned into a simple integer score that could be readily applied even at the bedside. This project was developed and implemented almost 15 years before shared decision-making became more formalized as a methodology to inform patient discussions. The score was validated in external databases and used to risk stratify patients to allow interindividual comparison of results.

To mitigate risk, inpatient populations with the highest risk, not necessarily those with cardiogenic shock from STEMI, but also those with severe left ventricular dysfunction combined with the need for a complex interventional procedure, required novel approaches and collaborations. Simply using an intra-aortic balloon pump was not enough for many of these patients, and numerous instances were encountered where the patient survived the complex interventional procedure but subsequently succumbed to the effects of systemic hypoperfusion, particularly with kidney and gut ischemia. Novel mechanical circulatory support devices allowed a window of opportunity to help such patients. The initial procedure using percutaneous bypass for mechanical support was performed in collaboration with cardiac surgery and the use of a cardiopulmonary bypass machine and surgical cutdown. Following a number of successful experiences with this approach, as previously mentioned, we turned our attention to utilization of the novel TandemHeart device. This device essentially provides left atrial to femoral artery bypass using percutaneous large bore cannula and allowed for an incremental 3–5 liters/minute of flow to augment cardiac output during often very complex interventional procedures. Operators had the initially harrowing experience of watching the left ventricle essentially go into standstill, and the pulsatile aorta pressure became flatline as, for example, a complex left main stenosis was being tackled and contrast pooled in the aorta. Interventionalists had to learn to think in terms of flow rather than pressure and focus on perfusion of vascular beds such as the kidney, extremities, and gut. Despite cardiac standstill that often lasted many minutes, with reperfusion of oxygenated blood into long-deprived myocardium, these ventricles, particularly in those patients with non cardiogenic STEMI, have been documented as having the ability to bounce back quickly, restoring the pulsatile flow that operators were used to seeing. Eventually Mayo Clinic became one largest users of this technology [49]. An advance in mechanical circulatory support was achieved with easier to use axial flow pumps that did not require transseptal access. This latter approach to mechanical circulatory support is now a staple of all complex interventional laboratories.

Radial Access

During this decade, an important technical innovation that has led to improved patient outcomes, increased laboratory efficiency, and more rapid ambulation following cardiac catheterization has been the adoption of the radial artery as the preferred route for coronary access. Developed in Canada by the pioneer Lucien Campeau, transradial catheterization was quickly adopted by European operators. While working in Canada, Rihal had the opportunity to learn and develop transradial catheterization from first principles working with senior colleagues who were Sones operators. It quickly became apparent that the radial artery was much too friable to cutdown in the classic Sones manner and that percutaneous access was preferred. Operators discovered that, having inserted a 6F vascular sheath, any coronary procedure that could be performed through a 6F femoral sheath could be performed from the radial site. The steady introduction of new sheaths and purpose-built devices and catheters in combination with data from randomized trials demonstrating the clear superiority of the transradial access site has resulted in it becoming the preferred access site around the world and at Mayo Clinic. Indeed trainees now garner much more experience with the radial access site then with the femoral. This in turn sets up new problems such as training for safe and effective femoral entry and exit with vascular access devices which have to be deliberately done.

Imaging Advances

Imaging continued to be an important focus. As procedures became more complex, by virtue of lesion complexity, efforts to provide approaches with new technology were developed. Information became available about stereotaxis, an approach which involved the use of magnetic guidance for the placement of specially constructed guide wires. These units combined conventional angiography with a magnetic interface. The cath lab working with electrophysiology explored the potential utility for complex coronary intervention, as well as for integration with EP imaging for complex ablation. From a forward-looking, visionary perspective, if such magnetic guidance of procedures could be demonstrated, this might form the platform for more remote guidance of procedures. Long-distance robotic guidance of procedures had been documented to be feasible. With such a magnetically guided system, the operator could be in a control room performing the procedure. For such long-term strategies, initial experience had to be gained. A specific cath lab room was developed with shielding for magnetic guidance. The room could also be used for conventional angiography and PCI. Early procedures with very complex coronary anatomy such as very severe angulation or chronic total occlusion were selected. The early magnetic guide wires proved to be rigid and inflexible with only a small radius of curvature that could be developed with magnetic control. Under the guidance of Guri Sandhu, early procedures were initiated. During this time, conventional guide wires became increasingly flexible and steerable with variable force characteristics, and as a result the need for magnetic control became less of an issue. In addition, from the EP standpoint, the mapping techniques evolved greatly such that magnetic guidance was also not needed. Finally, technical issues relating to the fact that patients with pacemakers could not be treated in that specific room led to decreasing use, and the potential for magnetic guidance was never realized. However, the concept of remote guidance has continued to be attractive, and Mayo Clinic has transmitted coronary procedures using remote guidance. Such an approach may have significant applications for laboratories in satellite facilities and may have great potential for patients with acute stroke. As has been found [50], current stent retrieval approaches for acute stroke in very carefully selected patients may result in dramatic improvement in outcome even out to 24 hours after onset of symptoms. In addition, IVUS advanced imaging may play an important role given the number of large vessel occlusion strokes in the United States and the relatively constrained number of neuroradiologists which represents an unmet clinical need [51]. Well-trained interventional cardiologists may be an important addition to the pool of physicians that could play an important role. Remote guidance could offer a great advantage in this setting. In a potential scenario, a cardiologist trained in carotid stenting could access the carotid in a patient with an acute large vessel ischemic stroke and then interface with another trained individual to navigate the cerebral vessels beyond the siphon to deliver a stent retriever.

Practice Advancements

There were other advances. The economics of patients admitted on Friday who would need early but not urgent procedures which by scheduling could not be performed on that Friday and who would then have to be admitted to hospital for the weekend were disadvantageous and related in patient delays. To address this, Saturday catheterizations at Mayo Clinic were initiated. These cases were scheduled the evening before as well as patients admitted during the evening. Such procedures often resulted in PCI, and the patients could then be dismissed after the procedure with either same-day discharge or on Sunday. This practice has been efficient and well received by clinical staff providing patient care; it has been very well accepted and received by patients who are always eager to avoid longer hospitalizations.

As part of the process of improving patient care, a strategy for outpatient angiographic procedures was implemented. Typically patients were seen as outpatients at the main Mayo Clinic facility which is approximately 1 mile away from St. Mary's Hospital where they would be admitted for angiography. The proposal for outpatient angiography was deliberated and approved by Mayo Clinic administration and involved construction of an angiographic procedure room at the outpatient building. Patients could be seen by their outpatient cardiologist, have appropriate early morning laboratory testing, and, then without the need for transfer, undergo angiography and if needed PCI. If the patient needed to undergo PCI, they would then be transferred to the hospital; however, many patients could be dismissed from the outpatient angiographic suite. This was well received by the attending physicians who could discuss face to face with the patient the results of testing and finalized care; in addition on-site surgical consultation could also be obtained. Despite the widespread acceptance, preprocedure imaging was often so helpful that patients probably requiring intervention were typically identified and scheduled electively at the hospital for their procedures. This led to refitting the angiographic outpatient suite for other applications. This process of evaluating new approaches and implementing some of them needs to be matched with rigorous study of the results of the new approach and decisions made on longer-term strategies based on the data which has been accumulated.

Traning and Education

Training and education both within Mayo Clinic and on a broader national level remained very important. Mayo Clinic (Holmes) was a member of the ACC Task Force 3: training in diagnostic and interventional cardiac catheterization [52], as well as continuing to serve on the test writing committee for the ABIM board for added qualifications in interventional cardiology. Mayo Clinic also focused on manuscript preparation and publication as well as participating in the development of a core curriculum for an interventional fellowship in structural and congenital heart disease for adults [53]. There was continued involvement in clinical competence statements from the professional societies on invasive electrophysiology studies, catheter ablation, and cardioversion. Finally, Mayo Clinic participated in the multinational recommendations for successful training on methods of delivery of biologics for cardiac regeneration, a report of the International Society for Cardiovascular Translational Research [54].

Leadership

Catheterization laboratory leadership changed in 2003. This was the result of a series of meetings based on time-limited leadership durations. At Mayo Clinic, administrative leadership roles such as CEO, CMO, and department and division chairs had an approximate 8-year term limit. This was based on the need for encouraging growth and the implementation of new ideas. That rule had never been applied to laboratory directors some of whom such as Holmes had served for 19 years. In 2002–2003, Mayo Clinic decided that the term limit rule should be applied across the laboratories. Accordingly in 2003, that was implemented in the cardiac laboratory, the echo laboratory, and the cardiac nuclear medicine laboratory. After deliberation for the cath lab position, two outstanding candidates, Chet Rihal and Kirk Garratt, were selected and discussed by a group convened for that purpose. At that point in time, Kirk was Head of the Mayo Clinic Health System in La Crosse, Wisconsin, cardiology practice, while Chet was continuing practice in Rochester. Chet was selected and agreed and subsequently, after 7 years, moved to become chair of the Division of Cardiology at Mayo Clinic. Garratt, after 17 years at Mayo Clinic, went on to work in New York at Lenox Hill Hospital as a Professor of Medicine, then subsequently to become President of the Society for Cardiovascular Angiography and Interventions, a Master Interventionalist of SCAI, and then Medical Director of Christiana Care for the state of Delaware. The transition was seamless. As part of the 10-year design, new approaches were brought in and new strategies of care established resulting in further build out of the mission for clinical care, research, and education. It included particularly robust growth in the field of structural heart disease, with development of new technologies such as TAVR and MitraClip and the design of and implantation of new families of RCTs and then FDA approval of new transformational technology which has had dramatic benefits for an increasingly diverse group of patients.

References

1. Holmes DR Jr, Califf RM, Topol EJ. Lessons we have learned from the GUSTO trial. Global utilization of streptokinase and tissue plasminogen activator for occluded arteries. J Am Coll Cardiol. 1995;25:10s–7s.
2. Hasdai D, Harrington RA, Hochman JS, et al. Platelet glycoprotein IIb/IIIa blockade and outcome of cardiogenic shock complicating acute coronary syndromes without persistent ST-segment elevation. J Am Coll Cardiol. 2000;36:685–92.
3. Hasdai D, Califf RM, Thompson TD, et al. Predictors of cardiogenic shock after thrombolytic therapy for acute myocardial infarction. J Am Coll Cardiol. 2000;35:136–43.
4. Hasdai D, Topol EJ, Califf RM, Berger PB, Holmes DR Jr. Cardiogenic shock complicating acute coronary syndromes. Lancet. 2000;356:749–56.
5. Dzavík V, Cotter G, Reynolds HR, et al. Effect of nitric oxide synthase inhibition on haemodynamics and outcome of patients with persistent cardiogenic shock complicating acute myocardial infarction: a phase II dose-ranging study. Eur Heart J. 2007;28:1109–16.
6. McFadden EP, Stabile E, Regar E, et al. Late thrombosis in drug-eluting coronary stents after discontinuation of antiplatelet therapy. Lancet. 2004;364:1519–21.
7. Sigwart U, Puel J, Mirkovitch V, Joffre F, Kappenberger L. Intravascular stents to prevent occlusion and restenosis after transluminal angioplasty. N Engl J Med. 1987;316:701–6.
8. Hannan EL, Wu C, Walford G, et al. Volume-outcome relationships for percutaneous coronary interventions in the stent era. Circulation. 2005;112:1171–9.
9. Holmes DR Jr, Berger PB, Garratt KN, et al. Application of the New York State PTCA mortality model in patients undergoing stent implantation. Circulation. 2000;102:517–22.
10. Hannan EL, Racz M, Holmes DR, et al. A comparison of mortality, myocardial infarction, and repeated revascularization for sirolimus-eluting and paclitaxel-eluting coronary stents. Am Heart J. 2007;154:545–53.
11. Hannan EL, Racz M, Holmes DR, et al. Comparison of coronary artery stenting outcomes in the eras before and after the introduction of drug-eluting stents. Circulation. 2008;117:2071–8.
12. Steinhubl SR, Talley JD, Braden GA, et al. Point-of-care measured platelet inhibition correlates with a reduced risk of an adverse cardiac event after percutaneous coronary intervention: results of the GOLD (AU-Assessing Ultegra) multicenter study. Circulation. 2001;103:2572–8.
13. Marks DS, Mensah GA, Kennard ED, Detre K, Holmes DR Jr. Race, baseline characteristics, and clinical outcomes after coronary intervention: The New Approaches in Coronary Interventions (NACI) registry. Am Heart J. 2000;140:162–9.
14. Jacobs AK, Johnston JM, Haviland A, et al. Improved outcomes for women undergoing contemporary percutaneous coronary intervention: a report from the National Heart, Lung, and Blood Institute Dynamic Registry. J Am Coll Cardiol. 2002;39:1608–14.
15. Holmes DR, Selzer F, Johnston JM, et al. Modeling and risk prediction in the current era of interventional cardiology: a report from the National Heart, Lung, and Blood Institute Dynamic Registry. Circulation. 2003;107:1871–6.
16. Rihal CS, Textor SC, Grill DE, et al. Incidence and prognostic importance of acute renal failure after percutaneous coronary intervention. Circulation. 2002;105:2259–64.
17. Prasad A, Singh M, Lerman A, Lennon RJ, Holmes DR Jr, Rihal CS. Isolated elevation in troponin T after percutaneous coronary intervention is associated with higher long-term mortality. J Am Coll Cardiol. 2006;48:1765–70.
18. Hasdai D, Rizza RA, Grill DE, Scott CG, Garratt KN, Holmes DR. Diabetes mellitus and outcome after successful percutaneous coronary revascularization: The Mayo Clinic Experience 1979-1998. Heart Drug. 2001;1:132–7.

19. Mathew V, Clavell AL, Lennon RJ, Grill DE, Holmes DR Jr. Percutaneous coronary interventions in patients with prior coronary artery bypass surgery: changes in patient characteristics and outcome during two decades. Am J Med. 2000;108:127–35.
20. Doyle BJ, Ting HH, Bell MR, et al. Major femoral bleeding complications after percutaneous coronary intervention: incidence, predictors, and impact on long-term survival among 17,901 patients treated at the Mayo Clinic from 1994 to 2005. JACC Cardiovasc Interv. 2008;1:202–9.
21. Ting HH, Garratt KN, Singh M, et al. Low-risk percutaneous coronary interventions without on-site cardiac surgery: two years' observational experience and follow-up. Am Heart J. 2003;145:278–84.
22. Holmes DR Jr, Firth BG, Wood DL. Paradigm shifts in cardiovascular medicine. J Am Coll Cardiol. 2004;43:507–12.
23. Gersh BJ, Stone GW, White HD, Holmes DR Jr. Pharmacological facilitation of primary percutaneous coronary intervention for acute myocardial infarction: is the slope of the curve the shape of the future? JAMA. 2005;293:979–86.
24. Ting HH, Rihal CS, Gersh BJ, et al. Regional systems of care to optimize timeliness of reperfusion therapy for ST-elevation myocardial infarction: the Mayo Clinic STEMI protocol. Circulation. 2007;116:729–36.
25. Singh M, Gersh BJ, Lennon RJ, et al. Outcomes of a system-wide protocol for elective and nonelective coronary angioplasty at sites without on-site surgery: the Mayo Clinic Experience. Mayo Clin Proc. 2009;84:501–8.
26. Hopkins LN, Holmes DR Jr, Ramee S. Turf wars and silos-joined at the hip: what can be done? Catheter Cardiovasc Interv. 2007;69:764–5.
27. Holmes DR Jr, Savage M, LaBlanche JM, et al. Results of Prevention of REStenosis with Tranilast and its Outcomes (PRESTO) trial. Circulation. 2002;106:1243–50.
28. Mathew V, Gersh BJ, Williams BA, et al. Outcomes in patients with diabetes mellitus undergoing percutaneous coronary intervention in the current era: a report from the Prevention of REStenosis with Tranilast and its Outcomes (PRESTO) trial. Circulation. 2004;109:476–80.
29. van der Giessen WJ, Lincoff AM, Schwartz RS, et al. Marked inflammatory sequelae to implantation of biodegradable and nonbiodegradable polymers in porcine coronary arteries. Circulation. 1996;94:1690–7.
30. Holmes DR Jr, Teirstein P, Satler L, et al. Sirolimus-eluting stents vs vascular brachytherapy for in-stent restenosis within bare-metal stents: the SISR randomized trial. JAMA. 2006;295:1264–73.
31. Mauri L, O'Malley AJ, Popma JJ, et al. Comparison of thrombosis and restenosis risk from stent length of sirolimus-eluting stents versus bare metal stents. Am J Cardiol. 2005;95:1140–5.
32. Holmes DR Jr, Kereiakes DJ, Laskey WK, et al. Thrombosis and drug-eluting stents: an objective appraisal. J Am Coll Cardiol. 2007;50:109–18.
33. Sandhu G, Doyle B, Singh R, et al. Frequency, etiology, treatment, and outcomes of drug-eluting stent thrombosis during one year of follow-up. Am J Cardiol. 2007;99:465–9.
34. Orford JL, Fasseas P, Melby S, et al. Safety and efficacy of aspirin, clopidogrel, and warfarin after coronary stent placement in patients with an indication for anticoagulation. Am Heart J. 2004;147:463–7.
35. Holmes DR Jr, Kereiakes DJ, Kleiman NS, Moliterno DJ, Patti G, Grines CL. Combining antiplatelet and anticoagulant therapies. J Am Coll Cardiol. 2009;54:95–109.
36. Mauri L, Kereiakes DJ, Normand SL, et al. Rationale and design of the dual antiplatelet therapy study, a prospective, multicenter, randomized, double-blind trial to assess the effectiveness and safety of 12 versus 30 months of dual antiplatelet therapy in subjects undergoing percutaneous coronary intervention with either drug-eluting stent or bare metal stent placement for the treatment of coronary artery lesions. Am Heart J. 2010;160:1035–41, 1041.e1.
37. Holmes DR Jr, Dehmer GJ, Kaul S, Leifer D, O'Gara PT, Stein CM. ACCF/AHA clopidogrel clinical alert: approaches to the FDA "boxed warning": a report of the American College of Cardiology Foundation task force on clinical expert consensus documents and the American Heart Association endorsed by the Society for Cardiovascular Angiography and Interventions and the Society of Thoracic Surgeons. J Am Coll Cardiol. 2010;56:321–41.

38. Liuzzo G, Goronzy JJ, Yang H, et al. Monoclonal T-cell proliferation and plaque instability in acute coronary syndromes. Circulation. 2000;101:2883–8.
39. Mathew V, Miller VM, Hasdai D, Barber DA, Holmes DR Jr, Lerman A. Increased coronary effects of stimulation of endothelin-B receptor in experimental hypercholesterolemia. Coron Artery Dis. 2000;11:585–92.
40. Herrmann J, Lerman LO, Rodriguez-Porcel M, et al. Coronary vasa vasorum neovascularization precedes epicardial endothelial dysfunction in experimental hypercholesterolemia. Cardiovasc Res. 2001;51:762–6.
41. Hamasaki S, Higano ST, Suwaidi JA, et al. Cholesterol-lowering treatment is associated with improvement in coronary vascular remodeling and endothelial function in patients with normal or mildly diseased coronary arteries. Arterioscler Thromb Vasc Biol. 2000;20:737–43.
42. Bayes-Genis A, Conover CA, Overgaard MT, et al. Pregnancy-associated plasma protein a as a marker of acute coronary syndromes. N Engl J Med. 2001;345:1022–9.
43. Singh M, Lennon RJ, Holmes DR Jr, Bell MR, Rihal CS. Correlates of procedural complications and a simple integer risk score for percutaneous coronary intervention. J Am Coll Cardiol. 2002;40:387–93.
44. Gössl M, Rihal CS, Lennon RJ, Singh M. Assessment of individual operator performance using a risk-adjustment model for percutaneous coronary interventions. Mayo Clin Proc. 2013;88:1250–8.
45. Singh M, Rihal CS, Roger VL, et al. Comorbid conditions and outcomes after percutaneous coronary intervention. Heart. 2008;94:1424–8.
46. Singh M, Rihal CS, Lennon RJ, Garratt KN, Holmes DR Jr. Comparison of Mayo Clinic risk score and American College of Cardiology/American Heart Association lesion classification in the prediction of adverse cardiovascular outcome following percutaneous coronary interventions. J Am Coll Cardiol. 2004;44:357–61.
47. Singh M, Rihal CS, Selzer F, Kip KE, Detre K, Holmes DR. Validation of Mayo Clinic risk adjustment model for in-hospital complications after percutaneous coronary interventions, using the National Heart, Lung, and Blood Institute Dynamic Registry. J Am Coll Cardiol. 2003;42:1722–8.
48. Singh M, Rihal CS, Lennon RJ, Spertus J, Rumsfeld JS, Holmes DR Jr. Bedside estimation of risk from percutaneous coronary intervention: the new Mayo Clinic risk scores. Mayo Clin Proc. 2007;82:701–8.
49. Alli OO, Singh IM, Holmes DR Jr, Pulido JN, Park SJ, Rihal CS. Percutaneous left ventricular assist device with TandemHeart for high-risk percutaneous coronary intervention: the Mayo Clinic experience. Catheter Cardiovasc Interv. 2012;80:728–34.
50. Holmes DR Jr, Hopkins LN. Patients, practice, practicality, and politics. JACC Cardiovasc Interv. 2019;12:1711–3.
51. Wehman JC, Holmes DR Jr, Hanel RA, Levy EI, Hopkins LN. Intravascular ultrasound for intracranial angioplasty and stent placement: technical case report. Neurosurgery. 2006;59:ONSE481–3; discussion ONSE483.
52. Jacobs AK, Babb JD, Hirshfeld JW Jr, Holmes DR Jr. Task force 3: training in diagnostic and interventional cardiac catheterization endorsed by the Society for Cardiovascular Angiography and Interventions. J Am Coll Cardiol. 2008;51:355–61.
53. Ruiz CE, Feldman TE, Hijazi ZM, et al. Interventional fellowship in structural and congenital heart disease for adults. Catheter Cardiovasc Interv. 2010;76:E90–105.
54. Dib N, Menasche P, Bartunek JJ, et al. Recommendations for successful training on methods of delivery of biologics for cardiac regeneration: a report of the International Society for Cardiovascular Translational Research. JACC Cardiovasc Interv. 2010;3:265–75.

Chapter 7
2000s: Structural Heart Disease

Charanjit S. Rihal, Trevor J. Simard, and David R. Holmes Jr.

Since the late 2000s, the advent of structural heart disease interventions for valve and other macro-abnormalities of the heart have gained increasing prominence. Novel procedures such as transcatheter aortic valve replacement (TAVR) have provided new hope and the ability to achieve minimally invasive treatment for severe symptomatic aortic stenosis. Hundreds of thousands of patients who previously would not have been candidates for any treatment or were extremely high-risk candidates for surgical aortic valve replacement, which was often accompanied by protracted and complicated postoperative courses, have benefitted. It is important to remember, however, that structural heart interventions stretch back much further in time than merely the advent of TAVR.

Percutaneous Balloon Mitral Valvuloplasty

For many years, the procedure second in importance only to percutaneous transluminal coronary angioplasty was balloon dilatation of the mitral valve for the treatment of rheumatic mitral stenosis. Known by a variety of names, this procedure more closely resembled closed mitral commissurotomy than it did any true valvuloplasty procedure. During the 1950s to 1960s, cardiovascular surgery had been very active in approaches to the treatment of rheumatic mitral stenosis, which was still a major health problem in the USA and even more so worldwide. Several approaches were developed using a left thoracotomy approach. Early approaches used a finger

C. S. Rihal (✉) · D. R. Holmes Jr.
Department of Cardiovascular Diseases, Mayo Clinic, Rochester, MN, USA
e-mail: rihal@mayo.edu; Holmes.david@mayo.edu

T. J. Simard
Mayo Clinic, Rochester, MN, USA
e-mail: Simard.trevor@mayo.edu

© Mayo Foundation for Medical Education and Research,
under exclusive license to Springer Nature Switzerland AG 2021
D. R. Holmes Jr., R. L. Frye (eds.), *The Mayo Clinic Cardiac Catheterization Laboratory*, https://doi.org/10.1007/978-3-030-79329-6_7

fracture operation, whereby the surgeon would palpate the mitral valve and then using his/her finger, mechanically dilate the valve. The procedure was difficult to teach because it was based on the tactile sense of the operator. It was not something that could be watched while the experienced surgeon performed the "finger fracturing," either directly or with imaging, as echocardiography had not yet been developed. Once fractured, if the results were suboptimal with the development of severe mitral regurgitation, they could not be taken back. This then led to the application of a different strategy using a graded dilator (Tubbs dilator), again, with a left thoracotomy, which was more reproducible. During this time, the potential for a less invasive approach was being developed.

To access the mitral valve, the left atrium would have to be entered. Approaches to access the LA had been explored at NIH beginning in the mid-1950s by Drs. John Ross and Eugene Braunwald working under the direction of the Dr. Andrew Morrow. Initial efforts focused on direct measurement of the LA pressure [1]. Several techniques were described, including transbronchial puncture, the Radner procedure with a direct suprasternal notch access, a posterior transthoracic strategy with direct puncture, and direct LV apical puncture. A series of experiments [2] during which transfemoral access through the intra-atrial septum was described and then perfected so that in addition to diagnostic pressure recording, therapeutic strategies could be developed.

As part of applying new and less invasive approaches, the visionary founder of Mansfield Meditech, John Abele, had been involved in the design of balloons. This design could be potentially used to duplicate the success of the Tubbs dilator surgical experience, which Rihal had reported on and found to be excellent and durable. For this, transseptal catheterization was required. Beginning in the 1980s in the cath lab, Seward had introduced the technique in pediatric cardiology in patients with pulmonary atresia. The application of this for mitral valve dilatation used the balloons developed by Abele. Initially, single balloons were used. But depending on the size of the annulus now able to be measured by echocardiography, a single balloon may not be sufficient, and so the double-balloon approach was used. Different formulas were developed in selecting the correct size of two balloons inflated together. These formulas were taped on the cabinets in the cath lab so that correct sizing with the mathematical formula of two circles in an oval structure was chosen. On one occasion, a cardiology trainee from India, Mandeep Singh, was scrubbed in with Holmes. When Holmes, facing the chart, is ready to select the appropriate size, Mandeep said quietly, "The appropriate size is…" He had identified this before any "real calculations" were performed. As it turned out, after the "official calculations by the chart taped to the wall in the lab" were performed, the strategy that Singh had laid out was identical. When the results of this interchange were discussed with Singh at the end of that successful procedure, he mentioned that he had been involved in multiple procedures because the high incidence of rheumatic heart disease (RHD) in India. Procedural performance there, based on many cases, was superb. He taught us all many lessons.

As the field developed, Mansfield worked closely with Mayo Clinic (Holmes) and, based on the results of multiple publications (Nishimura, Cannon, Rihal, Holmes, etc.), contacted Mayo Clinic to see if they would be able to present on the technology to the FDA panel for potential approval. After substantial regulatory practice sessions, that panel meeting led to device approval and then the multicenter Mansfield registry for this now-approved technology, as well as the development of excellent prediction scores used to identify optimal lesion selection criteria for treatment. In addition, new technology was developed in Japan, which made the procedure more predictable and straightforward.

Performed using antegrade transseptal techniques with one or two balloons ranging in size from 14 to 20 mm each, the double-balloon technique was initially deployed in an effort to generate maximum dilatation force to the fused commissures. When performing this complex procedure, operators had the experience of learning to manage sustained ventricular tachycardia while assessing hemodynamics and trying to avoid perforation of the cardiac apex; the procedure often took two or three operators. When a better alternative came about, it was hastily adopted by the interventional community. Developed by Kanji Inoue, a Japanese cardiac surgeon, the balloon which bears his name was a marvel of simplicity and engineering [3]. Having an interwoven mesh with differential weakness allowed inflation of the Inoue balloon in a stepwise manner. The weakest portion of the mesh, the distal third, was inflated first, followed by the proximal third, and finally, the middle of the balloon. This allowed precise placement and "locking" on to the stenotic mitral valve before dilatation took place. A major advantage of this device was avoidance of guide wires at the cardiac apex, thereby leading to a controlled and largely hemodynamically stable procedure in most patients [3]. In countries such as India with a very large population of patients with rheumatic mitral stenosis, including many young women of childbearing age, percutaneous mitral balloon valvuloplasty often proved an unaffordable Holy Grail, leading either to continued use of surgical commissurotomy or repeated use of the same balloon dilatation catheter [4].

At Mayo Clinic, Dr. Rick Nishimura led the charge in balloon valvuloplasty, ably assisted by Drs. David Holmes, Guy Reeder, and later, Rihal. It was quickly learned that advanced rheumatic morphologies, including marked chordal shortening, leaflet thickening, and calcification, impaired the ability to obtain ideal results [5]. The development of the echocardiographic Wilkins-Abascal score allowed for semi-quantitation of valve morphology and selection of ideal candidates for the procedure [6, 7]. The importance of morphology for the prediction of success solidified a key role for the echo lab not only in diagnosis but in procedural planning and execution (Table 7.1). Patients with a score less than 8 were deemed ideal, those with 8–10, intermediate risk, and those with scores greater than 10, generally not suitable for percutaneous commissurotomy [6–8]. Further refinement in patient selection came from the realization that since percutaneous balloon valvuloplasty is actually a commissurotomy, the presence of commissural calcification would make splitting the commissures difficult if not impossible. Studies from Mayo Clinic, first author Charles Cannan, at that time a fellow and now a practicing cardiologist, demonstrated the prognostic value of commissural calcification in obtaining ideal results at the time of the procedure (Fig. 7.1) [9]. Further studies from Mayo Clinic demonstrated that the long-term results of PBMV were dependent upon the acute results; thus, obtaining the final valve area greater than 1.5 with a gradient less than 5 mmHg without significant mitral regurgitation became an important goal. To further define long-term

Table 7.1 The outcome of mitral balloon valvuloplasty was dependent on the anatomic features. A common score involved evaluation of leaflet mobility, subvalvular thickening, leaflet thickening, and calcification, each of which was graded from 0 to 4. As the score increased, the outcome of the procedure varied. The optimal score for PMBV was ≤8 [7]

Grade	Mobility	Subvalvar thickening	Thickening	Calcification
1	Highly mobile valve with only leaflet tips restricted	Minimal thickening just below the mitral leaflets	Leaflets near normal in thickness (4–5 mm)	A single area of increased echo brightness
2	Leaflet mid and base portions have normal mobility	Thickening of chordal structures extending up to one-third of the chordal length	Mid-leaflets normal, considerable thickening of margins (5–8 mm)	Scattered areas of brightness confined to leaflet margins
3	Valve continues to move forward in diastole, mainly from the base	Thickening extending to the distal third of the chords	Thickening extending through the entire leaflet (5–8 mm)	Brightness extending into the mid-portion of the leaflets
4	No or minimal forward movement of the leaflets in diastole	Extensive thickening and shortening of all chordal structures extending down to the papillary muscles	Considerable thickening of all leaflet tissue (>8–10 mm)	Extensive brightness throughout much of the leaflet tissue

The total echocardiography score was derived from an analysis of mitral leaflet mobility, valvar and subvalvular thickening, and calcification, which were graded from 0 to 4, according to the above criteria. This gave a total score of 0–16.

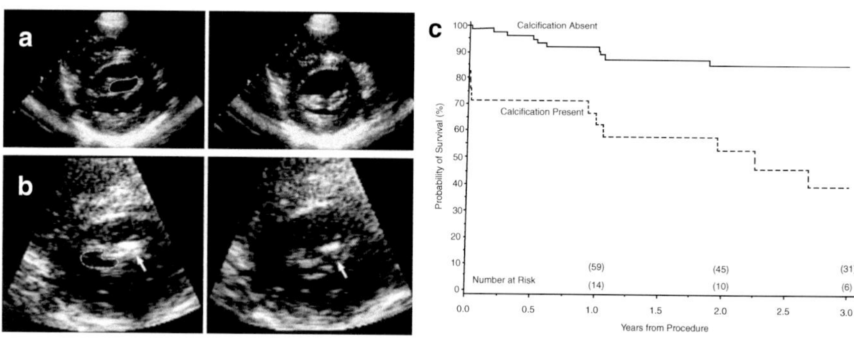

Fig. 7.1 Impact of commissural calcification on outcomes following percutaneous balloon mitral vavuloplasty. Parasternal short-axis view of rheumatic mitral stenosis during diastole (left) and systole (right) in patients without (**a**) and with (**b**) commissural calcification, as indicated by the white arrows. (**c**) Survival curves with freedom from death. Mitral valve replacement of repeat valvuloplasty demonstrates improved outcomes in patients without (solid line) versus with (dashed line) commissural calcium (*P*<0.001). (From Cannan et al. [9]; used with permission)

outcomes following percutaneous commissurotomy, Mayo investigators (Rihal et al.) looked at the long-term outcomes following closed mitral commissurotomy as performed surgically through a left thoracotomy [10]. Skilled surgeons, particularly proficient in the developing world, can perform this procedure within 45 minutes, leading to excellent results for their patients. Frequently, closed commissurotomy is more cost effective in the developing world than percutaneous valvuloplasty using expensive disposable catheters. To overcome some of the challenges of cost, in many countries Inoue balloons are reused up to a dozen times for PBMV. Moreover, prospective randomized trials demonstrated the superiority of percutaneous mitral valvuloplasty in comparison to surgery for the initial treatment of rheumatic mitral stenosis, further establishing it as a therapy of choice for this condition [11, 12].

International travel brings with it the opportunity for bilateral, experiential learning, and the author (CSR) recounts a visit to the Hanoi Heart Institute, where he participated in several balloon mitral valvuloplasty and coronary interventional procedures in the early 2000s. A particularly vivid memory is the first PBMV case where, following initial dilatation, the attending cardiologist asked the trainee to check for mitral regurgitation. Thinking there may be an echo instrument in the cath lab somewhere, the author was surprised and impressed when the fellow, unscrubbed, promptly grasped his stethoscope and inserted it into his ears. After carefully auscultating the patient's chest, he then pronounced, "No MR!" We then proceeded to perform another dilatation, resulting in an excellent result for the patient. This experience drove home the value of basic medical skills and delivering high-value care to patients rather than complete reliance upon technology. It is of interest to note that the Wilkins-Abascal score can largely be predicted through bedside physical examination (Table 7.1). A loud opening snap implies a mobile anterior mitral leaflet, whereas close coupling of the S2 and OS implies a high gradient. The absence of a systolic murmur makes significant mitral regurgitation unlikely, and the degree of pulmonary hypertension can be estimated from the relative intensity of the pulmonic closure sound. Structural interventions afford the opportunity to relearn and apply basic examination skills (more on this later).

In the cardiac cath lab now, PBMV has become a low-volume niche procedure, given the essential eradication of childhood rheumatic fever in North America. Occasional patients, largely from immigrant backgrounds, are still encountered for whom this is an excellent therapeutic option. More commonly seen, calcific mitral stenosis does not respond well to percutaneous dilatation with high risks of leaflet fracture and severe mitral regurgitation. As with any interventional procedure, there are inescapable risks, and operators quickly learn to recognize and treat severe regurgitation from tears of the anterior leaflet and calcium embolism from the leaflets, which if bad luck were to prevail, can result in acute occlusion of the left main coronary artery as we experienced (Figs. 7.2, 7.3, and 7.4) [13].

Balloon Aortic Valvuloplasty

Perhaps no interventional procedure held as much promise and as much frustration as balloon aortic valvuloplasty for the treatment of aortic stenosis. While efficacious and safe for congenital aortic stenosis, when applied to calcific aortic stenosis of the elderly, BAV proved an intensely frustrating experience, requiring healthy doses of

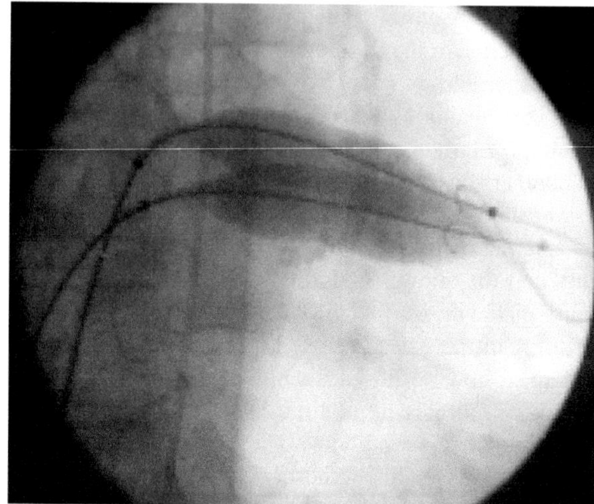

Fig. 7.2 Right anterior oblique view of double-balloon inflation in the stenotic mitral valve (patient X). (From Powell et al. [13]; used with permission)

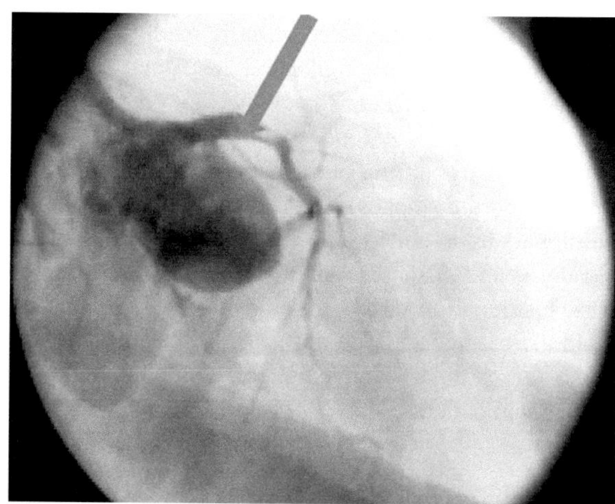

Fig. 7.3 Immediately after dilatation, patient X developed ST segment rhythms and then PEA. As can be seen, there is a filling defect in the distal LMCA that obstructs flow. (From Powell et al. [13]; used with permission)

optimism, verve, and perseverance to overcome its many obstacles. Given its successes in the pediatric population, it was inevitable that BAV would be attempted in adult patients, particularly among those in whom surgery was considered high risk. The symptoms of aortic stenosis have been known since the original classic description by Braunwald of angina, dyspnea, and syncope [14]. Importantly, that initial description involved patients aged in their mid-40s. Information on patients with this disease continued to accrue during the 1980s and 1990s. Passik et al. documented changes in the pathophysiology of aortic stenosis in 646 surgical cases at Mayo Clinic [15]. They found that the majority of patients were in their seventh or eighth decade of life; in this group, the mechanism was typically senile degeneration of a tricuspid valve with large calcific deposits at the bases of the cusps (Fig. 7.5a). At that time, surgical valve replacement was the treatment of choice.

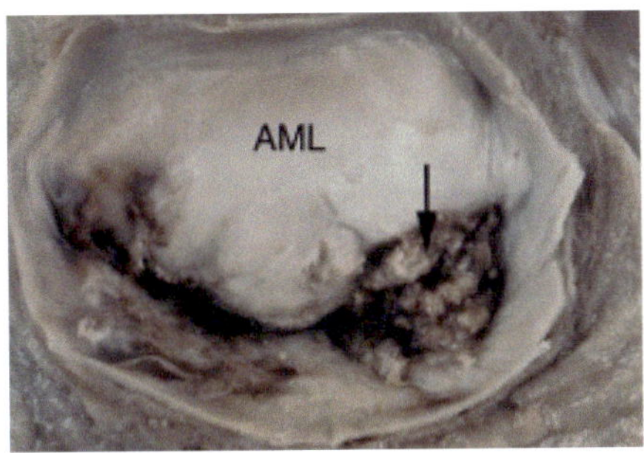

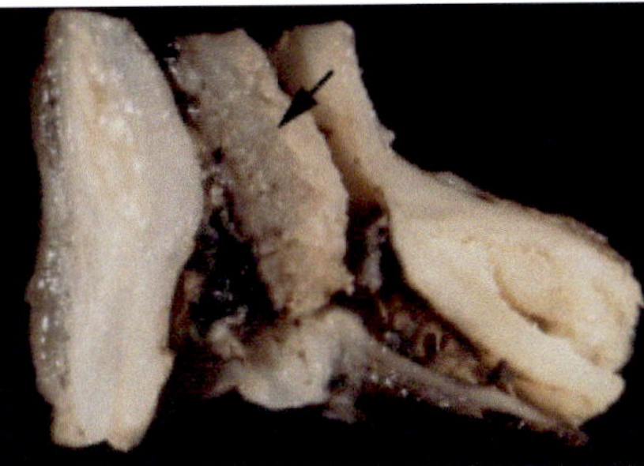

Fig. 7.4 Patient X, as seen in Figs. 7.2 and 7.3, could not be successfully resuscitated. At the time of postmortem examination, the mitral valve viewed from the left atrial side documents a severely calcified lesion near the posteromedial commissure (*arrow*). This was responsible for the embolic calcific nodule that embolized to the LMCA (*arrow, right panel*), occluding flow to the LAD and circumflex. (From Powell et al. [13]; used with permission)

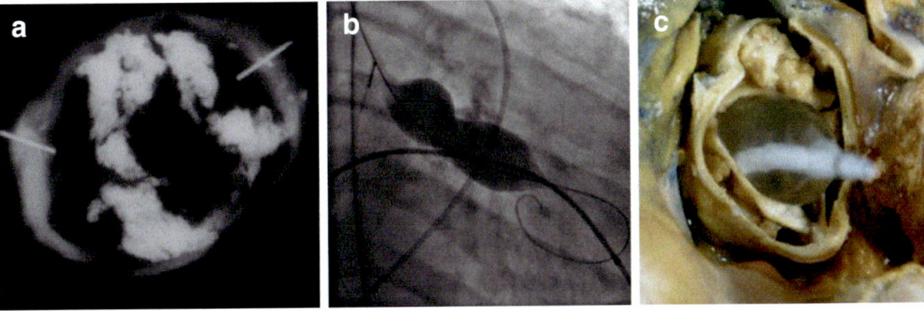

Fig. 7.5 The presence of severe AS related to senile calcific disease was the most common indication for balloon aortic valvuloplasty. As seen, the bulky calcium nodule involves all three leaflets (**a**). With balloon inflation (**b**), the waist of the balloon results from immobile calcific nodules. Under direct visualization (**c**), calcific nodules often remained intact. (Courtesy of Dr. W.E. Edwards, Department of Pathology, Mayo Clinic)

However, there were some patients treated medically, typically. with dismal results. O'Keefe et al. evaluated 50 Mayo patients with at high operative risk severe aortic stenosis between 1975 and 1983 who were treated medically [16]. They identified a mortality rate of 3.8% per month such that over a 3-year period of time, follow-up survival was only 25% (Fig. 7.6a, b). The overwhelming (97%) cause of death was cardiac.

Against this background, three elderly patients at high operative risk with severe symptomatic aortic stenosis had dramatic symptomatic improvement with balloon aortic valvuloplasty; the 1986 report detailing these successful procedures was enthusiastically embraced (Fig. 7.5b, c) [17]. Although complications such as restenosis were identified, this approach was felt to be a huge improvement in select patients over the next several years. At that time, the center of attention focused on the hospital in Rouen where Cribier and his associates practiced. With relatively unbridled enthusiasm, live courses were developed there which were typically

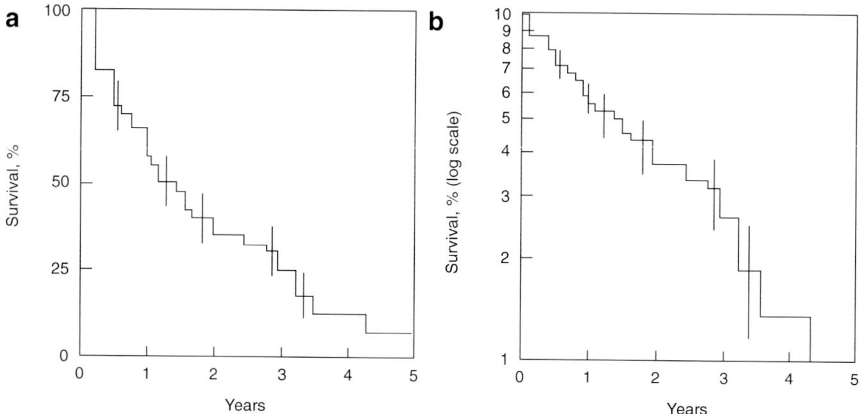

Fig. 7.6 Survival curve of 50 patients with severe aortic stenosis treated with conservative medical therapy documented the dismal inexorable outcome (**a**). In another analysis, the mortality is nearly linear (**b**). (From O'Keefe et al. [16]; used with permission)

oversubscribed. Nishimura and Holmes had developed protocols for adopting this at Mayo Clinic. As part of their effort, they enrolled in the course. Set in the cathedral town of Rouen, it was an extremely impressive classic European setting. An unusual winter had brought snow which greeted us. A side trip to the classic Rouen Cathedral involved wearing our heavy, winter, Rochester, Minnesota, coats. The Cathedral, which was not heated, made services chilly. The atmosphere of the meeting was exciting as the techniques pioneered by Cribier and colleagues were written down by all the attendees for implementation at home. Attendee dinners were held in magnificent baroque settings. Nishimura had trouble with accommodations as the meeting was so crowded, so he roomed in a rather Spartan garret room. Unfortunately, by unconfirmed report, the roommate appeared to have significant OSA, particularly after French wine, that resulted in only a brief respite of poor sleep for Nishimura.

After returning to Mayo Clinic, protocols were developed and equipment brought in. The approach was transfemoral with large 16 French sheaths for delivery of the balloons. Sizing was based on echo assessment of annulus size. Although in France, transmitral approaches were often used for dilatation, we concentrated on a transfemoral approach. In some patients, two simultaneous balloons were used, one from each femoral vessel. In those patients, calculation involved the use of two balloons to result in ideal size without over dilating the valve and annulus to avoid the potential for rupture, which, while infrequent, was catastrophic. For each case, there was excitement but also at least some unease. During that time, rapid pacing had not yet been described, and the balloons would often migrate with uncontrollable "watermelon seeding" motion during inflation despite the use of 4.0-cm-long balloons selected to enhance stability. During inflation, there was typically loss of patient consciousness and sometimes seizures. Procedures were guided by echo to assess the results as well as by transvalvular gradients before and afterward. Typically, the hemodynamic results were, at best, modest. That being the case, we usually chose the best result to report in our records.

Post procedure, there were multiple issues, mainly depending on the forearm, hand, and wrist strength. The sheaths were 16 French, and vascular closure devices had not yet been developed or implemented. Patients were taken to 4DS, the CCU, for sheath removal. Certain housekeeping arrangements had to be done because manual holds were used. Typically, gaining hemostasis might involve 3 hours. As Nish and I had introduced the technique, we were the designees chosen: a wonderful sort of bonding. Later during the project, advanced trainees were selected, typically with large forearms. Of concern was the fact that even with those approaches, at least one fellow developed carpal tunnel syndrome.

From a national perspective, the number of patients treated increased more than might have been expected as the selection criteria and enthusiasm broadened. Toward the end of the 1980s, a National BAV Registry was developed in Seattle, which enrolled approximately 1000 patients in a relatively short period of time. However, during this time, the complication rates and, even more importantly, the only modest hemodynamic results and the almost uniform appearance of restenosis within 6 months were increasingly recognized. This led to a dramatic reduction in procedural performance, and its subsequent position as a potential bail-out approach in patients being scheduled for major surgical procedures. However, also during this time, there was great focused interest and attention paid to the development of an implantable heart valve, which became the truly transformational technology that had been dreamed of.

Requiring large caliber balloons, 14–22 mm in diameter, with large arterial access sheaths, BAV in the early days was not for the fainthearted. Heavily calcified valves, with multiple cusp involvement, stenotic and calcific aortas notwithstanding, valves would always yield under the onslaught of a high-pressure balloon catheter. Frustratingly, the calcium, of course, would result in immediate recoil in the catheterization laboratory. As a result, often all the best operators could do was to take critical aortic stenosis to severe aortic stenosis. Final valve areas were rarely, if ever, greater than 1.0 cm^2. Operators would wait anxiously for echo colleagues to pronounce the verdict, anxiously gazing at the continuous wave Doppler envelopes. Careful attention to the development of aortic regurgitation was necessary, as there was generally no good treatment. If it were to occur, it was usually poorly tolerated given the small hypertrophic left ventricles that patients with aortic stenosis frequently have. Large multicenter registries, like the Mansfield Registry, established the basic framework and data regarding success and complication rates, which remained static over time without significant temporal improvement. Trainees, while initially enthusiastic about participating in these procedures, quickly learned the importance of careful manual arterial compression and the strength it took to persevere, at times, for hours, in the era before closure devices were available! Tips and tricks such as allowing a small squirt of blood facilitated earlier closure. Careful attention always had to be given to the exit wound, as a slip could result in a multiunit bleed very easily.

In more recent years, BAV has made somewhat of a comeback as a potential diagnostic procedure among patients with severe aortic stenosis who also have severe pulmonary disease. If BAV results in some symptomatic improvement, then one may suppose the patient would respond favorably to TAVR. The absence of improvement, however, does not exclude aortic stenosis as an important contributor to symptomatology. BAV has never managed to garner a class I indication under any circumstances, instead being largely confined to TAVR pre-dilatation. Although, even there its use is becoming increasingly rare. Perhaps the greatest importance of BAV in recent years has been in the run-up phase to TAVR, which essentially emulates the BAV procedure but for the presence of a balloon-expandable valve. Thus, operators who were comfortable and experienced offering BAV to their patients made the ready transition to the next phase of treatment for severe symptomatic aortic stenosis – transcatheter aortic valve replacement.

Transcatheter Aortic Valve Replacement

Perhaps no procedure hats had such an immediate and profound impact on the field of interventional cardiology since the original advent of balloon angioplasty as transcatheter aortic valve replacement (previously implantation). A true disruptive innovation, TAVR was the brainchild of Dr. Henning Rud Andersen of Arhus, Denmark. Dr. Andersen was attending an interventional symposium in Scottsdale, Arizona, in 1989, listening to speakers talk about coronary stenting when he realized that a much larger stent could be made within which a valve could be sewn and potentially applied to the treatment of aortic stenosis. Like with all disruptive innovations – and in his own words – initially no one believed this could be done and that it was simply too unrealistic an idea for it to ever work. Initially, the concept gained little traction, and Dr. Andersen had difficulty finding funding, resulting, remarkably in retrospect, in the idea stalling for many years. Dr. Andersen himself performed the first animal studies in pigs in 1989 and presented and published the first abstracts and papers on a balloon expandable aortic valve prosthesis [18]. He was granted two US patents in 1995 and 1998. Following the initial animal work, his concept did garner attention from industry and, through an iterative process of innovation and investment, eventually resulted in the first human procedure performed by Dr. Alain Cribier in Rouen, France, April 16, 2002 (Fig. 7.7). The procedure gained worldwide attention and was widely reported in the news media such as *The New York Times*. The patient fortunately survived and was discharged home on day 8 post implantation. Had the patient not survived, the setback could have been irretrievable. The original Cribier transcutaneous heart valve eventually gave way to subsequent generations of the SAPIEN prosthesis manufactured by Edwards LifeSciences (Irvine, California, USA), followed by numerous other designs that have entered the market.

Perhaps what is very important about TAVR is the impact it had beyond the procedure itself. Application of this disruptive new technology required new ways of working together and developing new standard operating procedures. Often rivals, friendly or otherwise, the initial pivotal trials forced a marriage between the often

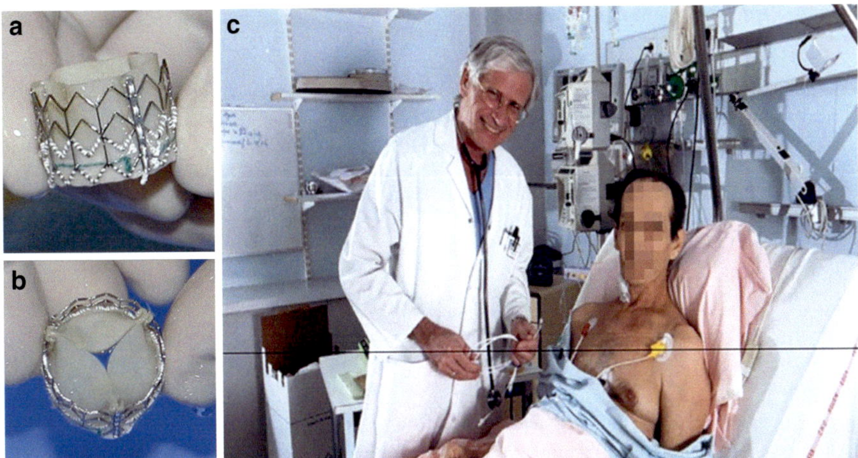

Fig. 7.7 The first patient treated with a TAVR prosthesis (**a**, **b**) by Dr. Alain Cribier (**c**), the innovator who developed the procedure. (From Cribier et al. GCSP 2017; used with permission)

rivals, friendly or otherwise, interventionalists and cardiac surgeons, along with their imaging colleagues, in what became known as the Heart Team. Physicians and surgeons of different professional backgrounds learned to communicate, learned about each other's fields and concerns, and learned a common language. For example, both interventionalists and surgeons became rapidly conversant with the criteria for severity of aortic stenosis as defined echocardiographically and became familiar with previously unfamiliar obscure terms such as "dimensionless index" and technology such as CT imaging.

The procedures themselves instilled a new way of working together, where, for the first time, surgeons and interventionalists worked side by side in bringing their expertise for the benefit of the patient. Of course, the usual jockeying for position occurred, but ultimately TAVR has become a widely accepted, incredibly safe, and highly efficacious treatment for severe aortic stenosis.

Mayo Clinic was involved in the PARTNER series of pivotal trials that started enrolling patients at the extremes of risk and then gradually marched down the risk spectrum. The PARTNER 1B Trial enrolled patients considered inoperable and randomly assigned them to TAVR versus usual care. Remarkably, at 12 months, absolute 20 percentage point risk reduction was observed, with control group mortality of 50.7% versus treatment group mortality of 30.7% (still high however) [19]. This 20% ARR, without exaggeration, was the highest absolute risk reduction observed in any cardiovascular treatment trial to date. A 20% ARR of course would translate to 200 lives saved for 1000 patients treated, whereas in comparison, beta-blockers post-myocardial infarction would be expected to save 6 lives per 1000 patients treated and reperfusion with aspirin, approximately 50–60 lives per 1000 patients treated.

Death From Any Cause, All Patients

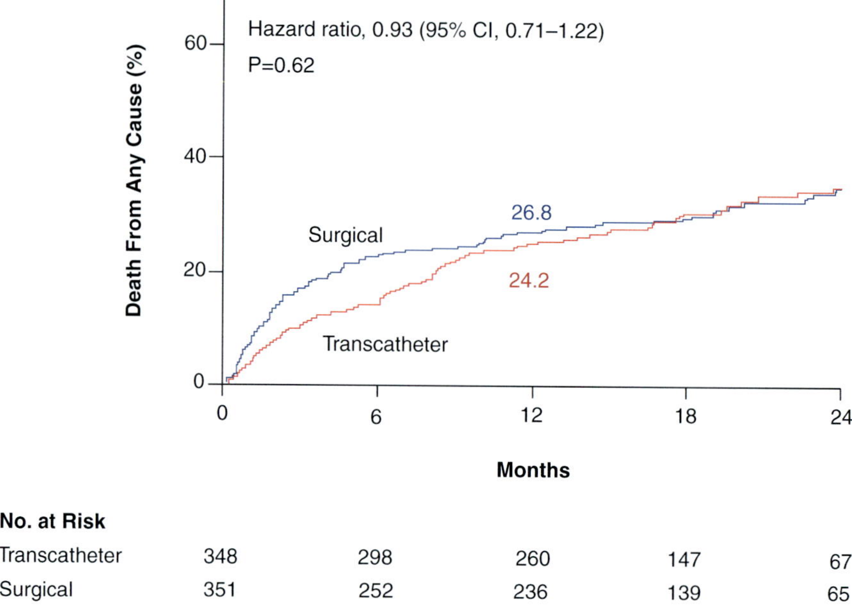

No. at Risk

Transcatheter	348	298	260	147	67
Surgical	351	252	236	139	65

Fig. 7.8 Pivotal trials were the basis for approval of TAVR technology. Seen here, the PARTNER 1A Trial in high-risk surgical patients in whom there was similar 2-year mortality irrespective of whether patients were treated with surgical aortic valve replacement (blue) or TAVR (red). (From Smith et al. [20]; used with permission)

The PARTNER 1A Trial enrolled patients considered at high-risk for open surgery and randomized them to TAVR or open aortic valve replacement [20]. The results at 1, 2, and 3 years (Fig. 7.8) demonstrated almost identical mortality for the two groups. Importantly, parameters of functional improvement such as NYHA class and 6-minute walk test improved dramatically in both groups. For example, by 1 year, patients treated either with TAVR or open AVR were able to walk almost 100 m (about the length of a Canadian football field) further on the 6-minute walk test than at baseline, representing a significant functional improvement in this patient population.

Other novel valve designs, such as the self-expanding CoreValve prosthesis marketed by Medtronic (Galway, Ireland), also came to clinical application and demonstrated efficacy in comparison to surgical valve replacement [21, 22]. Numerous valve designs have been developed, with less than a handful coming to clinical practice and some programs being terminated after clinical launch [23].

Following the demonstration of safety and efficacy among patients at extreme risk for surgery, as well as those at high risk, further prospective randomized clinical trials demonstrated the similar outcomes of TAVR and open aortic valve replacement in patients at intermediate risk for surgery, as defined by the Society of

Thoracic Surgeons (STS) risk calculator [24, 25]. In these intermediate-risk patients, both procedures are similar in terms of the incidence of death and disabling stroke over 2 years of follow-up, and, in fact, transfemoral (as compared to transapical) TAVR was superior to open surgery. Finally, a series of pivotal trials in patients at low risk for open surgery have now been published, further expanding indications for this procedure [26, 27].

Numerous challenges exist, although some have been overcome. For example, the incidence of stroke was high in the PARTNER 1B cohort, raising important concerns about the safety of the TAVR procedure itself [28]. With time, however, the risk of stroke has gradually decreased, and now the advent of embolic protection devices promises to lower it even further. These devices are currently undergoing prospective evaluation, and while some centers have adopted them routinely, others have decided to take a more selective approach. Data from large prospective randomized trials will ultimately define the role of these devices, which add procedural complexity and cost but also hold a promise of adding safety in routine clinical practice [29]. The design of endpoints for these trials will be of particular importance; will the primary endpoints be clinical neurologic events detected by prospective neurologic evaluation or brain imaging, such as DWMRI abnormalities, which may not correlate with changes in clinical outcome? Valve durability has been questioned from the start of the procedure, particularly since balloon expandable valves are forcefully inserted into position. It should be noted the manufacturing process mirrors that of surgical valves with the same deceleration and fixation processes. Careful clinical follow-up has confirmed medium-term (perhaps 10 years) valve durability, with gradients for balloon expandable valves typically about 10 mmHg and effective orifice areas typically about 1.6 cm^2, which is slightly larger than surgical prostheses [30].

The introduction of computed tomographic (CT) imaging to the study of patients who are potential TAVR candidates has been revolutionary; CT imaging is now routinely used for sizing of valves and determination of optimum access sites and has resulted in important observations related to valve durability. Subclinical leaflet thrombosis has been observed both in surgical and percutaneous valves and is a relatively common finding, 13–40% [31]. Importantly, when warfarin is administered early after bioprosthetic valve insertion, subclinical leaflet thrombosis is almost unheard of. The optimal anticoagulation and antiplatelet therapy strategy following TAVR and surgical AVR is evolving, but in most centers at least a short-term course of warfarin is now routine.

The next important challenge that was encountered in TAVR was that of paravalvular regurgitation. Since the native aortic leaflets remain in situ, potential spaces (neosinuses) developed between the stent of the TAVR valve and the interstices of the valve itself. With the original valve designs, paravalvular leak (PVL) was not uncommon and was directly related to long-term outcome [32]. Once again, however, this problem has diminished under the onslaught of innovation and investment, resulting in improved valve designs that include skirts to fill these potential spaces and interstices, thereby minimizing the risk of PVL. Significant PVL is now very rare following TAVR procedures, and separate PVL closure procedures following

TAVR are rarely performed. All of these represent important advances from the standpoint of both the patient and the healthcare system. Similarly, the catastrophic complications that may potentially occur with TAVR, such as annular rupture, coronary obstruction, valve embolization, and tamponade, now have become exceedingly rare and are seen less than 1% of the time. A corollary to this is that trainees may not see these during the entire period of structural training and will need special training modules and case review sessions to learn how to manage them if they are encountered in future patients.

Despite the important advances in the field, numerous challenges remain in the field of TAVR. This includes defining its role in bicuspid aortic valve stenosis under unique anatomic circumstances that present, such as aortopathy. The role of TAVR for younger patients, the mean age even in the low-risk trials being in their mid-70s, for moderate aortic stenosis and for aortic regurgitation, remains undefined. Based on recent history, however, our expectation is that each of these conditions will eventually be amenable to TAVR either with modifications of current prostheses or with novel designs such that only patients who cannot be treated with TAVR will need to undergo surgical AVR. This in and of itself raises issues related to the training of cardiovascular surgeons. In an analogous way and discipline, the now standard percutaneous treatment of abdominal aortic aneurysm has resulted in current vascular surgical trainees who have minimal or even no experience with open repair.

Early TAVR

At Mayo Clinic, we were approached by Edwards LifeSciences (Irvine, California, USA), to participate in the initial PARTNER series of pivotal prospective randomized clinical trials. As at all centers, this necessitated a development of a Heart Team and unique circumstances and experiences. The initial TAVR procedures were much different than they are now when we can reliably complete four procedures by noon. In the original experience, procedures were intensive and emulated what happened in the operating room in terms of lines and intubation. Cardiopulmonary bypass machines and perfusionists were on standby, and an air of uncertainty and risk hung in the atmosphere. Worrying and, at times, disapproving, glances from operating room staff when the interventionalists would walk into the room occurred, but with time and familiarity, gave way to looks of approval.

The learning curve for TAVR was formidable in the era of 26 French sheaths, and little experience with percutaneous access. Surgical cut downs were routine, whereas now percutaneous closure is the standard. The large caliber of introducer sheaths was an important challenge, particularly among patients with calcified iliofemoral systems that were prone to rupture or, even worse, avulsion. A particularly unforgettable experience occurred on Case No. 4 which was the quickest time to deployment, approximately 45 minutes. This was followed by an increase in the systolic pressure by 50 points as the gradient was relieved. The operators, immensely pleased with their technical prowess, were suddenly dismayed when the 26 French sheath was rapidly expelled from the femoral artery, bottle rocket like, and landed at the patient's foot! Blood under new high pressure squirted over 2 feet into the air, and Dr. Kevin Greason, surgeon, worked frantically to clamp the femoral artery. In the meantime, to their horror, Drs. Holmes and Rihal working on the contralateral side discovered the CODA balloons do not fit within an 8 French sheath! In the midst of the frenetic situation, Dr. Holmes who had experience working with simulation with the US Navy made a memorable comment, "This is why arterial war wounds are uniformly fatal," and the term "the red sea" came into use. Fortunately, skilled and rapid teamwork salvaged the situation, and the patient not only survived but was symptomatically better. Such is the learning curve of new procedures and such is the bonding experience brought on by participating as a team.

Paravalvular Leak Closure

The development of procedures designed to allow safe and effective paravalvular leak closure represents an interesting study in teamwork, collaboration, and innovation rising to meet the challenges of an important unmet clinical need. While Mayo Clinic may not have been the first center to successfully perform PVL (paravalvular leak) closure, Mayo Clinic led the way in developing standardized reliable techniques that can be taught, learned, and translated to other centers around the country and the world. PVL historically has represented an important clinical challenge and can occur around any prosthetic heart valve of any type in any position. In adult cardiology, of course, mitral and aortic PVL are commonly encountered in up to 15% of patients with surgical prostheses. In a minority of these, PVL may manifest clinically with symptoms of heart failure, hemolytic anemia, or both. The underlying causes are diverse and include extensive annular calcification, particularly common around the mitral annulus, and often the posterior aortic annulus, making the placement of sutures technically challenging. These technical factors would sometimes necessitate reoperation immediately after coming off pump. Other rare causes include tissue friability from prior or recent endocarditis, the recent initiation of corticosteroids, any underlying systemic inflammatory disorder, or simply age as tissues weaken. Paravalvular leak most commonly occurs early following operation but can develop years later, and we have seen instances of new leaks arising up to 10 years following index surgery. Historically, treatment was supportive with diuretics for heart failure and no specific treatment for hemolysis other than support of transfusion and epoprostenol as required. Reoperation was frequently necessary, with its attendant higher risks.

Accordingly, when Dr. Maurice Sarano was discussing a case with Dr. Rihal, and threw out the clinical challenge, "Why can't you just put a plug in it?" Rihal quickly realized a gauntlet had been thrown. A quick scan of the literature in the late 2000s revealed scant reports only frequently using coils, which were prone to embolization. What followed was a process of iterative procedural innovation building on techniques   in   interventional   cardiology,   borrowing   equipment   from electrophysiology and leveraging closure devices typically used by pediatric cardiologists – all of this while striving to develop a standardized approach that could be taught and learned by others.

The procedure was broken down and approached in a stepwise fashion. Thus, for mitral paravalvular leak, interventional cardiologists were already highly accustomed to obtaining transseptal left ventricular access for balloon mitral valvuloplasty (as above), but challenges remained in terms of identifying and accessing mitral PVL. Observing how electrophysiology colleagues used deflectable left atrial sheaths gave us the idea that these would be extraordinarily useful for mitral PVL closure, and we rapidly adopted the use of the Agilis sheath (Abbott, Minneapolis, Minnesota, USA). This sheath has a deflectable tip, which allows an operator to quickly flex, rotate, and translate around the mitral annulus. Commensurate with this was the necessity to develop imaging support to facilitate the procedures. Around the same time, the advent of real-time, three-dimensional transesophageal echocardiography proved a boon to structural heart interventions. Drs. Charles Bruce and Rihal initiated the first interventional imaging service consisting of dedicated echocardiologists with an interest in operating room and cath lab imaging. Certain things became rapidly apparent, such as the fact that we viewed the world from different angles and used different terminology. For example, echocardiologists used to working in the operating room use the surgeon's view, which is a left atrial view of the mitral valve, whereas interventional cardiologists use the left anterior oblique view with caudal angulation. These views are right-left flipped and imaging software did not allow autocorrection. Therefore, we realized that the surgeon's view and the interventionalist's view were, perhaps not unironically, 180 degrees opposite! The second important observation was the realization that we cannot use terms such as 12 o'clock and 3 o'clock to identify where leaks are. Again, this was due to the different perspectives, and often the interventionalists and echocardiographer were in different time zones. Thus, we standardized using anatomically correct language such as anterior, medial, posterior, inferior, intervalvular fibrosa, at the base of the appendage, and by the septum. The use of anatomically precise language greatly facilitated performance of these procedures and was mutually satisfactory and beneficial to all concerned [33–35].

Following the implementation of a left atrial deflectable sheath, a delivery catheter had to be placed across the leak. This led to more challenges, as the standard delivery sheaths that came with Amplatzer delivery systems were neither flexible nor did they fit within the deflectable left atrial sheaths, which provided the backbone for these procedures. Thus, through an iterative trial and error process, we developed a mother-child technique of a 125-cm, 5 French, multipurpose diagnostic catheter placed within a 100-cm, 6 French, multipurpose coronary guiding catheter, in turn placed within the deflectable left atrial sheath. Through the center of these three coaxial catheters ran a guide wire. Ultimately, we favored using a 0.035-inch hydrophilic wire, either stiff or floppy, with which to cross these defects. Crossing the defect, of course, was dependent upon imaging and the precise geometry unique to each patient, all facilitated by the common lexicon. However, having crossed with the wire was no guarantee of being able to cross with catheters. Thus, we had to relearn techniques of snaring the wires in the ascending or descending thoracic aorta to create venoarterial rails, which in turn allowed the necessary support to push and pull catheters across the leaks. We then learned again by trial and error which plugs would fit within which delivery catheters. Dr. Mario Goessl, the interventional fellow, developed what we affectionately call the "smiley face" compatibility chart that is still used to this day (Fig. 7.9) [36].

Developing and improving each of the sequential procedural steps has led to a situation where we can now close the most complex mitral PVL within 60–90 minutes using any one of several techniques to deploy multiple plugs as necessary. These techniques include the simple antegrade single-plug approach without rail, simultaneous deployment, or using a venoarterial rail to rapidly deploy two or more plugs as necessary. At Mayo Clinic, we always favored the thin nitinol braid arterial vascular plug (AVP) II devices as opposed to the thicker braid, muscular VSD

Compatibility table of catheter-only technique (no anchor wire during deployment, part a)

	AVP II 6 mm	AVP II 8 mm	AVP II 10 mm	AVP II 12 mm
6F coronary guide	☺	☺	☺	☺
7F coronary guide	☺	☺	☺	☺
8F coronary guide	☺	☺	☺	☺
4F Shuttle	☺	☺	X	X
5F Shuttle	☺	☺	☺	☺
6F Shuttle	☺	☺	☺	☺
7F Shuttle	☺	☺	☺	☺
8F Shuttle	☺	☺	☺	☺

AVP II = Amplatzer vascular plug II

☺ = AVP II fits into delivery catheter (coronary guide or Shuttle catheter)

X = AVP II does not fit into the delivey catheter

Example: the 12-mm AVP fits in all delivery catheters but the 4F Shuttle

In an extremely difficult case, you can cut the proximal hub of a 4F Shuttle sheath and use up to a 10-mm AVP II.

A 6F Shuttle catheter fits through an 8.5F Agilis sheath (not 7F nor 8F Shuttles); one can start the case with this system if needed.

6, 7, and 8F MPA2 guides fit through an 8.5F Agilis sheath

Fig. 7.9 (**a–c**) Development of strategies of catheters for closure of paravalvular leak included consideration of specific guiding catheter requirements for specific techniques, such as anchor techniques and guide wire type. (From Mario Gossl et al. [36]; used with permission)

Compatibility table of anchor technique with 0.032 extra stiff
Amplatzer <u>within</u> guide/shuttle, part b

	AVP II 6 mm	AVP II 8 mm	AVP II 10 mm	AVP II 12 mm
6F coronary guide	X	X	X	X
7F coronary guide	☺	☺	X	X
8F coronary guide	☺	☺	☺	☺
4F Shuttle	X	X	X	X
5F Shuttle	☺	☺ (hard)	X	X
6F Shuttle	☺	☺	☺	☺
7F Shuttle	☺	☺	☺	☺
8F Shuttle	☺	☺	☺	☺

AVP II = Amplatzer vascular plug II

☺ = AVP II fits into delivery catheter with anchor wire

X = AVP II does not fit into the delivery catheter with anchor wire

Example: the 12-mm AVP II and a 0.032 Amplatzer extra stiff wire fit
both in an 8F coronary guide as well as 6,7, and 8F Shuttles but not in
6 and 7F coronary guides or 4 and 5F Shuttles

Fig. 7.9 (continued)

Compatibility table of anchor technique with 0.035 extra stiff
glide wire <u>within</u> guide/shuttle, part c

	AVP II 6 mm	AVP II 8 mm	AVP II 10 mm	AVP II 12 mm
6F coronary guide	X	X	X	X
7F coronary guide	☺	☺	X	X
8F coronary guide	☺	☺	☺	☺
4F Shuttle	X	X	X	X
5F Shuttle	☺	☺ (hard)	X	X
6F Shuttle	☺	☺	☺	☺
7F Shuttle	☺	☺	☺	☺
8F Shuttle	☺	☺	☺	☺

AVP II = Amplatzer vascular plug II

☺ = AVP II fits into delivery catheter with anchor wire

X = AVP II does not fit into the delivery catheter with anchor wire

Example: the 12-mm AVP II and a 0.0325 Amplatzer extra stiff wire fit
both in an 8F coronary guide as well as 6,7, and 8F Shuttles but not in a
6 and 7F coronary guide or a 4 and 5F Shuttles

Fig. 7.9 (continued)

(ventricular septal defect) closure devices or ductal closure devices. The thinner devices are much easier to fit within delivery catheters and are a fraction of the cost of the thick grade devices. It was observed early on that hemolysis can worsen with placement of intracardiac plugs due to the presence of small high-velocity jets traversing through the plugs themselves. Fortuitously, we experienced a very low rate of acceleration of hemolysis with the thinner braid devices (in comparison to a 15–20% incidence with the thick braid devices), and these have now become standard for these procedures.

The development of new procedures such as PVL (paravalvular leak) closure was greatly aided and abetted by the annual presence of highly talented structural heart fellows. Each year the trainees were given a challenge to improve our procedures, and each graduating class has risen to that challenge providing iterative improvements that have ultimately led to better patient care.

Developing new procedures is often a trying effort, and numerous challenges were encountered. We estimate that we did 75–100 cases before we could reliably perform these procedures in less than 2 hours, while early on in the learning curve, procedures would often take 3–4 hours. Now most aortic PVL (paravalvular leak) closures can be done in less than 1 hour and even the most complex mitral closure procedures in less than 2 hours. The collaboration between skilled physicians of different professional backgrounds (IC, EP, pediatric and congenital, imaging, surgery) and the interaction with trainees with fresh eyes on an annual basis led to this becoming a standardized first-line treatment for paravalvular regurgitation.

Mitral Edge-to-Edge Repair

Building on the above techniques, the adoption of mitral edge-to-edge repair was natural in the evolution of the cath lab. The first device approved for this, the MitraClip (Abbott Cardiovascular, Plymouth, MN, USA), was approved for clinical use in 2013 and has become a standard treatment for carefully selected patients with mitral regurgitation. The skills necessary to safely and effectively undertake clip implantation emulate those required for other mitral interventional procedures, such as mitral PVL closure, and include transseptal catheterization at the appropriate site, 3D image interpretation, a detailed knowledge of normal and abnormal mitral valve anatomy, and the ability to learn a complex new device and use it safely. Given the large valve and surgical practice at Mayo Clinic, the clip procedure rapidly found a place in the therapeutic armamentarium for patients who had symptomatic mitral regurgitation despite medical therapy yet were not good candidates for surgical repair or valve replacement. For this procedure, surgeons act as a gatekeeper, consult on every patient, and preferentially offer operation to those felt to be good surgical candidates and with a high likelihood of successful repair or replacement. What has become apparent is that the population of patients with mitral regurgitation is huge, and the practices have grown accordingly. A successful clip procedure

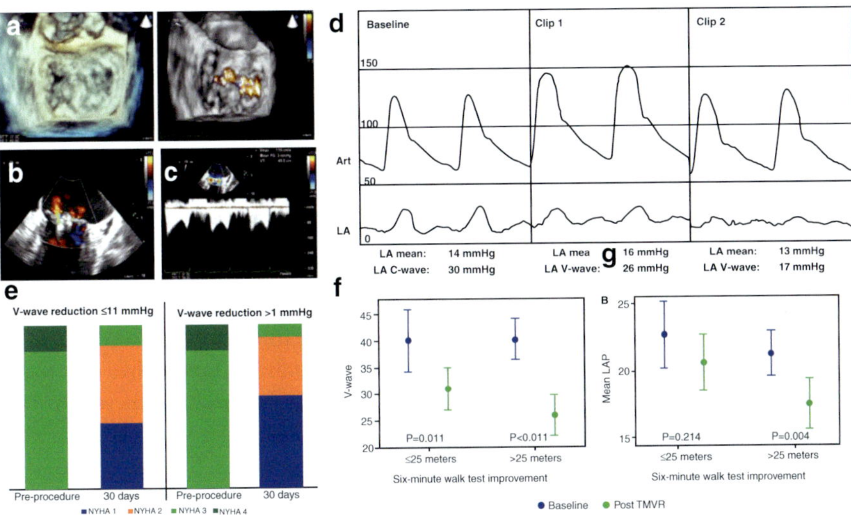

Fig. 7.10 Left atrial pressure predicts clinical outcomes following transcatheter mitral valve edge-to-edge repair. (**a**) Three-dimensional transesophageal echocardiography (TEE) without (*left*) and with (*right*) color flow Doppler following the placement of two MitraClip devices with successful reduction in mitral regurgitation (MR) and only mild residual MR confirmed on two-dimensional color flow assessment (**b**). (**c**) Continuous-wave Doppler assessment of mitral valve post intervention demonstrating no significant post-procedural stenosis (mean gradient, 3 mmHg). (**d**) Continuous arterial (Art) and left atrial (LA) pressure monitoring demonstrates progressive decline in LA V-wave from 30 mmHg at baseline to 26 mmHg and then 17 mmHg following the placement of the first and second MitraClips, respectively. (**e**) Change in New York Heart Association (NYHA) class striated by those with V-wave reductions ≤11 mmHg versus >11 mmHg following MitraClip. Acute changes in LA V-wave (**f**) and mean LA pressure (**g**) predict improvement in a 6-minute walk distance with more marked improvements observed in those with >25-meter improvement in 6-minute walk distances. (Panels a–d from Lloyd et al. [37], Figures 10, 11; used with permission. Panels e–g from Maor et al. [38], Figures 2A & B, 3; used with permission)

can immediately result in symptomatic improvement, particularly if the left atrial V-wave falls dramatically during the procedure (Fig. 7.10) [37–39].

Importance of Hemodynamic Assessment

The storied hemodynamic expertise and history of the Mayo Clinic Cath Lab, dating back to the time of Dr. Earl Wood (indeed the lab is now called the Earl H. Wood, MD Cardiac Cath Lab) proved invaluable in assessing the results of PVL (paravalvular leak) closure and other interventional procedures. We quickly realized, for example, that even a relatively modest amount of regurgitation into a stiff noncompliant left atrium would give rise to not only a higher mean LA pressure but also sometimes dramatically elevated V-waves and moderate to severe secondary pulmonary hypertension, due to pressure reflection back through the cardiopulmonary circuit [40]. Using color flow Doppler to assess the results of PVL closure and its severity can be challenging due to splaying of the color jet into the receiving chamber (garden hose effect), and we learned early on to use hemodynamic assessment of the results as an important adjunctive or primary tool. Many years later, these same principles were applied to assessment of the results following mitral clip implantation. Initially, we developed a double-wire technique, the brainchild of Dr. Guy S Reeder. Over the second wire, we inserted a 4 French diagnostic catheter into the left atrium for continuous pressure monitoring [41]. These pressure catheters lead to important observations, particularly in patients with a discrepancy between color flow and pressure. Dr. Elad Maor, interventional trainee, published an important paper demonstrating patients with the best results, and follow-up had important reductions of both color flow and pressure. Those that had reductions of just one parameter, Doppler or hemodynamic, had intermediate results, whereas those that had no improvement either with color flow or hemodynamics, of course, had poor outcomes (Fig. 7.11) [42]. Invasive pressure monitoring also taught us the importance of the noncompliant left atrium as is frequently seen following radiofrequency ablation or radiation therapy [43]. Often no therapeutic maneuvers can significantly reduce left atrial pressure or V-wave height in these patients. The importance of

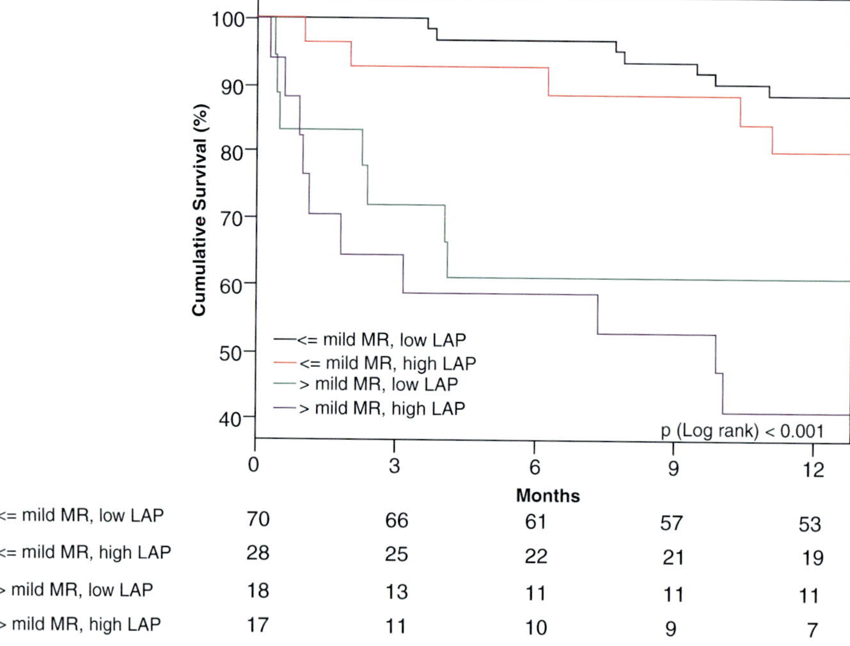

	0	3	6	9	12
<= mild MR, low LAP	70	66	61	57	53
<= mild MR, high LAP	28	25	22	21	19
> mild MR, low LAP	18	13	11	11	11
> mild MR, high LAP	17	11	10	9	7

Fig. 7.11 Twelve-month outcome of mitral paravalvular leak closure was dependent on the residual mitral regurgitation and left atrial pressure. As seen, there is progressive increased mortality depending on amount of residual MR and increase in MR pressure. (From Maor et al. [42]; used with permission)

hemodynamic monitoring was recognized by the manufacturer, who has now added a monitoring port to the latest generation of device.

Left Atrial Appendage Occlusion

An important structural initiative focused on the field of stroke prevention in patients with non-valvular atrial fibrillation, which had started in the late 1990s. It had been fueled, in large part, by a study from Mayo Clinic's campus in Jacksonville, Florida, by Blackshear et al. on the pathophysiology of stroke; in patients with non-valvular atrial fibrillation, the left atrial appendage (LAA) was the source of thrombus, resulting in stroke/systemic embolism (S/S) in approximately 90% of patients (Fig. 7.12). This contrasts with those patients in whom atrial fibrillation occurred in the setting of valvular heart disease (mitral stenosis related to either rheumatic heart fever or mitral annular calcification with a significant diastolic gradient). In this latter group of patients, the thrombus often may come from the body of the left atrium itself. Differentiating those two groups was essential in developing local site-specific therapy that focused on the LAA. With that information, the number of patients

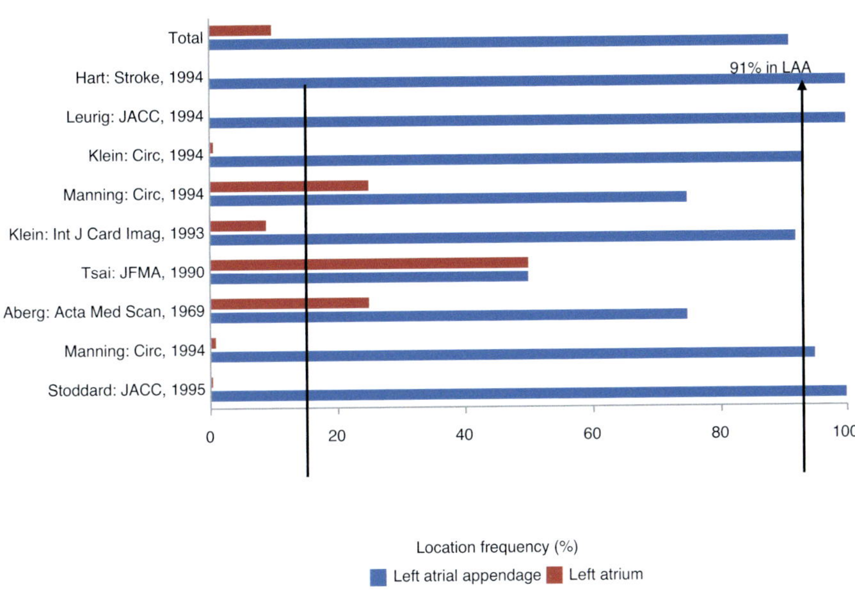

Fig. 7.12 The relationship between the underlying anatomy of the left atrium and location of thrombus, which resulted in stroke/systemic embolism being of great importance. In patients with non-valvular atrial fibrillation, the source of the thrombus was the left atrial appendage in 90%, in contrast to patients with structural mitral valve disease with a mitral gradient in whom the thrombus may have come from the body of the left atrium itself. (Adapted from Blackshear et al. Ann Thoracic Surg 61, 1996)

with non-valvular atrial fibrillation at risk for stroke or systemic embolism and the increasing data that noncompliance with oral anticoagulants or absolute or relative contraindications to oral anticoagulants resulted in inadequate treatment for many patients and presented an excellent opportunity for device-based strategies.

The animal laboratory working with Schwartz and Holmes in concert with Mayo Clinic Medical Ventures and a small company (Atritech, Plymouth, Minnesota) developed a series of prototypes designed to occlude the left atrial appendage percutaneously that were tested in a porcine model. Issues that were addressed included fixation anchors to ensure stable position optimizing, how many anchors, what design, etc., and a biocompatible, semipermeable polymer surface membrane to promote and provide a scaffold for endothelial sealing and healing – which polymer? And how much of the surface to cover with the polymer – 25%, 50%, or even 75%?

In the full and final iteration of the initial device, an open-end design was chosen with a semipermeable PET fabric covering (Fig. 7.13a, b). There were important questions related to sizing, placement strategies, and adjunctive postprocedure medications. Of interest was the fact that the preclinical animal study had used warfarin for 6 weeks post procedure designed to enhance sealing and prevent thrombus formation. That approach was never subjected to rigorous testing nor was it mentioned in any of the three panel meetings but became part of the lexicon and eventual instructions for use (IFU) approved by the FDA. A large number of design issues for the program were addressed [44]. After discussions with the FDA, the company developed an early feasibility and first-in-human study, which was designed and implemented [45]. The first US patient underwent placement of the "Watchman" device on Halloween, October 31, 2003, in a patient referred by Dr. Tom Munger. The procedure was performed by Holmes and Dr. Doug Packer with a very interested audience in the cath lab control room and resulted in an excellent success with a stable position, with no leak and no complications to everyone's relief. This set the stage for the very first multicenter randomized clinical trial – PROTECT AF (Fig. 7.14). This trial randomized patients to either the Watchman or the control group who were treated with long-term warfarin with a two device:one control

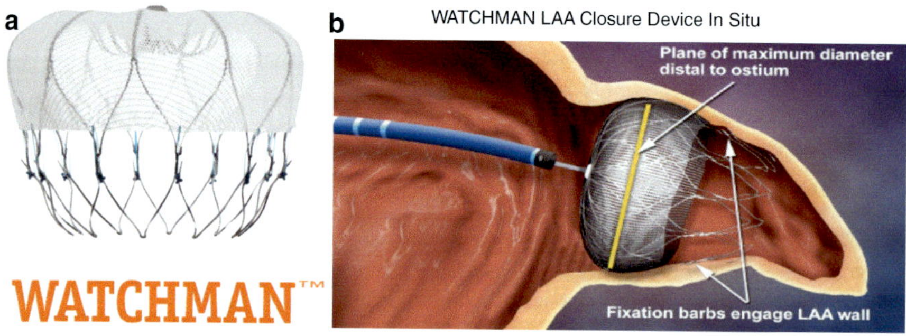

Fig. 7.13 (**a**) The initial design of the Watchman device includes a semipermeable PET fabric as seen with a row of fixation devices. (**b**) As can be seen, the device is positioned at the ostium, and stability is enhanced by the fixation barbs

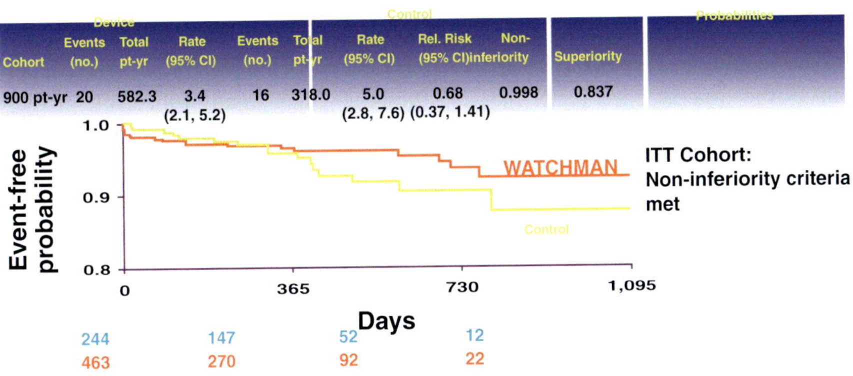

Fig. 7.14 The primary efficacy intention to treat results evaluated event-free probability. The relative risk of a primary efficacy event with Watchman was 0.68 (95% CI, 0.37, 1.41), and the posterior probability for non-inferiority was 0.998

allocation. At the time when this study was initiated, DOACs were not available for general use. This had important subsequent implications, namely, that when the device was approved, it was only approved in patients in whom long-term warfarin was not felt to be optimal or feasible. Again, Mayo Clinic (Holmes, Packer, Munger) implanted their first trial patient on October 31, 2006. Following this, there would be a second randomized clinical trial – PREVAIL – mandated by the FDA to more fully explore the safety of the device. As was true with PROTECT AF, this trial also mandated warfarin as the control long-term therapy. For these two randomized clinical trials, there were two accompanying registries evaluating the device in patients in a larger, more real-world experience. These two registries now contain the longest follow-up data in the field with this specific device. For each randomized clinical trial, Mayo Clinic was the principal investigator for the multicenter trials, which substantiated the hypothesis that the left atrial appendage was the source of clots that result in stroke/systemic embolization in patients with non-valvular atrial fibrillation.

The journey from there was convoluted [44] with three separate FDA panel meetings focused on the same device and the same indication at each panel meeting. At that time, there was no historical FDA perspective with any other device, which while interesting, was not of great comfort to the investigators or device manufacturers. During this extended period, Boston Scientific Corporation became the sponsor absorbing the intellectual property and technology from Atritech (Plymouth, Minnesota), as well as hiring the key employees and developers. Some of the earliest employees of Atritech continued with Boston Scientific as key individuals for this device and its application. Examples include George Latus who was the 14th overall hire and the first clinical hire for Atritech who seamlessly transitioned to Boston Scientific where he became the most experienced clinical specialist and teacher in the world for Watchman implantation and now has added Territory Manager to his menu. The continuity and collaboration between the clinical community, which involved electrophysiologists, invasive cardiologists, echocardiography working with industry, and the FDA, continue to be essential for developing strategies for the treatment of unmet clinical needs.

The regulatory responses for the submissions were interesting and not concordant at the time of each panel meeting; however, they finally did result in FDA approval on March 13, 2015. Additional processes included CMS evaluation, which culminated in CMS reimbursement approval on February 8, 2016. As part of the process, all patients were required to be enrolled in a national registry, and all patients had to have a more formal shared decision-making process as a requirement for approval. This series of events resulted in now still the only device approved in the USA for stroke prevention in this patient group and is now been placed in more than 150,000 patients worldwide at the time of this writing. This intellectual property and the development of a device for a new indication have set the stage for the increasing field of approaches for local site therapy to prevent stroke. As is true with any new technology, device modifications have continued with the most recent addition being a modified device (FLX) (Fig. 7.15a, b), which includes different

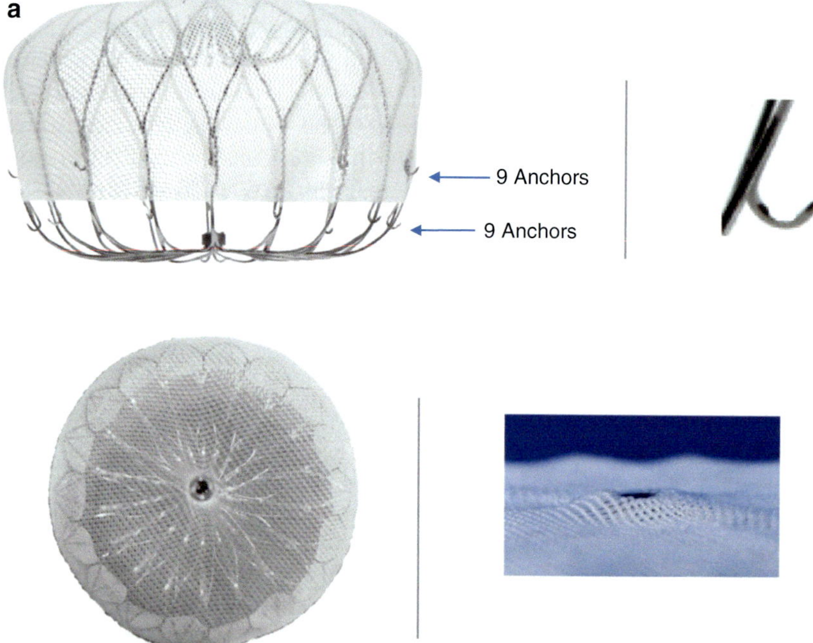

Fig. 7.15 (a) The FLX device has several features to improve the outcome and expand the number of patients who could benefit. There is a dual row of anchors to enhance long-term stability. The deployment connection has been modified to have minimal exposure of metal. This has been designed to reduce healing time and thrombus formation. (b) It also has an increased size range to accommodate a wide range of LAA sizes compared with the initial device

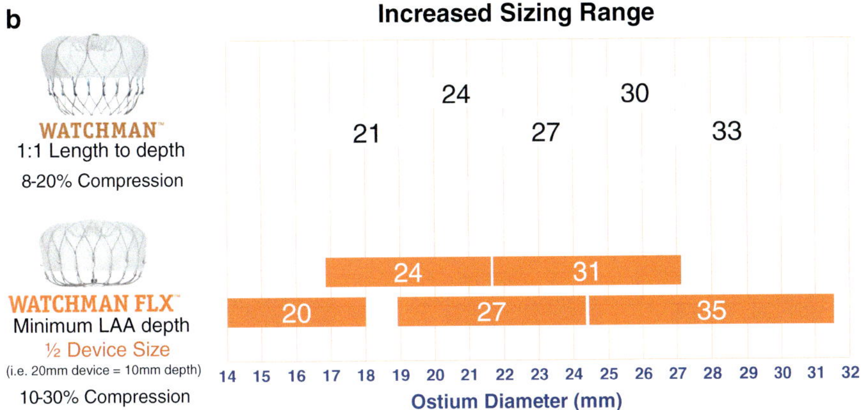

Fig. 7.15 (continued)

sizes, different anchoring designs, and configuration, all of which have improved success rates, decreased complications, and improved the number of patients who can be successfully treated compared to the initial Watchman device. This current device is the focus of the largest randomized clinical trial in the field which uses as the comparator DOACs. Other manufacturers are also involved with addressing the question of devices versus anticoagulation with DOACs for patient at risk of stroke with non-valvular atrial fibrillation. The results of these studies will be pivotal for bringing this technology to a Guideline 1 recommendation and which would allow patients to be offered either a device or drug approach for stroke prevention at the time of their initial evaluation.

The Building Block Approach to SHD Interventions

Training in structural interventions presents unique challenges. Whereas in standard interventional or operative procedures, such as PCI and TAVR, case numbers predict outcomes and can be used as a surrogate for competency and expertise in training and practice. In many SHD interventions, however, the numbers of any individual procedure type are often too low to mandate specific numbers for training purposes. For example, a trainee may see only one or two significant coronary artery fistulas over the course of his or her training and yet must be conversant and competent in closing fistulas, particularly if senior colleagues with more experience are not readily available. Many structural procedures fall into this category, such as pseudoaneurysm closure and PVL closure among others.

At Mayo Clinic, we realized that complex structural procedures are generally composed of specific "building blocks" that are translatable from procedure to procedure. For example, the ability to perform safe and reliable transseptal puncture is applicable not only to mitral clip but for every left atrial-based interventional

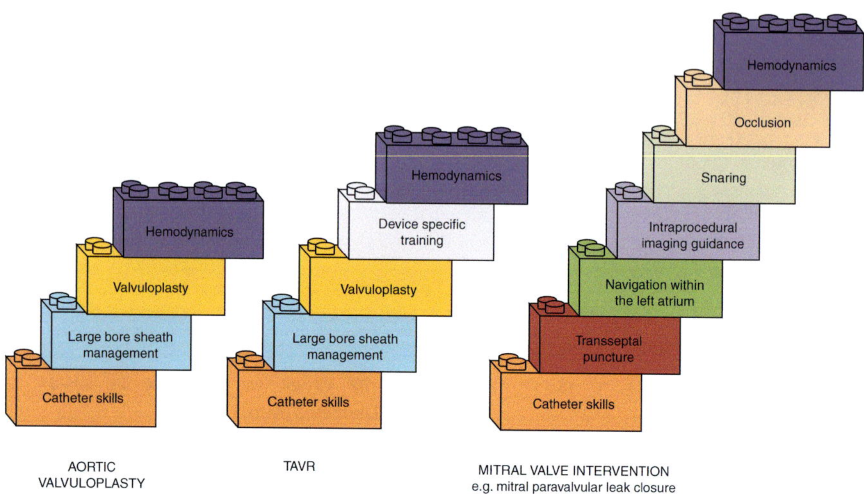

Fig. 7.16 The concept of building block approach demonstrated with colored blocks denoting specific fundamental skills, which when combined in a sequential fashion enables the performance of increasingly complex procedures. Examples provided include aortic valvuloplasty, transcatheter aortic valve replacement (TAVR), and mitral valve intervention for paravalvular leak closure. (From Raphael et al. [46]; used with permission)

procedure. We identified ten key building blocks and promulgated the concept of a novel modular approach to structural interventional training (Fig. 7.16) [46]. Breaking down complex structural procedures into their constituent building blocks allows achievement of competency within 1 year of advanced training. These building blocks include prior full training in coronary interventions, proficiency in safe large bore arterial and venous access, left ventricular apical entry, transseptal puncture, valvuloplasty, understanding 3D relational anatomy, image interpretation, guiding devices in three-dimensions, closure techniques, and learning new devices as they become available. One can readily understand how the new procedures can be constructed and performed using the basic building block techniques that are learned and acquired during structural interventional training.

Translatability of Procedures

Whether a new procedure ultimately is useful and has utility depends, of course, on the ability to teach it and translate its effectiveness to other centers. At Mayo Clinic, we had a regular train of visitors joining us from around the world to observe PVL (paravalvular leak) closure procedures, and, in turn, we had the opportunity to travel to many highly skilled centers around the world in countries such as Korea, Vietnam, India, and Israel and to many domestic centers demonstrating our procedural techniques. It was gratifying to see the enthusiasm for this new procedure by many highly skilled cardiologists, and this procedure has now become a standard in the repertoire of structural heart interventionalists.

References

1. Ross J, Braunwald E, Morrow AG. Transseptal left atrial puncture: new technique for the measurement of left atrial pressure in man. Am J Cardiol. 1959;3(5):653–5.
2. Ross J. Transseptal left heart catheterization. J Am Coll Cardiol. 2008;51(22):2107–15.
3. Inoue K, Owaki T, Nakamura T, Kitamura F, Miyamoto N. Clinical application of transvenous mitral commissurotomy by a new balloon catheter. J Thorac Cardiovasc Surg. 1984;87(3):394–402.
4. Cribier A, Rath PC, Letac B. Percutaneous mitral valvotomy with a metal dilatator. Lancet. 1997;349(9066):1667.
5. Rihal CS, Nishimura RA, Holmes DR Jr. Percutaneous balloon mitral valvuloplasty: the learning curve. Am Heart J. 1991;122(6):1750–6.
6. Abascal VM, Wilkins GT, O'Shea JP, Choong CY, Palacios IF, Thomas JD, et al. Prediction of successful outcome in 130 patients undergoing percutaneous balloon mitral valvotomy. Circulation. 1990;82(2):448–56.
7. Wilkins GT, Weyman AE, Abascal VM, Block PC, Palacios IF. Percutaneous balloon dilatation of the mitral valve: an analysis of echocardiographic variables related to outcome and the mechanism of dilatation. Heart. 1988;60(4):299–308.
8. Nishimura RA, Otto CM, Bonow RO, Carabello BA, Erwin JP 3rd, Guyton RA, et al. AHA/ACC guideline for the management of patients with valvular heart disease: a report of the American College of Cardiology/American Heart Association Task Force on Practice Guidelines. J Am Coll Cardiol. 2014;63(22):e57–185.
9. Cannan CR, Nishimura RA, Reeder GS, Ilstrup DR, Larson DR, Holmes DR, et al. Echocardiographic assessment of commissural calcium: a simple predictor of outcome after percutaneous mitral balloon valvotomy. J Am Coll Cardiol. 1997;29(1):175–80.
10. Ommen SR, Nishimura RA, Grill DE, Holmes DR Jr, Rihal CS. Comparison of long-term results of percutaneous mitral balloon valvotomy with closed transventricular mitral commissurotomy at a single north American institution. Am J Cardiol. 1999;84(5):575–7.
11. Turi ZG, Reyes VP, Raju BS, Raju AR, Kumar DN, Rajagopal P, et al. Percutaneous balloon versus surgical closed commissurotomy for mitral stenosis. A prospective, randomized trial. Circulation. 1991;83(4):1179–85.
12. Reyes VP, Raju BS, Wynne J, Stephenson LW, Raju R, Fromm BS, et al. Percutaneous balloon valvuloplasty compared with open surgical commissurotomy for mitral stenosis. N Engl J Med. 1994;331(15):961–7.
13. Powell BD, Holmes DR, Nishimura RA, Rihal CS. Calcium embolism of the coronary arteries after percutaneous mitral balloon valvuloplasty. Mayo Clin Proc. 2001;76(7):753–7.
14. ROSS J, Braunwald E. Aortic stenosis. Circulation. 1968;38(1s5):V-61–V-7.
15. Passik CS, Ackermann DM, Pluth JR, Edwards WD. Temporal changes in the causes of aortic stenosis: a surgical pathologic study of 646 cases. Mayo Clin Proc. 1987;62(2):119–23.
16. O'Keefe JH Jr, Vlietstra RE, Bailey KR, Holmes DR Jr. Natural history of candidates for balloon aortic valvuloplasty. Mayo Clin Proc. 1987;62(11):986–91.
17. Cribier A, Savin T, Saoudi N, Rocha P, Berland J, Letac B. Percutaneous transluminal valvuloplasty of acquired aortic stenosis in elderly patients: an alternative to valve replacement? Lancet. 1986;1(8472):63–7.

18. Andersen HR, Knudsen LL, Hasenkam JM. Transluminal implantation of artificial heart valves. Description of a new expandable aortic valve and initial results with implantation by catheter technique in closed chest pigs. Eur Heart J. 1992;13(5):704–8.
19. Leon MB, Smith CR, Mack M, Miller DC, Moses JW, Svensson LG, et al. Transcatheter aortic-valve implantation for aortic stenosis in patients who cannot undergo surgery. N Engl J Med. 2010;363(17):1597–607.
20. Smith CR, Leon MB, Mack MJ, Miller DC, Moses JW, Svensson LG, et al. Transcatheter versus surgical aortic-valve replacement in high-risk patients. N Engl J Med. 2011;364(23):2187–98.
21. Adams DH, Popma JJ, Reardon MJ, Yakubov SJ, Coselli JS, Deeb GM, et al. Transcatheter aortic-valve replacement with a self-expanding prosthesis. N Engl J Med. 2014;370(19):1790–8.
22. Popma JJ, Adams DH, Reardon MJ, Yakubov SJ, Kleiman NS, Heimansohn D, et al. Transcatheter aortic valve replacement using a self-expanding bioprosthesis in patients with severe aortic stenosis at extreme risk for surgery. J Am Coll Cardiol. 2014;63(19):1972–81.
23. Meredith IT, Worthley SG, Whitbourn RJ, Antonis P, Montarello JK, Newcomb AE, et al. Transfemoral aortic valve replacement with the repositionable Lotus valve system in high surgical risk patients: the REPRISE I study. EuroIntervention. 2014;9(11):1264–70.
24. Leon MB, Smith CR, Mack MJ, Makkar RR, Svensson LG, Kodali SK, et al. Transcatheter or surgical aortic-valve replacement in intermediate-risk patients. N Engl J Med. 2016;374(17):1609–20.
25. Reardon MJ, Van Mieghem NM, Popma JJ, Kleiman NS, Søndergaard L, Mumtaz M, et al. Surgical or transcatheter aortic-valve replacement in intermediate-risk patients. N Engl J Med. 2017;376(14):1321–31.
26. Mack MJ, Leon MB, Thourani VH, Makkar R, Kodali SK, Russo M, et al. Transcatheter aortic-valve replacement with a balloon-expandable valve in low-risk patients. N Engl J Med. 2019;380(18):1695–705.
27. Popma JJ, Deeb GM, Yakubov SJ, Mumtaz M, Gada H, O'Hair D, et al. Transcatheter aortic-valve replacement with a self-expanding valve in low-risk patients. N Engl J Med. 2019;380(18):1706–15.
28. Schaff HV. Transcatheter aortic-valve implantation — at what price? N Engl J Med. 2011;364(23):2256–8.
29. Kapadia SR, Kodali S, Makkar R, Mehran R, Lazar RM, Zivadinov R, et al. Protection against cerebral embolism during transcatheter aortic valve replacement. J Am Coll Cardiol. 2017;69(4):367–77.
30. Søndergaard L, Ihlemann N, Capodanno D, Jørgensen TH, Nissen H, Kjeldsen BJ, et al. Durability of transcatheter and surgical bioprosthetic aortic valves in patients at lower surgical risk. J Am Coll Cardiol. 2019;73(5):546–53.
31. Makkar RR, Fontana G, Jilaihawi H, Chakravarty T, Kofoed KF, De Backer O, et al. Possible subclinical leaflet thrombosis in bioprosthetic aortic valves. N Engl J Med. 2015;373(21):2015–24.
32. Généreux P, Head Stuart J, Hahn R, Daneault B, Kodali S, Williams Mathew R, et al. Paravalvular leak after transcatheter aortic valve replacement. J Am Coll Cardiol. 2013;61(11):1125–36.
33. Alkhouli M, Sarraf M, Maor E, Sanon S, Cabalka A, Eleid MF, et al. Techniques and outcomes of percutaneous aortic paravalvular leak closure. JACC Cardiovasc Interv. 2016;9(23):2416–26.
34. Eleid MF, Cabalka AK, Malouf JF, Sanon S, Hagler DJ, Rihal CS. Techniques and outcomes for the treatment of paravalvular leak. Circ Cardiovasc Interv. 2015;8(8):e001945.
35. Rihal CS, Sorajja P, Booker JD, Hagler DJ, Cabalka AK. Principles of percutaneous paravalvular leak closure. J Am Coll Cardiol Intv. 2012;5(2):121–30.
36. Gössl M, Rihal CS. Percutaneous treatment of aortic and mitral valve paravalvular regurgitation. Curr Cardiol Rep. 2013;15(8):388.
37. Lloyd JW, Rihal CS, Eleid MF. Hemodynamics rounds: hemodynamics of mitral valve interventions. Catheter Cardiovasc Interv. 2020;96(3):712–24.

38. Maor E, Raphael CE, Panaich SS, Reeder GS, Nishimura RA, Nkomo VT, et al. Acute changes in left atrial pressure after MitraClip are associated with improvement in 6-minute walk distance. Circ Cardiovasc Interv. 2017;10(4):e004856.
39. Stone GW, Lindenfeld J, Abraham WT, Kar S, Lim DS, Mishell JM, et al. Transcatheter mitral-valve repair in patients with heart failure. N Engl J Med. 2018;379(24):2307–18.
40. Pilote L, Hüttner I, Marpole D, Sniderman A. Stiff left atrial syndrome. Can J Cardiol. 1988;4(6):255–7.
41. Eleid MF, Reeder GS, Rihal CS. Comparison of left atrial pressure monitoring with dedicated catheter versus steerable guiding catheter during transcatheter mitral valve repair. Catheter Cardiovasc Interv. 2018;92(2):374–8.
42. Maor E, Raphael CE, Panaich SS, Alkhouli M, Cabalka A, Hagler DJ, et al. Left atrial pressure and predictors of survival after percutaneous mitral paravalvular leak closure. Catheter Cardiovasc Interv. 2017;90(5):861–9.
43. Gibson DN, Di Biase L, Mohanty P, Patel JD, Bai R, Sanchez J, et al. Stiff left atrial syndrome after catheter ablation for atrial fibrillation: clinical characterization, prevalence, and predictors. Heart Rhythm. 2011;8(9):1364–71.
44. Holmes DR Jr, Schwartz RS, Latus GG, Van Tassel RAA. History of left atrial appendage occlusion. Interv Cardiol Clin. 2018;7(2):143–50.
45. Holmes DR, Reddy VY, Turi ZG, Doshi SK, Sievert H, Buchbinder M, et al. Percutaneous closure of the left atrial appendage versus warfarin therapy for prevention of stroke in patients with atrial fibrillation: a randomised non-inferiority trial. Lancet. 2009;374(9689):534–42.
46. Raphael CE, Alkhouli M, Maor E, Panaich SS, Alli O, Coylewright M, et al. Building blocks of structural intervention. Catheter Cardiovasc Interv. 2017;10(10):e005686.

Chapter 8
2010–2020s

Gurpreet S. Sandhu

Bookended by the 2008 recession and the 2020 COVID-19 pandemic, this was a head-spinning decade in which extensive technological breakthroughs and medical advances occurred and the Mayo Clinic Cardiac Catheterization Laboratory truly thrived and made unprecedented progress. Deeply influenced by societal expectations and technological breakthroughs, incessant and dynamic changes became the norm, and some preceding history is important from a contextual perspective. My family's association with Mayo Clinic began decades before my birth, and ironically it was during the global influenza pandemic of 1918 that this story begins. Soldiers returning home after serving in Europe during World War I had carried the lethal virus back to their countries, and a similar situation unfolded in India with returning British Indian Army veterans spreading this contagion throughout the Indian subcontinent and adding to the death toll of millions worldwide. Dr. Randhir Singh Sandhu, my grandfather, was born in the Sikh holy city of Amritsar, India, in 1898. Following the death of his parents in this pandemic, this young man joined early Indian Sikh migrants to California where farming and the railroad had opened up new opportunities in the United States. He initially earned a degree in pharmacy at the University of California at Berkeley, followed by medical school at the University of Kansas Medical Center (KUMC), where he graduated in the class of 1928. This was followed by time as a visiting physician at Mayo Clinic in 1930, where he met both Mayo brothers as well as Dr. Plummer and was deeply influenced by their work. My association with Mayo Clinic started in 1987 when as a freshly graduated physician from the University of Delhi, I came to Rochester to earn a PhD in molecular biology. My grandfather shared his experiences at Mayo Clinic, which he described as one of the world's leading centers of excellence in the 1930s, and this deeply influenced

G. S. Sandhu (✉)
Department of Cardiovascular Diseases, Mayo Clinic, Rochester, MN, USA
e-mail: Sandhu.gurpreet@mayo.edu

D. R. Holmes Jr., R. L. Frye (eds.), *The Mayo Clinic Cardiac Catheterization Laboratory*, https://doi.org/10.1007/978-3-030-79329-6_8

187

my commitment toward strengthening the humanitarian legacy of this iconic institution.

From a personal perspective, the late 1980s and 1990s had led to an explosion of new scientific discovery and innovation, fueled in part by the Internet and a rapid sharing of novel discoveries, and it was an amazing experience to be a part of this wave. With technologies like polymerase chain reaction (PCR) that sparked novel diagnostics and therapeutics, the ability to rapidly sequence and synthesize DNA, make genetic alterations, and develop new strategies for previously untreatable conditions became a reality. I spent 5 years earning my PhD under the mentorship of Dr. Bruce Kline, with other national experts including Drs. Tom Spelsberg, Eric Wieben, and Larry Pease on my thesis steering committee. This was followed by 4 years as a postdoctoral fellow developing DNA-based molecular diagnostics for atypical pathogens that impacted immunocompromised patients such as those with HIV or posttransplant immunosuppression. I resumed my clinical training with an internal medicine residency at the University of Minnesota in Minneapolis where I also continued scientific research under the mentorship of Dr. David Ingbar. My association with cardiology at Mayo Clinic started in the year 2000 when I was recruited as a cardiology fellow by Dr. Guy Reeder. During my 3 years of general cardiology fellowship and 1 year of interventional fellowship, I had the privilege of working closely with and learning from academic cardiologists such as Dr. Rob Simari, Dr. David Holmes, Dr. Chet Rihal, Dr. Bob Frye, Dr. John Bresnahan, Dr. David Hayes, and many others. I continued my basic and translational science research in close partnership with Dr. Simari and worked with many wonderful colleagues in his laboratory in the Guggenheim building. During this time I was invited by Dr. Eric Wieben to join the Mayo Genomics Advisory group that initiated the University of Minnesota-Mayo Clinic research partnership, and with support from Drs. David Hayes, Amir Lerman, and Rob Simari, cardiology became a key partner in the development of the new Stabile research building. Dr. Simari generously provided great opportunity for many cardiologists to continue their research in his laboratory with Drs. Rajiv Gulati, Sorin Pislaru, Ripu Singh, Barry Boilson, and I being amongst his many mentees and collaborators. Some of my research included creating transgenic models for natriuretic peptide-based heart failure studies, superparamagnetic nanoparticle-targeted cellular therapeutics, endothelial cell-capturing stents, electrospun and bioprinted vascular conduits, and several interventional cardiology devices. These led to numerous patents with Drs. Simari, Holmes, Gulati, and Rihal being co-inventors on several of these.

A few additional things happened along the way that played a key role in the shaping of events between 2010 and 2020. I was recruited to join the consulting staff as an interventional cardiologist by Dr. Chet Rihal in 2004. Drs. Bob Frye, David Holmes, David Hayes, Bernard Gersh, Rob Simari, and John Bresnahan also played key roles in my recruitment, with the final words of wisdom coming from Dr. Bresnahan over a cup of coffee, "There will be the same issues at all institutions, at least you know what you are getting into out here." During Dr. Rihal's leadership years in the cath lab, I became a part of the cath lab education committee in 2005 and the clinical practice committee and research committee in 2007. This insight into the operational management of an academic medical practice provided additional building blocks toward leadership training.

Dr. David Hayes subsequently invited me to lead the Marketing committee for the Division of Cardiovascular Diseases in 2009, opening the door towards understanding the dynamics of external public, regulatory and competitive influences, and efforts required to support the robust growth of the clinical and academic practice. It also became clear that providing the outstanding Mayo Clinic model of clinical care was necessary, but inadequate to ensure enduring success, and that it was increasingly important to ensure that our outstanding quality and safety metrics were fully highlighted and that we embraced transparency and public reporting in the growing number of external registries. The United States had entered a pivotal recession in 2008, and this impact would be felt throughout the organization for the next several years. The cath lab was faced with declining patient volumes and a significant reduction in reimbursements, and it rapidly became clear that due to the recession patients were delaying care, or seeking care closer to home instead of traveling long distances to Mayo Clinic. Historically, Mayo Clinic had been very conservative in its approach toward public affairs and had not participated in any direct-to-patient initiatives or direct public marketing. This all changed as cardiology decided to volunteer for new public-facing initiatives. With support from Dr. David Hayes and our administrator Ron Menaker, the CV marketing team initiated public screening events and lipid checks at baseball games and marathons in the Minneapolis and Saint Paul area, developed videos that ran every 30 minutes on all screens at the Mall of America, and the institution even briefly explored building a hospital at this location. Educational events were developed for patients similar to the continuing medical education events for physicians, and several cardiologists and cardiovascular surgeons participated in these including Drs. Sam Asirvatham and Sharonne Hayes. Prioritized access was established for US patients to reach a cardiology officer of the day, and Drs. David Hayes, Tom Behrenbeck, Abhi Prasad, and I carried a cardiology cell phone that was a direct line provided to 200 VIP international patients. Around this time I was invited by Dr. Rajeev Chaudhry to help develop the first Mayo Clinic-Cisco telemedicine pilot, and CV took the lead with both Dr. Scott Wright and I piloting remote care at Cannon Falls, Minnesota. Additionally, I also had the privilege of working closely with Mr. Jeff Bolton who was then Mayo Clinic's chief financial officer, as well as institutional leaders Dr. Mike Harper and Dr. John Noseworthy, as we explored building an international joint-venture hospital, and the learnings from this played a substantial role during subsequent international initiatives.

In 2010, I was invited by Dr. Rihal to develop a business plan and build a Cardiovascular Innovation Laboratory (CVIL) that would bring us to the cutting edge of bench-to-bedside research and innovation. As the founding director of the CVIL, I worked closely with our major proponents Dr. Rihal, Dr. Simari, and Dr. Lerman, as well as institutional leadership that included Mr. Jeff Bolton and Dr. John Noseworthy, to develop a business plan and oversee the construction of a hybrid cath lab, electrophysiology lab, and robotic-equipped surgical operating room. This facility was operationalized in November 2011 and became instrumental in facilitating large animal research as well as external partnerships, with numerous scientific discoveries, first-in-human technologies, and innovative intellectual property being developed here. Novel cellular, molecular, and nanotechnology-based therapeutics, and other futuristic devices, as well as innovations in surgical and procedural technologies, now became feasible as cutting-edge technologies were made available for the first time in a translational setting. In parallel, with support from institutional leadership and great help from our business development and legal team led by Mr. Jim Rogers III, we also established Mayo Clinic's first large partnership with a commercial organization, Boston Scientific. This collaboration subsequently expanded to cover numerous departments and led to the establishment of a joint company named Motion Medical that became a partner in Mayo Clinic's new Discovery Square research building.

With Dr. Rihal stepping down as director of the cath lab to become the division chair for cardiology in 2009, there was a 3-year period where the cath lab was ably managed through difficult times and downsizing by our Interim director Dr. John Bresnahan. Dr. Bresnahan always provided a calm and reassuring presence throughout his career at Mayo Clinic and was always someone who could be counted upon to help other colleagues during challenging high-risk and complex procedures. He was also instrumental in helping behind the scenes with virtually every major initiative in the cath lab until he retired in 2019.

Following a formal search and interview process in 2012, I was offered the position of director of the cath lab at Rochester, and followed in the footsteps of Drs. Frye, Holmes, Rihal, and Bresnahan. After personal meetings with every member of the cath lab consulting staff as well as allied health staff, it became very clear that major reorganization was needed to stem the post-recession decline and to prepare for future challenges that would include declining reimbursement, bundled payments, increasing regulatory burden, time-consuming documentation inefficiencies, declining morale, and staff burnout. Transparency, collegiality, and a team approach were the only way forward, and extensive support was forthcoming from the entire team during my tenure as director. Getting to know each other on a personal basis was important, and this included reducing the hierarchical barriers between physicians and allied health staff. Besides including nurses and technicians on all cath lab committees including clinical practice (CPC), education, staff satisfaction, research, etc., we also opened up the annual cath lab holiday party to entire families including the children and parents of all cath lab personnel. The party planning now included volunteers from the nursing, technical, and administrative staff, and attendance increased from the previous 40–50 attendees to almost 150 people during the first year.

Our vision for the cath lab was to be number one in the world in the breadth and depth of our procedural expertise, as well as in our research and innovation that spanned basic science, translational, and clinical research. Our educational offerings including invasive diagnostics, hemodynamics, and interventional and structural cardiology fellowships would be unrivaled, as would our CME and Board Review Programs, and teaching at national and international meetings. Each new member recruited to our team became part of our diverse and collegial family and led the entire group to higher levels of accomplishment. Drs. Alkhouli, Barsness, Bell, Best, Eleid, Guerrero, Gulati, Holmes, Prasad, Reeder, Rihal, Sandhu, Sandoval, Singh, and Tilbury were the interventional cardiologists during 2020, with Drs. Alkhouli, Eleid, Guerrero, Prasad, and Sandoval being recruited to the group during my tenure. Drs. Behfar, Borlaug, Frantz, Herrmann, Lerman, Miranda, Nishimura, and Reddy were the invasive cardiologists, out of whom Drs. Behfar, Miranda, and Reddy were also recruited during my tenure. Our friend Dr. Rob Simari left to pursue a wonderful opportunity as the Dean of the University of Kansas Medical Center. This was a bitter sweet moment for the entire team but came with a personal silver lining as he made the discovery that my grandfather was a KUMC graduate and sent me his photograph from the class of 1928 that was displayed in the halls of the Medical School. Five pediatric colleagues, Drs. Anderson, Cabalka, Cetta, Hagler, and Taggart, along with our medical physicist Dr. Fetterly, rounded off our cath lab team. In addition, Dr. Rihal had initiated enterprise-wide integration of cardiology that led to the creation of specialty councils, followed by an enterprise-wide cardiology department. This led to my personal area of responsibility extending to support colleagues at five additional cath labs in Mayo Clinic facilities at Arizona, Florida, Mankato, Eau Claire, and La Crosse, and all were a close-knit part of the team with people rotating and helping across sites. The entire group was ably supported by Ms. Sue Eastman, MBA, as the operations manager, and Brent Konz, RN, and Moises Aguilar, RCIS/RT, as the leaders of the nursing and technical staff, with all three and their teams contributing in immense ways to support the institution. In fact, each one of the individuals mentioned above has left an indelible imprint in the history of the greatest cath lab in the world.

Achieving this vision while recovering from recession would require team building, shared decision-making and responsibilities, standardizing the practice, improving efficiencies, and strategically planned investments towards reversing the downsizing, and building a practice that all of us would be honored to be a part of. Reinvigorating clinical, research, education, and administrative excellence would necessitate an enduring and sustainable team effort, and all members of the lab stepped forward to help.

My personal philosophy was to have the right mix of individuals on the team, fully engaged and empowered to achieve their personal professional goals, and to give them the space and resources to grow, with complete transparency instead of micromanagement, ensuring that we were pulling together for the common good of patients and the organization. In order to ensure fairness and respect for the entire team, all physicians were invited to participate in any procedure of their choice so that no one would be left out of the emerging structural heart disease innovations. The entire group was trained in TAVR and two-thirds continued this procedure long-term. Over time the entire group had self-selected three to four procedure types that were aligned with their academic and personal procedural interests. This provided everyone an opportunity to innovate and to be a part of tightly knit subspecialist teams of three to four colleagues that would work together to grow a cutting-edge referral practice. All consultants shared nightly and weekend on-call duty, as well as routine interventional and hemodynamics responsibilities, while participating in complex coronary interventions and emerging structural heart disease interventions of their choice. Technologies such as stereotaxis, lasers, rotational atherectomy, robotics, and various hemodynamic support devices including ECMO, balloon lithotripsy, and complex valvular interventions were expanded to become a routine part of our daily practice. Double-scrubbing by two consultants in complex cases was encouraged as this fostered innovation, collegiality, personal education, and enhanced our ability to offer high-risk and complex procedures with a greater margin of safety for our patients. New technologies were proactively and ably supported by the cath lab technical and nursing staff, several of whom were instrumental in providing additional clinical and technical innovation. Proctors were invited from across the world to help us develop new capabilities, and cath lab consultants participated in leadership roles on national societies and advisory boards to further share our knowledge with the rest of the world.

Sharing each individual consultant's procedural volumes, waste reports, quality and safety metrics, personal and patient radiation exposures, and quarterly PCI database reports was also transitioned to an open and nonjudgmental setting. This allowed each one of us to see how we compared with peers who did similar procedures and allowed us to learn from each other for the greater benefit of our patients. It also became clear to the team that everyone was contributing equally and in several different manners. While some people would do seven or eight procedures in a day, others would do two or three high-risk and long cases, and some would do four or five procedures while taking on the additional responsibility of educating junior fellows. Similarly, research and education were encouraged, with accomplishments highlighted and celebrated by the entire group.

Scheduling individual physicians was done in a systematic manner, with all interventional cardiologists receiving 40%–50% time in the cath lab and all invasive cardiologists receiving 20%–30% time. A review of the annual volumes of each consultant and the procedure types done by them was used to assign days of the week to ensure that a full spectrum of capabilities was available for patient care throughout the week. In addition, the entire group participated in supporting the inpatient as well as the outpatient practice and continued to pursue independent research funding for clinical as well as basic and translational science initiatives. Great success was achieved in obtaining both intramural and extramural national and international grants, with the cath lab group publishing approximately 200 peer-reviewed articles each year. Dr. Amir Lerman established the Cardiovascular Research Center for Mayo Clinic, leading to further support for research within Cardiology and the cath lab.

In 2013, the cath lab was formally named the Dr. Earl H. Wood Cardiac Catheterization Laboratory as part of our acknowledgment of the amazing history of the pioneers in our field at Mayo Clinic. Dr. Wood had carried out extensive invasive hemodynamics research to study human physiology and was the inventor of the G-suit used by fighter pilots since World War II. A generous research endowment had been provided by one of his former cardiology trainees and was commemorated by the lab being named after Dr. Wood. This took place at a wonderful ceremony attended by Mayo Clinic leadership and many emeritus cardiologists, as well as the family of Dr. Earl Wood (Fig. 8.1).

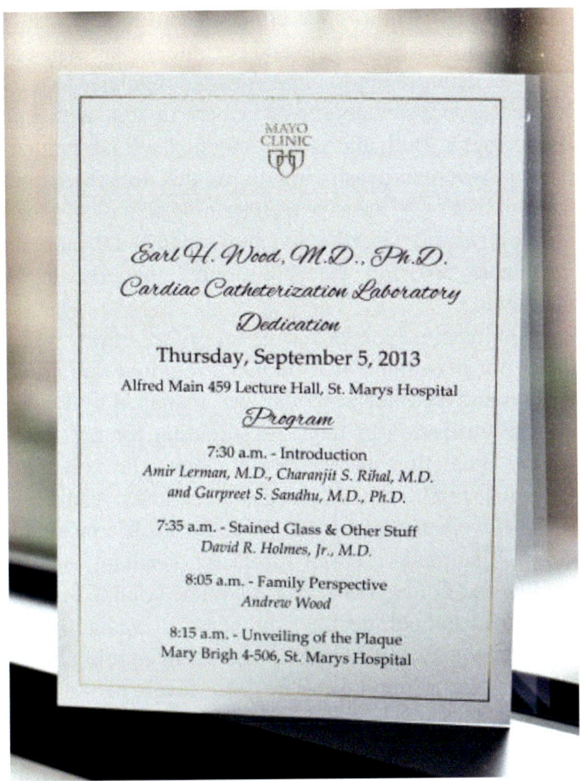

Fig. 8.1 The dedication of Earl H. Wood, MD, PhD, the Mayo Clinic Cardiac Catheterization Laboratory, was an extremely important milestone celebrated Thursday, September 5, 2013. It involved multiple key figures coming together to honor the legacy of Dr. Wood

The cardiovascular innovation laboratory continued to provide excellent bench-to-bedside support and facilitated Mayo Clinic-developed first-in-human studies within the cath lab. Examples of a few studies include percutaneous pericardotomy, autologous cell therapy for coronary vasospasm, stenotic aortic valve crossing devices, and novel pharmacologics for acute MI and circulatory failure among others. Collaboration with device companies also led to an expansion of early feasibility studies for structural heart disease innovations, leading to greater academic opportunities and cutting-edge technologies being made available to help patients who lacked other therapeutic options.

Education continued to be a very strong focus with Dr. Andre Lapeyre establishing a highly organized level 1 and level 2 general cardiology training pathway for fellows. All consultants in the lab contributed in numerous ways toward the technical, clinical, and research mentorship of our trainees. In parallel, Dr. Abhi Prasad and the cath lab education committee established one of the first formal 2-year fellowships for teaching interventional cardiology and structural heart disease in an academic setting. Besides an outstanding and well-rounded education, departing fellows continued to be provided mentorship several years after graduating from Mayo Clinic. Drs. Greg Barsness, Guy Reeder, and John Bresnahan made valuable contributions as former program directors, with Drs. Patti Best, Barry Borlaug, and Rajiv Gulati providing consistent support for the programs and mentorship for the trainees.

The Mayo Clinic interventional cardiology board review course continued to strengthen over the decade and became the premier course for interventional cardiologists, including those who attended regularly to refresh their clinical knowledge. Numerous physicians played a part in this with enduring contributions by Dr. Barsness, Dr. Bell, and several others. Cath lab grand rounds went online and were recorded for external sharing during this decade. A rarely known fact is that the cath lab also had a CV invasive tech training school and this was expanded to include EP training, with Dr. Reeder and subsequently Dr. Best serving as the directors of this invaluable program that contributes toward supplying high-quality graduates nationwide.

Simultaneously, educational and other efforts were made to improve radiation safety for personnel. This included required radiation safety education for all new fellows and technical staff that was managed by Dr. Ken Fetterly. Besides optimizing the utilization of physical shielding for proceduralists, we also incorporated similar protection in new labs for our echo colleagues to improve safety during extended structural heart disease procedures. Additionally, personal radiation exposure, as well as patient radiation, for each consultant was shared with the entire group. This made it easier for each consultant to compare their numbers with the numbers of colleagues doing a similar volume and complexity of procedures and led to substantial declines in personal radiation exposure for all consultants. Simultaneously, efforts were made on an ongoing basis to optimize image quality in all rooms using the lowest possible levels of radiation. Adjustments optimized at Mayo Clinic were shared with manufacturers for deployment at other centers. Radiation protection aprons and vests from vendors were also systematically studied to identify the best balance of maximally protective lightweight garments. In parallel Dr. Mandeep Singh studied and published the impact on occupational safety and musculoskeletal injury in personnel.

The entire invasive cardiology team contributed strongly toward all aspects of the outstanding clinical and academic performance of the group. Dr. Nishimura continued his work with external societies to develop guidelines and spearheaded institutional "Ask Mayo Clinic Expert" repositories of information, and mentored advanced fellows interested in honing their hemodynamics skills. Other colleagues had great success leading large independent research teams and obtaining leadership roles internally and externally. Dr. Borlaug was an integral member of the CPC and led numerous heart failure and innovative device initiatives, while Dr. Behfar advanced cutting-edge basic science, regenerative medicine, and hemodynamic innovations. Dr. Frantz played a key role in developing a large referral practice of patients suffering from severe pulmonary hypertension due to chronic thromboembolic disease. Working closely with Japanese experts over several years, Dr. Frantz and I developed a cutting-edge pulmonary angioplasty practice with excellent outcomes for our patients. Additionally, Dr. Frantz also played a key role in developing the invasive follow-up of cardiac transplant patients. Meanwhile Dr. Herrmann continued to advance his cardio-oncology research and also led the quality and registry teams for the cath lab. He played a key role in improving safety and outcomes working closely with Dr. Gulati who was the CPC Chair. Dr. Lerman in his CV research leadership role mentored numerous consultants and fellows and helped connect individuals with resources for research grants. He also provided a continuous push for incorporating new clinical technologies and for creating structure around the research opportunities for fellows in training.

While a majority of this chapter is dedicated to the clinical practice, all interventional colleagues played a hands-on role across all aspects of the clinical and academic advances. Dr. Barsness who led many educational initiatives including the fellowship program and board review courses was a leader in peripheral and CTO interventions and served as the director of the Cardiac Intensive Care Unit (CICU). Dr. Prasad brought great academic oversight and mentorship as the director of the 2-year interventional fellowship and also reorganized cath lab grand rounds to include surgical colleagues and regional practices. He was integral in the development of a complex CTO referral practice along with Dr. Rajiv Gulati. Dr. Patti Best led the lab in the highest average number of PCIs per day, and never met a complex coronary lesion that she did not like. Besides being an integral member of the CICU, she was deeply involved in the selection of candidates for fellowships and faculty positions, and served as the director of the CVIS tech training school. Drs. Bresnahan and Reeder were the pragmatic superstars who were involved in virtually all initiatives going back three decades, and it was impossible to go through the history of the lab and not find numerous examples of procedures ranging from first stent placement to first gene therapy where they were not involved. Both played key roles in fellowship programs and educational initiatives and were part of virtually every procedural innovation in the lab. Dr. Reeder served as the Program director for the CV fellowship and CVIS program, while Dr. Bresnahan served as interim cath lab director and the interventional fellowship director during this decade. Dr. Tilbury was the strong voice of reason that advocated for selecting the highest-quality fellows and faculty for ensuring long-term success of the group and, besides being known for his exceptionally high procedural outcomes, spent a significant time in the CICU practice. Parts of his vacation and trip time were spent on humanitarian efforts in underdeveloped countries. Dr. Alkhouli brought unprecedented quality and efficiencies in the structural heart disease practice and was a leader in peer-reviewed publications. Dr. Guerrero was recruited as a national expert in mitral heart disease and quickly developed a robust referral practice and had great success in expanding her national presence as a leader in structural heart disease trials. Several new procedures including transcaval TAVR were added to the practice by her. Dr. Bell served multiple roles in the cath lab and the cardiology department, including Chair of the Ischemic Heart Disease Division and enterprise-wide IHD council, and most recently as Vice Chair for cardiology. Besides oversight for the CICU, he was closely involved in all aspects of the fellowship programs, board review and CME programs, high-risk PCI practice, facility development, and numerous practice initiatives. Dr. Eleid was recruited as faculty after completing his fellowship in the cath lab and became the go-to person for structural heart disease procedures. Besides being a highly experienced interventionalist with skills that include a large array of structural devices, he provided great mentorship for fellows and was closely involved in all aspects of practice optimization with Drs. Gulati and

Sandhu. Dr. Holmes and Dr. Rihal as previous directors of the lab, and by virtue of their subsequent national and institutional roles, supported every aspect of the cath lab practice with their guidance for the entire team and limitless commitment toward fellow education, support for research, and unbridled enthusiasm for technological innovations. Dr. Rihal's efforts at developing the educational aspects of the SHD program also culminated in the publication of his handbook outlining the building blocks of the SHD practice. Along with contributions mentioned elsewhere, Dr. Mandeep Singh was a high-volume interventionalist, and also led the entire regional ACS and STEMI network for the cath lab and the department, with significant improvements in quality and outcomes. Dr. Sandoval was the newest addition to the Rochester group having successfully served as the lab director at our La Crosse regional facility, and added to our academic strengths in ischemic heart disease. Last but not least were the extensive contributions of Dr. Rajiv Gulati, my successor as the next Chair of Interventional Cardiology and director of the cardiac cath lab. Our association started in Dr. Simari's research lab when I was a cardiology fellow and Dr. Gulati came from the United Kingdom to complete his research training under the mentorship of Rob Simari. From jointly developing basic science and innovative translational technologies during our early careers to working closely in developing a cutting-edge and academic cath lab procedural practice, Dr. Gulati has played an outstanding role that has been recognized by the entire group. Besides his role as the CPC Chair, Dr. Gulati made major contributions toward board review courses, CME events, mentoring of fellows, academics, and advancing the complex and high-risk procedural practice (Figs. 8.2 and 8.3).

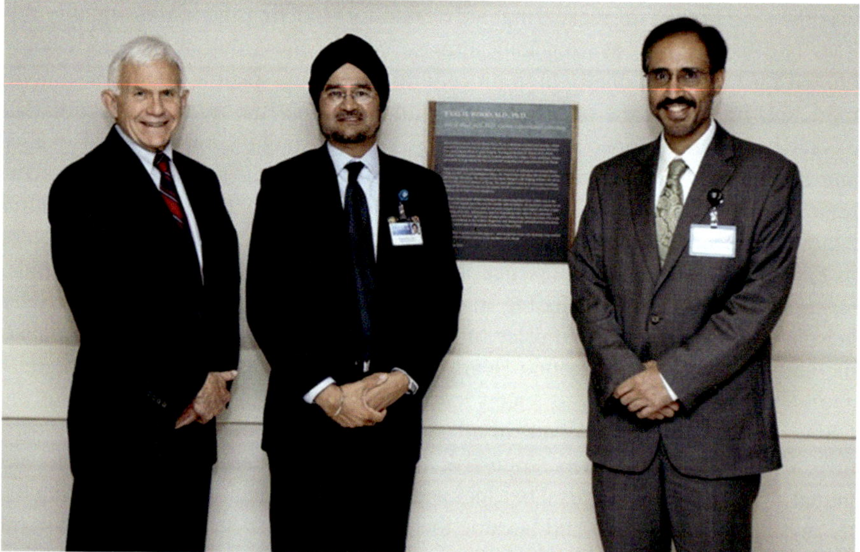

Fig. 8.2 The three most recent catheterization laboratory directors, Drs. Holmes, Rihal, and Sandhu at the Earl H. Wood, MD, PhD, Cardiac Catheterization Laboratory plaque unveiling in 2013

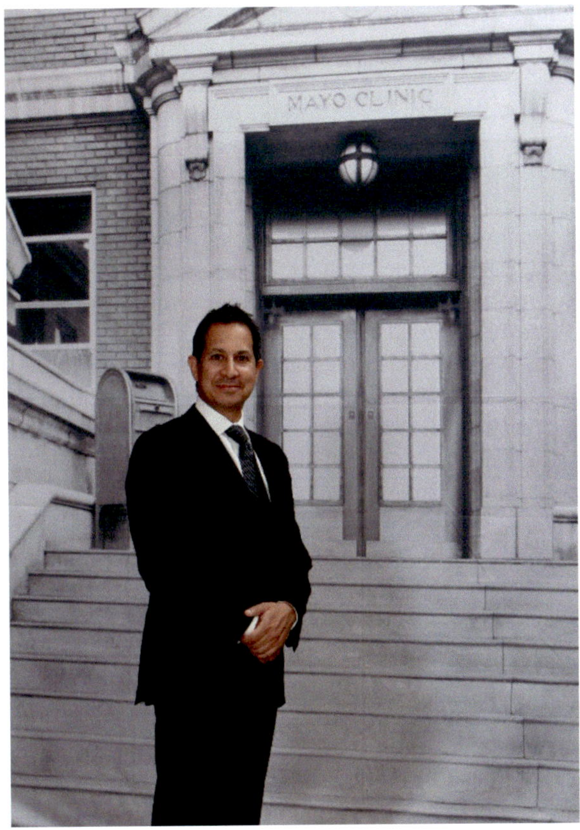

Fig. 8.3 The current laboratory director, Dr. Rajiv Gulati, also participated in the celebration

The expansion of all aspects of the structural heart disease practice, complex coronary interventional practice, and invasive hemodynamics expansion was critical for the success of the lab. With Drs. Rihal and Holmes pioneering some of the early perileak, TAVR, and LAA expansion described in other chapters, Dr. Reeder and the pediatric group contributed to ASD, PFO, and other structural interventions. High-risk PCI (Bell, Gulati, Prasad, Sandhu), pulmonary artery implantable sensors and posttransplant hemodynamic support (Behfar, Borlaug, Sandhu), pulmonary artery interventions (Frantz, Sandhu), CTOs (Barsness, Gulati, Prasad, Sandhu), peripheral interventions (Barsness, Gulati), and mitral and tricuspid innovations (Alkhouli, Eleid, Guerrero, Reeder, Rihal) grew strongly as well. The partnership with CV surgery was critical during this expansion and led to improved patient care, successful "manage to reimbursement" initiatives, new intellectual property, shared clinics, and a high degree of comfort with scrubbing in each other's areas.

TAVR expansion and the extreme risk posed by unfavorable financial consequences had caused significant concern as the volumes increased. Even though Mayo Clinic was an early adopter and started TAVR in the cath lab in 2008, we were not immune to market trends promoting the building of hybrid operating rooms to support this new practice. Two hybrid ORs were constructed, and the entire TAVR practice migrated to the OR almost immediately. Within the first year, it became apparent that performing TAVR in the OR was financially nonviable as the complete operating room environment was being brought to bear upon a percutaneous procedure. Percutaneous cutdown for routine femoral artery access, a large number of transapical access cases, general anesthesia for all patients, 1–2 day ICU stay, opening of surgical equipment trays, routine use of transesophageal echo, priming of bypass machines for possible emergencies, high pacemaker rates, and the large number of personnel in the space were contributing toward inefficiency and excessive costs. The ORs were being tied down for the entire day for two TAVRs, and access for open surgical cases was being restricted. With institutional support and in collaboration with CV surgery, Drs. Sandhu, Greason, and Nkomo led an extensive enterprise-wide effort to change the practice over the next 2 years. We transitioned appropriate cases in a graduated manner back to the cath lab, reduced personnel, eliminated general anesthesia and switched to RN-mediated moderate sedation, replaced TEE with transthoracic echo, discontinued percutaneous cutdown access, standardized equipment, and optimized all steps of the procedure. Improved supply chain contracts helped partially offset high device costs. There were significant improvements in safety, quality, and patient outcomes. Hospital length of stay declined from 5 days down to 1.5 days, and ICU stay was eliminated for uncomplicated cases. Pacemaker rates were reduced substantially by developing guidelines that included extended monitoring for borderline indications. With further de-escalation, we were able to complete four TAVR procedures by 10:00 or 11:00 a.m., with next-day discharge for the majority of patients. Ensuring sustainable financials for revenue-losing SHD procedures will continue to be an ongoing priority for all structural heart disease procedures that require expensive devices. Lessons from these efforts helped mitigate the need to build expensive hybrid ORs by systematically and safely expanding the types of SHD cases treated using minimally invasive and percutaneous access in the cath lab procedure rooms. These lessons were also shared and implemented at other Mayo Clinic sites including Arizona, Florida, and Eau Claire, Wisconsin.

We were early adopters of most new technologies, and the great scientific expertise of the group ensured that we were able to quickly determine the clinical utility as well as the societal and financial impact of emerging technologies fairly quickly. This enabled us to avoid jumping on the bandwagon with numerous pharmaceutical and device technologies that were later found to have a lot less utility than was initially reported. Additionally, we found value in including manufacturer specialists and external proctors in the procedure room for guidance during the early stages. This was especially helpful in numerous instances with devices such as TAVR valves, atrial appendage occlusion devices, and mitral valve repair technologies. Additionally, there were likely benefits for external practices, as company representatives often share patient safety and efficiency strategies being utilized by larger centers.

Enterprise integration was another major focus during this decade. I had previously led the NSTEMI practice standardization process for all 6 sites, and the team had included approximately 50 representatives spanning physicians, nurses, quality, administrative, and other staff across the enterprise. Various aspects such as diagnosis, procedural prioritization, medications, quality, etc, were delegated among five teams, and within 2 weeks each team leader presented their guidelines and best practice-based recommendations. These leaders of each team were then charged with developing a consensus document that was presented to the entire group at the end of another 2 weeks. Within 30 days a completed document was shared with physicians and nurses across the enterprise using a variety of settings, including grand rounds, as well as small group informational sessions. Once there was adequate awareness among the six enterprise sites, this was operationalized with close follow-up of quality and safety outcomes. With ongoing updates over the past decade, this effort provided a template for enduring quality improvement initiatives across the enterprise.

Supply chain management (SCM) had become as increasingly important part of the practice with new structural devices costing $20,000–$30,000 each, and increasing financial pressures placed by declining reimbursements from both government and private insurance sources. We partnered very closely with Mayo Clinic SCM while working with major device and pharmaceutical companies to obtain the best possible evidence-based technologies for our patients, at the most reasonable cost. This included ensuring pragmatic and long-term relationships with suppliers, keeping in mind that technology evolved constantly and that backup options were required for patient safety in the event of any product recall. We also led efforts as subject matter experts in the Captis/Vizient consortium to ensure that Mayo Clinic's best practice recommendations would also help other medical organizations and patients across the nation.

Financial transparency was achieved within the cath lab, by ensuring that consultants, technical staff, and nurses saw monthly as well as annual financial reports and were an active part of all initiatives. Nurses played a key role in developing and optimizing same-day dismissal policies for outpatient procedures and further improved safety by following up with patients via phone calls the next morning. Technical staff members were empowered to identify and offer cost-effective and equivalent devices to consultants during procedures.

We volunteered to participate in the CMS bundled payments BPCI-A program in 2018 as we had done substantial ground work with optimizing coronary devices and acute coronary care pathways, including same-day dismissal and follow-up management. This proved invaluable when the initial financial results from 2019 became available and provided quality as well as financial data to support our continued participation. Working closely with revenue analysts and the fee review committee helped ensure greater value for society and our patients. Supporting charity care, including for international referrals, continued to be a hallmark of the cath lab practice as the team tried to provide care for those who would not otherwise have access.

Payer mix continues to be a concern for all organizations, and it was clear that over the longer term private insurance payments would continue to decline and approach government payment levels. Improving efficiency and patient outcomes, as well as identifying emerging revenue sources from international and remote-care initiatives, would be important over the longer term. The cath lab continued to play a leading role with the international practice, providing outreach visits for international patients and participating in emerging artificial intelligence-based technologies to maintain our cutting edge. Additionally, in my additional role as Vice Chair, Department of Cardiovascular Medicine (International), we actively assisted in the development of a cardiology practice at Mayo Clinic Healthcare at London, and at the Mayo Clinic joint venture in Abu Dhabi, the Sheikh Shakhbout Medical City.

Quality, safety, and patient experience continued to be on the forefront with numerous initiatives being undertaken to ensure accuracy for various database and registry reporting. The database and registry team was expanded to include the five other cath lab sites and, upon the successful completion of this stage, to integrate with teams managing other aspects of the Cardiovascular Department databases. At this point the operations were transitioned to the department, with Ms. Sue Eastman continuing to provide support as the enterprise operations manager. Dr. Joerg Herrmann played a key role as the Chair of Quality for the Interventional Cardiology Division and the Ischemic Heart Disease Division. The quarterly M&M conferences were also reformatted to include updates on quality and outcomes for both the PCI and structural heart disease metrics.

Leadership development and succession planning is critically important for any organization, and it is the cath lab director's responsibility to ensure that the next leader stepping into the role and the lab support systems is primed for success. Toward that objective, we engaged the institutional leadership development team at an early stage and also identified candidates for leadership training aligned with their area of clinical, research, and educational interest. This was done across the enterprise cath labs with one or two individuals selected at all sites. All identified individuals underwent a leadership 360 review and also received feedback and mentorship, with some receiving additional formal coaching as well. Leadership roles were provided on the clinical practice committee, educational committee, and research committee for individuals to understand the functioning of Mayo Clinic's matrix organization, and this allowed individuals to interact outside the department with institutional groups. Those interested in clinical practice received graduated education in finance, working with teams, and more autonomy in leadership decision-making. I had personally benefited from being a part of numerous cath lab, department, and institutional opportunities over the past two decades and ensured that others would receive similar opportunities for personal development. My role on the Rochester Surgical and Procedural committee had also allowed me to learn and contribute toward developing pragmatic policies for the institution.

Staff satisfaction is crucial for the success of any organization, and understaffing to maximize financial margins is a recipe for failure at multiple levels. In order to ensure success, physician staffing was arranged in an equitable manner keeping in mind that the lab needed to provide our entire spectrum of complex interventional and hemodynamic procedures on all 5 days of the week, as well as 24/7 emergency care. Vacation and trip time was never denied to any physician, and under staffing was covered by either asking for volunteers, or by operating the lab with one less consultant, with the other assigned consultants covering the gap.

Staff safety and patient safety are closely interlinked, and ensuring a safe working environment and minimizing the potential for burnout were always kept front and center. There were challenging periods where due to unexpected retirements and illnesses, our nursing and technical team personnel fell short for extended periods. Extensive efforts were made to fill the gaps by having nurses come in from other units to help with nonprocedural tasks. This was more challenging in the case of the technical staff as even new hires would require a minimum of 3 months of supervised training to manage the unusually demanding and complex procedural requirements. Numerous staffing models were developed with input from personnel, including staggered early and late shifts to try and ensure that personnel were able to leave at a predictable time to look after their children and families. Team briefings, shared decision-making with referring physicians, standardization of policies, and a close partnership with anesthesiology were also helpful in creating a collegial, safe, equitable, and efficient environment.

A proactive and independent cath lab CPC, with strong AHS participation, provided ownership of the practice and a voice for all team members. The RNs were authorized to establish a large charge nurse team with fully delegated responsibility for daily operations. Interpersonal respect and valuing the contributions of all personnel fostered long-term success. All issues dealt with immediately and effectively in a very transparent manner, and this included utilizing institutional resources wherever necessary. Nurse practitioners were added to the practice in 2018 to streamline the overnight observation practice for patients who did not require full hospital admissions. This led to improved quality, efficiencies, and standardization of patient care. This also improved the educational experience for our senior follows as they now had more time for procedures and academic pursuits.

Over the past 10–15 years, the cath lab had developed robust internal software systems that allowed management of daily patient schedules, and linked with our research and quality registry teams. These systems also had report generation capabilities that would then feed into Mayo Clinic's electronic medical records. Significant disruption was anticipated when it was announced that the institution would be changing electronic medical record systems in 2018. Upon reviewing with Mayo Clinic IT, as well as with colleagues at other institutions that had undergone EMR conversions, it quickly became apparent that the new EMR did not have modules that would provide high-quality functionality similar to our own cath lab systems. The additional work required to manage daily tasks was conservatively estimated to result in a 15%-20% reduction in efficiencies. This would have been an existential challenge as the cath lab had been on a strong trajectory of growth. The team made a decision of partnering closely with the institutional IT teams and invited EMR vendor personnel to shadow our cath lab teams to observe our practice requirements. These three groups worked extremely closely for 2 years with oversight by cath lab leadership to identify every potential obstacle and developed solutions that would allow critical functionality of our existing systems to operate in the new environment. This required extensive efforts with numerous IT, compliance, regulatory, legal, and practice-related committees at all Mayo Clinic sites to achieve consensus, as well as approval to standardize cath lab imaging and reporting systems across the enterprise. The cath lab had one of the most trouble-free transitions on the new EMR go-live date in 2018, thanks to the extensive work done by the entire team, especially the nursing and technical teams. Within 1 month, our efficiencies and patient volumes rebounded to our preconversion levels, and the subsequent year (2019) saw the highest cath lab volumes ever recorded in terms of both absolute numbers and procedural complexity.

Numerous other challenges arose unexpectedly including a state law that would prevent highly trained RCIS-certified cath lab techs from switching on and repositioning cath lab tables. This could have effectively shut down all cath labs in the state for being out of compliance with this rule that required hiring radiology techs. Correcting this situation required working with institutional experts in government policy, regional hospitals, medical societies, organizations that certify RCIS/RCES techs, local radiology groups, the state health department, and state legislators. Dr. Ken Fetterly played a key role in managing this process for the cath lab, and this work led to a consensus proposal being passed that preserved the interests of all groups and allowed continuation of patient care in cath labs. Other transient challenges have included shortages of critical medications such as intravenous heparin, nitroglycerin, and acetylcholine, as well as nonavailability of interventional devices after Hurricane Maria damaged dozens of device-manufacturing facilities in Puerto Rico in late 2017. All of these events required significant short-term innovation so that we could continue to provide safe procedural care.

Long-term strategic planning and facilities development are critical for supporting the mission and vision of the institution. Master-space planning was initiated around 2016 and led to the approval of a modern 32-bed patient intake and recovery unit attached to the cath lab. This was opened in November 2020 and was a tremendous help with supporting same-day dismissal for outpatient procedures. Having opened in the midst of the COVID-19 pandemic, this also helped reduce the number of patients requiring admission to a hospital bed for postprocedure observation. This new unit provided long-term stability and resources for ongoing growth into the next decade. Resources were also obtained from the institution to build an additional five procedural labs that would expand the current set of six cath and six electrophysiology labs.

As the COVID-19 pandemic started unfolding in January 2020, we followed closely with increasing concern as an increasing number of nations reported outbreaks. It became very clear early on that this was not simply a respiratory ailment. Colleagues in Europe and Asia were reporting patients coming in with acute myocarditis, acute coronary events, shock, and conduction system disturbances. During the early days, this led to numerous overseas cath lab personnel being exposed to the virus and either falling ill or being placed under quarantine. Entire cath labs were shut down in many cities around the world, and in the midst of this was increasing misinformation circulating within the media, public, medical professionals, and political interest groups. We faced the same critical shortage of personal protective equipment as the rest of the country, and it was clear that even the best-intentioned and best laid-out pandemic plans did not include awareness that the cath labs were also first responders like emergency room personnel, and presented an open front door for COVID-19 entry into any hospital. On February 19, 2020, after reflecting on the global state of chaos, I wrote "Intensely reflected sunlight can lift the veil of darkness, while blinding one to reality…G. S. Sandhu, MD, PhD."

The most important steps for me personally were to protect our entire team and to continue to provide timely and exceptional care for our patients. This meant ensuring that we did whatever we could to remain operational throughout the pandemic. Dr. Rajiv Gulati, Sue Eastman, Brent Konz, and Moises Aguilar were critical partners who worked tirelessly along with numerous nurses, physicians, and technicians to get us through these difficult times. Having decided that we would maintain 24/7 operations, and with limited personal protective equipment, we set forth to plan for a worst-case scenario and that estimated placing more than half of our team in quarantine. It was very clear that our close working quarters did not allow for enough separation between patients and staff, so we operationalized wearing masks at all times well before universal masking was mandated. With an impending state-mandated halt to elective procedures and surgeries, we took the opportunity to practice disaster plans and divided the entire cath lab team of interventional cardiologists, nurses, and technicians into three groups. Each group would come in for 1 week rotations to do procedures, with the second group being kept in reserve to come in immediately if the first group was placed in quarantine, or if lab volumes were high. The third group would isolate at home and utilize that week for providing remote care, or to continue remote research and education activities. Some consultants who were in a high-risk group volunteered to cover outpatient clinics and provided telemedicine consults. Since there were no elective diagnostic cases, the invasive group volunteered to cover inpatient hospital services and the CICU. This was an incredible team effort, and the technical staff refined the donning and doffing procedures for our limited supplies of personal protective equipment. Meanwhile the nurses voluntarily came in on nights and weekends to make calls to reschedule several hundred planned procedures and to keep in touch with patients so that they could be brought back when it was safe to do so. Working closely with our surgical and procedural committee, hospital incident command teams, infection control, and supply chain management, we were able to adequately prioritize N95 respirators and PAPRs to maintain operations for supporting urgent and emergent procedures. Air exchange rates for all procedure rooms were estimated by facilities engineers, and later measured so that we could post aerosol clearance times on the doors and develop room turnover protocols. Working closely with colleagues in ischemic heart disease, circulatory failure, heart rhythm, and the CICU, we developed protocols for managing COVID-19 patients with cardiac presentations. This helped streamline pathways for evaluation by the emergency room and cardiology consult service physicians. Once we had adequate systems in place, we were able to restart the practice safely, and the three teams were merged to support normal operations.

Drs. Prasad and Eleid provided invaluable support during this team-based pilot, and we retained the ability to rapidly revert back to smaller teams in order to provide uninterrupted services if the pandemic threatened to overwhelm hospitals in the region. These learnings and protocols were also shared with our cath labs at five other sites with the United States, as well as our newly established hospital at Abu Dhabi. While we had a few staff members become infected with COVID-19 during

2020, there was no transmission between personnel, and at no time was the lab at risk of widespread loss of services. By the time COVID-19 cases started spiking in late fall, the entire team was very comfortable in safely caring for all patients. There was a rapid restoration to pre-pandemic procedural volumes after restrictions on the scheduling of surgeries and procedures were eased.

Additional factors became increasingly important around the time of the pandemic, and one was the ability to provide timely care from a distance. Telemedicine was expanded substantially, and a large proportion of preprocedural evaluation was done without the patient traveling for a face-to-face visit. Drs. Eleid, Lerman, Sandhu, and Gulati had previously initiated research into remote coronary stent placement, and the importance of developing these remote technologies was clearly highlighted during this pandemic. Having previously demonstrated the world's first live case of a preclinical coronary stent placement from a building located over a mile away (Dr. Sandhu at TCT 2018), the team continued to accelerate research and development of novel capabilities (Fig. 8.4).

Artificial intelligence-based research had been initiated in 2018 with Drs. Fetterly, Barsness, and Sandhu leading the first project where autonomous algorithms would identify and assess significant coronary artery lesions based upon morphology and flow characteristics. Numerous additional projects were added with contributions from several cath lab consultants in late 2020, with funding established to hire a full-time AI engineer dedicated toward cath lab projects.

As with any other large group of 30 highly accomplished consultants, there were numerous personal and professional accomplishments, and what truly highlighted this decade was the strong team spirit and collegiality. This was even more evident outside work with shared interests, hobbies, and impromptu gatherings, including during CME trips worldwide. Many of us volunteered to travel and teach in underserved areas in Asia, Africa, and Central and South America. Longstanding traditions of a summer golf competition were kept alive by Dr. Rihal and others. Dr. Reeder and I shared tools as we worked on his classic sports cars and my vintage WW2 jeeps, and we would make an occasional motorcycle trip during summer weekends. Numerous other cardiology colleagues were an integral part of our cath lab accomplishments, with Drs. Bernard Gersh, Naser Ammash, Sam Asirvatham, Vuyisile Nkomo, Wells Askew, Sorin Pislaru, and numerous others being a part of the social, practice, and academic fabric of the team. Anchoring the entire practice was the tireless, steadfast, and highly organized management support provided by my administrative partner Sue Eastman, MBA. There was literally no small or large issue that she couldn't address with her limitless knowledge, wisdom, and connections within or outside the institution. Mr. Bob Cole is another individual who was the glue that kept operations running when small or large infrastructure gremlins would strike without warning, and his sense of humor and electronic gold stars sent randomly to consultants were much sought after.

As with any field, there is continual renewal and evolution, and achieving diversity and inclusion is critical for enduring success. These principles were

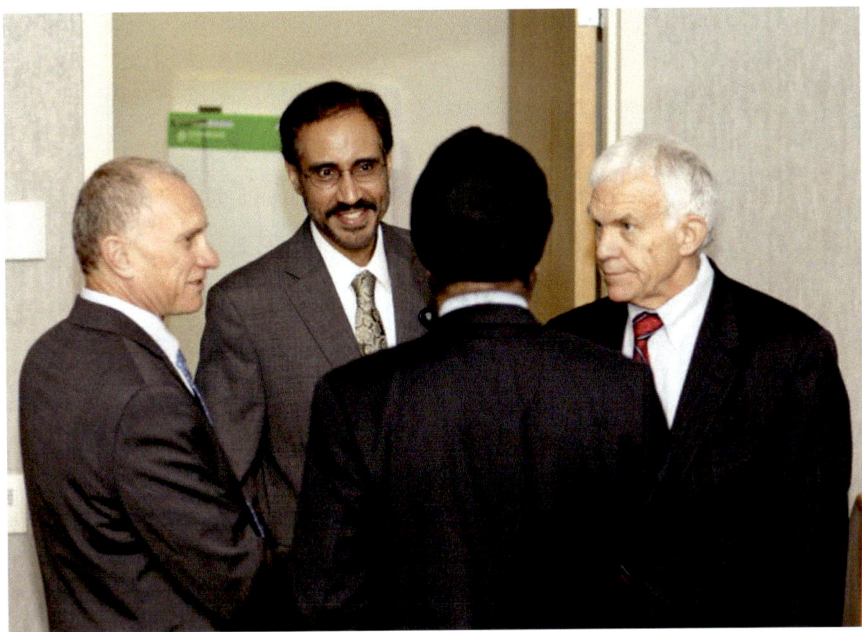

Fig. 8.4 Drs. Lerman, Sandhu, Holmes, and Rihal represented some of the scientific and outreach programs under the direction of the catheterization laboratory

front and center during all cath lab initiatives as we recruited an outstanding group of five interventional and three invasive cardiologists. Female representation among interventional cardiologists is extremely low at 7%–8% nationwide, and we made sustained efforts to recruit female physicians to our interventional training programs and achieved a 35% level during the past several years, and reached 50% in 2019–2020. With three female consultants in the cath lab, there is substantial opportunity for progress as the practice grows and senior consultants transition out of the procedural practice. Drs. Bresnahan and Lapeyre, two of the most accomplished and humble contributors toward the success of our clinical and educational excellence, retired in 2019. With each person, transition is a deeply personal decision, and some elected to reduce cath lab time, while continuing to participate in a rich and rewarding clinical practice, and mentored fellows and faculty. The latest leadership transition occurred in November 2020 with Rajiv Gulati, MD, PhD, an outstanding academically and technically accomplished interventional cardiologist, continuing this chain as the next Chair of the Division of Interventional Cardiology. In reflecting back upon the changes during each previous decade, it is clear that all our cath lab leaders more than accomplished what my mother Dr. Inderjeet Sandhu, a retired cardiologist, has always taught me to do, "Leave every place in much better condition than when you found it," and we did (Fig. 8.5).

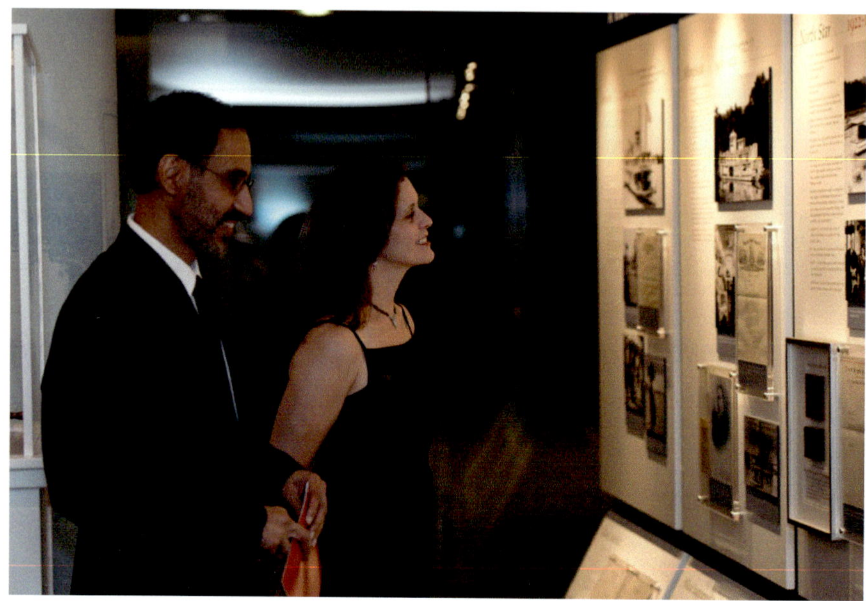

Fig. 8.5 Drs. Gurpreet and Nicole Sandhu viewing historical pieces of information and early mementos at the 100th Anniversary of Cardiology at Mayo Clinic celebrations

Chapter 9
Coronary Endothelial and Microvascular Function Testing

Amir Lerman and Michel T. Corban

One of the original and landmark observations on the role of vascular wall in the regulation of coronary vascular tone in humans from our cardiac catheterization laboratory described the in vitro vasoconstrictor activity of coronary sinus blood taken from patients with atheromatous coronary artery disease and blunted initial vascular relaxation phase during exercise potentially due to impaired release of vasodilating factor or factors [1]. The combination of plasma vasoconstrictor factors (unknown yet at that time) along with impaired endothelial function was hypothesized to potentially provoke flow-limiting stenosis and myocardial ischemia, leading the authors to conclude that the vascular wall potentially releases vasodilator and vasoconstrictor factors that mediate vascular tone [1]. The story of nitric oxide (NO) discovery and its role in endothelial cell-mediated regulation of vascular tone emerged shortly after July 10, 1986. The historical announcement on the major role of NO in the regulation of vascular tone was held at a Willow Creek Middle School in Rochester, Minnesota, during one of Mayo Clinic's symposiums (Fig. 9.1). Previously, RF Furchgott – who received later the Nobel Prize for the discovery – and JV Zawadzki had demonstrated an obligatory role of functional endothelial cells in inducing relaxation of arterial smooth muscle in response to acetylcholine, through a yet undiscovered mediator substance initially termed "endothelium-derived relaxation factor" (EDRF) [2, 3]. Furchgott's announcement in Rochester, Minnesota, Mayo Clinic's home, that EDRF may indeed be NO was particularly interesting at that time, since NO was not known to be produced in mammals and more importantly was not previously known to have any specific role in vascular tone regulation.

A. Lerman (✉) · M. T. Corban
Department of Cardiovascular Diseases, Mayo Clinic, Rochester, MN, USA
e-mail: Lerman.amir@mayo.edu; Corban.michel@mayo.edu

D. R. Holmes Jr., R. L. Frye (eds.), *The Mayo Clinic Cardiac Catheterization Laboratory*, https://doi.org/10.1007/978-3-030-79329-6_9

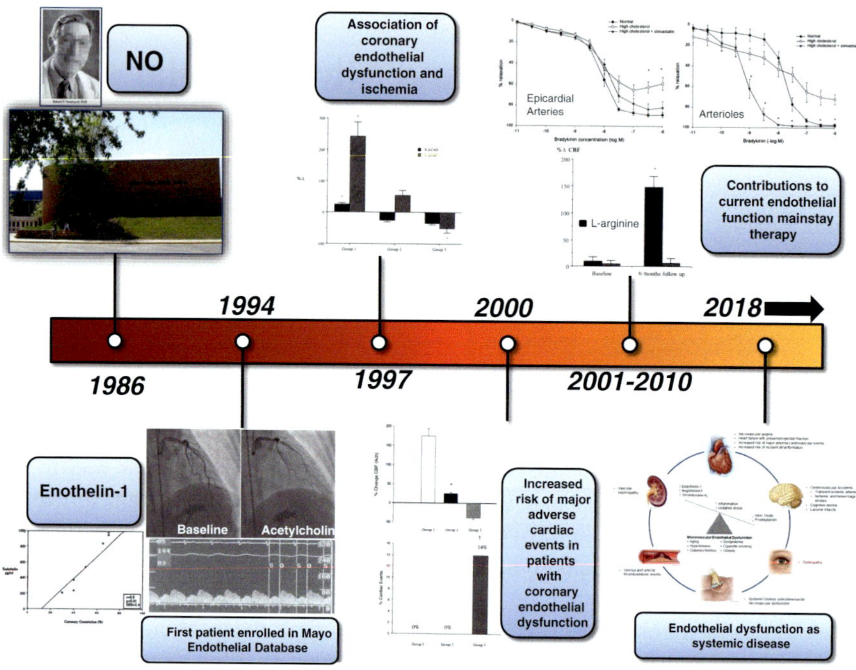

Fig. 9.1 Illustrative summary of discoveries and events at Mayo Clinic Cardiac Catheterization Laboratory that significantly contributed to our understanding of pathophysiology, diagnosis, prognosis, and treatment of coronary endothelial dysfunction. NO indicates nitric oxide

Over the next decade, Mayo Clinic and other institutions have significantly contributed to our current understanding of the complex regulation of vascular tone by endothelial cells and to the discovery of potent vasoconstrictor molecules opposing NO vasodilatory response in hypercholesterolemia. Working on the hypercholesterolemia porcine model, A Lerman, V Fuster, JH Chesebro, JC Burnett Jr., and others extended the concept of the role of endothelium-derived factors (such as endothelin-1) in the regulation of coronary vascular tone and in mediating an endothelial-dependent vasoconstriction response to intracoronary acetylcholine infusion [4]. Indeed, it has become more evident that the functional and structural integrity of the vascular endothelium is not only important to maintain the balance between circulating endothelium-derived vasodilator and vasoconstrictor molecules, but also confers protection from arterial atherosclerosis and thrombosis [5].

In parallel, translation of the assessment of endothelial function utilizing intracoronary acetylcholine infusion protocol from animal models to humans was underway at Mayo Clinic. Initial studies for endothelial function assessment in our lab focused on the evaluation of coronary epicardial angiographic vasoconstriction in response to acetylcholine consistent with epicardial endothelial dysfunction. While multiple studies from other institutions back then suggested that endothelial dysfunction only occurs in patients with diffuse or local angiographically significant atherosclerosis, R Nishimura and colleagues demonstrated in 1995, using intravascular ultrasound imaging, that epicardial vasoconstriction in response to acetylcholine is not dependent on the presence or absence of atherosclerosis and thus may proceed plaque development [6]. Moreover, their observation of greater vasoconstrictive response to acetylcholine infusion in patients with versus without risk factors for coronary artery disease was consistent with animal studies and among the earliest findings strongly suggestive that endothelial impairment is the earliest detectable form of coronary atherosclerosis in humans – a hypothesis that was subsequently validated [7]. This concept was later extended with serial studies from our laboratory using more sophisticated intracoronary imaging tools demonstrating the association between segmental epicardial endothelial dysfunction, plaque progression [8], and vulnerable plaque phenotype [9, 10].

However, coronary circulation is anatomically comprised of not only epicardial arteries but also of microvascular arterioles. In fact, coronary blood flow is mostly regulated by the resistance pre-arterioles and arterioles, while the epicardial arteries are mostly conductance vessels. Thus, for comprehensive evaluation of coronary physiology, it was crucial to also interrogate microvascular endothelial function with acetylcholine. Nevertheless, in contrast to epicardial coronary vasculature, the microcirculation has always been – and remains – elusive to conventional invasive and noninvasive imaging techniques. Therefore, introduction of innovative invasive direct evaluation of functional changes in coronary blood flow, rather than visual changes in epicardial anatomy in response to acetylcholine, was needed to evaluate microvascular function in the cardiac cath lab. Accordingly, the introduction and validation of coronary blood flow assessment using a combination of Doppler wire measurement of blood velocity and quantitative coronary angiography for changes in coronary artery diameter in response to escalating doses of intracoronary adenosine (as a non-endothelium-dependent microvascular vasodilator) and acetylcholine infusion, as surrogate for coronary microvascular endothelial function evaluation, in patients with no obstructive epicardial coronary artery disease (NOCAD) was undertaken. This protocol was initiated as an integral part of an NIH grant that was awarded and initiated in 1994 in our cath lab (Fig. 9.1). Following successful completion of the NIH study, it became apparent that there was an unmet clinical need for a protocol to assess the coronary microcirculation in patients with chest pain and nonobstructive CAD – a population that accounts for up to 40% of our patients undergoing clinically indicated coronary angiography. Thus, the protocol that was used in the NIH grant was approved as a clinical practice protocol in our cardiac catheterization laboratory in 1997 (Fig. 9.2). In addition, the establishment of an outpatient chest pain and coronary physiology clinic as a part of our cath lab enhanced our referral base and our ability to provide care for this challenging patient population.

Nevertheless, the importance of any new clinical tool lies in its diagnostic, prognostic, and treatment-guidance role in patient care; invasive coronary endothelial function testing is not different. Indeed, as described in detail below, cutting-edge research studies and high-impact papers published by our lab helped pave the way for clinical coronary endothelial function testing in the realm of coronary

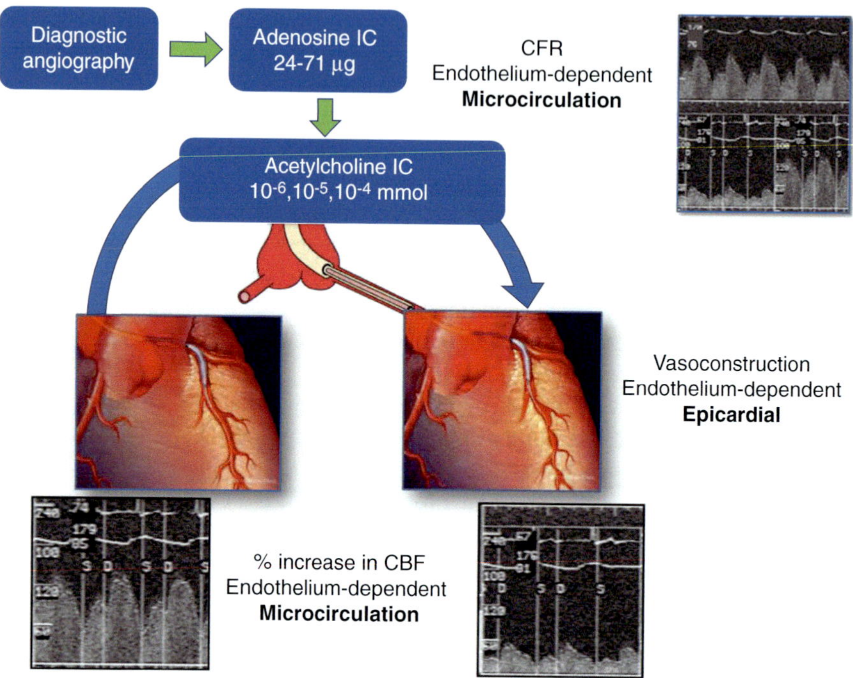

Fig. 9.2 Clinical protocol for coronary endothelial and microvascular function assessment. CBF indicates coronary blood flow, CFR coronary flow reserve, IC intracoronary

physiology. In a series of studies, we demonstrated the association between coronary microvascular function, myocardial ischemia, and cardiovascular events (Fig. 9.1). We initially demonstrated that coronary endothelial dysfunction in the left anterior descending coronary artery (LAD) of symptomatic NOCAD patients, resulting in decreased coronary blood flow, was indeed associated with ischemic myocardial perfusion defects within the LAD territory on ^{99m}Tc-sestamibi SPECT imaging [11] and ischemic electrocardiographic (ECG) changes on 80-lead body surface ECG mapping [12]. These results are underscored by the demonstrated lack of correlation between multimodality noninvasive stress tests and invasively diagnosed coronary microvascular dysfunction in symptomatic NOCAD patients [13]. Moreover, we were also the first to show that NOCAD patients with coronary endothelial dysfunction are at increased risk of not only major adverse cardiac events, including myocardial infarction, heart failure, and surgical and percutaneous coronary revascularization [14], but also cerebrovascular events [15], extending the concept to other vascular beds.

One of the challenging aspects of treating this patient population is the lack of novel effective therapies. We have designed, executed, and published multiple NIH, AHA, and Mayo Foundation-funded animal and human trials investigating new therapeutic options for coronary endothelial dysfunction that either constitute current mainstay clinical therapy for this challenging disease entity such statins [16] and NO precursor L-arginine [17] (Fig. 9.1) or cornerstone early studies of potentially promising investigational therapies such as endothelin-1 antagonists [18] and most recently autologous intracoronary CD34+ cell therapy (unpublished work, currently under review).

Finally, we were among the first to introduce and advance the concept that endothelial dysfunction is a systemic disease with not only cardiac but also numerous clinical manifestations beyond the heart [19]. Indeed, our recent supporting data links systemic endothelial dysfunction and microvascular endothelial dysfunction to increased risk of incident atrial fibrillation [20] and heart failure with preserved ejection fraction [21, 22], in addition to its association with erectile dysfunction [23], antiphospholipid syndrome, and venous and arterial thromboembolism [24, 25] (Fig. 9.1).

In conclusion, the role of the Mayo Clinic Cardiac Catheterization Laboratory in understanding the pathophysiology, establishing the diagnosis, predicting the prognosis, and advancing treatment of coronary endothelial dysfunction has been, and in fact remains, crucial. The Mayo Clinic Microvascular Database, the largest current database of invasive coronary endothelial function tests worldwide, includes more than 2,000 patients presenting with angina and/or ischemia and undergoing clinically indicated coronary angiogram and endothelial function testing. Invasive wire-based mediated functional angiography remains the only definitive diagnostic tool for coronary microvascular dysfunction today, and the cath lab remains an example of the translation of basic science principles to simplifying diagnostic techniques and ultimately finding a safe, disease-modifying, and effective therapy for coronary and peripheral endothelial dysfunction.

References

1. Rubanyl GM, Frye RL, Holmes DR Jr, Vanhoutte PM. Vasoconstrictor activity of coronary sinus plasma from patients with coronary artery disease. J Am Coll Cardiol. 1987;9(6):1243–9.
2. Furchgott RF, Cherry PD, Zawadzki JV, Jothianandan D. Endothelial cells as mediators of vasodilation of arteries. J Cardiovasc Pharmacol. 1984;6(Suppl 2):S336–43.
3. Furchgott RF, Zawadzki JV. The obligatory role of endothelial cells in the relaxation of arterial smooth muscle by acetylcholine. Nature. 1980;288(5789):373–6.
4. Lerman A, Webster MW, Chesebro JH, Edwards WD, Wei CM, Fuster V, et al. Circulating and tissue endothelin immunoreactivity in hypercholesterolemic pigs. Circulation. 1993;88(6):2923–8.
5. Badimon L, Badimon JJ, Penny W, Webster MW, Chesebro JH, Fuster V. Endothelium and atherosclerosis. J Hypertens Suppl. 1992;10(2):S43–50.
6. Nishimura RA, Lerman A, Chesebro JH, Ilstrup DM, Hodge DO, Higano ST, et al. Epicardial vasomotor responses to acetylcholine are not predicted by coronary atherosclerosis as assessed by intracoronary ultrasound. J Am Coll Cardiol. 1995;26(1):41–9.
7. Gutiérrez E, Flammer AJ, Lerman LO, Elízaga J, Lerman A, Fernández-Avilés F. Endothelial dysfunction over the course of coronary artery disease. Eur Heart J. 2013;34(41):3175–81.
8. Yoon MH, Reriani M, Mario G, Rihal C, Gulati R, Lennon R, et al. Long-term endothelin receptor antagonism attenuates coronary plaque progression in patients with early atherosclerosis. Int J Cardiol. 2013;168(2):1316–21.

9. Godo S, Corban MT, Toya T, Gulati R, Lerman LO, Lerman A. Association of coronary microvascular endothelial dysfunction with vulnerable plaque characteristics in early coronary atherosclerosis. EuroIntervention. 2020;16(5):387–94.

10. Lavi S, Bae JH, Rihal CS, Prasad A, Barsness GW, Lennon RJ, et al. Segmental coronary endothelial dysfunction in patients with minimal atherosclerosis is associated with necrotic core plaques. Heart. 2009;95(18):1525–30.

11. Hasdai D, Gibbons RJ, Holmes DR Jr, Higano ST, Lerman A. Coronary endothelial dysfunction in humans is associated with myocardial perfusion defects. Circulation. 1997;96(10):3390–5.

12. Summers MR, Lerman A, Lennon RJ, Rihal CS, Prasad A. Myocardial ischaemia in patients with coronary endothelial dysfunction: insights from body surface ECG mapping and implications for invasive evaluation of chronic chest pain. Eur Heart J. 2011;32(22):2758–65.

13. Cassar A, Chareonthaitawee P, Rihal CS, Prasad A, Lennon RJ, Lerman LO, et al. Lack of correlation between noninvasive stress tests and invasive coronary vasomotor dysfunction in patients with nonobstructive coronary artery disease. Circ Cardiovasc Interv. 2009;2(3):237–44.

14. Suwaidi JA, Hamasaki S, Higano ST, Nishimura RA, Holmes DR Jr, Lerman A. Long-term follow-up of patients with mild coronary artery disease and endothelial dysfunction. Circulation. 2000;101(9):948–54.

15. Targonski PV, Bonetti PO, Pumper GM, Higano ST, Holmes DR Jr, Lerman A. Coronary endothelial dysfunction is associated with an increased risk of cerebrovascular events. Circulation. 2003;107(22):2805–9.

16. Wilson SH, Simari RD, Best PJ, Peterson TE, Lerman LO, Aviram M, et al. Simvastatin preserves coronary endothelial function in hypercholesterolemia in the absence of lipid lowering. Arterioscler Thromb Vasc Biol. 2001;21(1):122–8.

17. Lerman A, Burnett JC Jr, Higano ST, McKinley LJ, Holmes DR Jr. Long-term L-arginine supplementation improves small-vessel coronary endothelial function in humans. Circulation. 1998;97(21):2123–8.

18. Reriani M, Raichlin E, Prasad A, Mathew V, Pumper GM, Nelson RE, et al. Long-term administration of endothelin receptor antagonist improves coronary endothelial function in patients with early atherosclerosis. Circulation. 2010;122(10):958–66.

19. Corban MT, Lerman LO, Lerman A. Ubiquitous yet unseen: microvascular endothelial dysfunction beyond the heart. Eur Heart J. 2018;39(46):4098–100.

20. Corban MT, Godo S, Burczak DR, Noseworthy PA, Toya T, Lewis BR, et al. Coronary endothelial dysfunction is associated with increased risk of incident atrial fibrillation. J Am Heart Assoc. 2020;9(8):e014850.

21. Ahmad A, Corban MT, Toya T, Verbrugge FH, Sara JD, Lerman LO, et al. Coronary microvascular dysfunction is associated with exertional haemodynamic abnormalities in patients with heart failure with preserved ejection fraction. Eur J Heart Fail. 2021;23(5):765–72.

22. Borlaug BA, Olson TP, Lam CS, Flood KS, Lerman A, Johnson BD, et al. Global cardiovascular reserve dysfunction in heart failure with preserved ejection fraction. J Am Coll Cardiol. 2010;56(11):845–54.

23. Reriani M, Flammer AJ, Li J, Prasad M, Rihal C, Prasad A, et al. Microvascular endothelial dysfunction predicts the development of erectile dysfunction in men with coronary atherosclerosis without critical stenoses. Coron Artery Dis. 2014;25(7):552–7.

24. Corban MT, Duarte-Garcia A, McBane RD, Matteson EL, Lerman LO, Lerman A. Antiphospholipid syndrome: role of vascular endothelial cells and implications for risk stratification and targeted therapeutics. J Am Coll Cardiol. 2017;69(18):2317–30.

25. Prasad M, McBane R, Reriani M, Lerman LO, Lerman A. Coronary endothelial dysfunction is associated with increased risk of venous thromboembolism. Thromb Res. 2016;139:17–21.

Chapter 10
The Mayo Clinic Hemodynamic Cath Lab: A 70-Year Journey

William R. Miranda and Rick A. Nishimura

Given the widespread and foundational presence of cardiac cath labs in today's medical practice, it might be difficult to imagine that for many years only a few institutions in the United States were able to perform invasive cardiac catheterization procedures or even have the ability to accurately measure and record central cardiac pressures. It is important to remember that the epidemiology of cardiac pathologies was also markedly different 70 years ago. Following the report of the right heart catheterization by Cornaund in 1945 [1], this procedure was predominantly applied to the evaluation of individuals with congenital heart disease. The pivotal importance of hemodynamic assessment in the care of patients with congenital heart disease also contributed to the geography of cardiac catheterization centers during that time. It was not unexpected that cath labs at Johns Hopkins and the former Peter Bent Hospital (led by Dr. Richard Bing and Dr. Lewis Dexter, respectively) emerged while supporting their clinical and surgical practices; these laboratories rapidly became an integral part in the management of these patients. Similarly, with the introduction of cardiopulmonary bypass during surgical repairs for complex congenital heart disease by Dr. John Kirklin and his colleagues, who included physiologists, pediatric and adult cardiologists, biomedical engineers, and anatomists, there was a need for a cardiac cath lab at Mayo Clinic that paralleled the inventiveness and progress of brilliant surgical peers. This was the birth of Mayo's catheterization practice and the beginning of a journey of excellence in clinical care, research, and education that forged our current practice and values. This chapter summarizes this journey, with particular emphasis on its evolution.

W. R. Miranda (✉) · R. A. Nishimura
Department of Cardiovascular Diseases, Mayo Clinic, Rochester, MN, USA
e-mail: miranda.william@mayo.edu

© Mayo Foundation for Medical Education and Research,
under exclusive license to Springer Nature Switzerland AG 2021
D. R. Holmes Jr., R. L. Frye (eds.), *The Mayo Clinic Cardiac Catheterization Laboratory*, https://doi.org/10.1007/978-3-030-79329-6_10

The 1950–1960s: Birth Defects and Rheumatic Heart Disease

Like any new technique, the introduction of catheterization into clinical practice mandated an understanding of expected findings in normal individuals before being applied to diseased states. Selection bias in series of patients undergoing invasive hemodynamic studies remains inevitable in today's practice, as healthy individuals are not typically subjected to invasive procedures. Certainly, individuals with cyanotic heart disease could not be used to derive normative values. Under the guidance of Dr. Earl Wood, a true pioneer and visionary, Mayo Clinic played a central role in describing the normal hemodynamic findings at the time of cardiac catheterization [2]. The observations of his seminal work "Cardiac output and related measurements and pressure values in the right heart and associated vessels, together with an analysis of the hemodynamic response to the inhalation of high oxygen mixtures in healthy subjects" [3] are used worldwide each time a right heart catheterization is performed. The intimate relationship between cardiac physiology and cardiac surgery is also illustrated in this manuscript. The first author, Dr. Barratt-Boyes, at the time a mentee of Dr. Kirklin's, went on to become an internationally renowned congenital surgeon and one of the fathers of cardiac surgery in New Zealand.

One aspect of the methodology in the derivation of normative values in these early studies in healthy individuals deserves mentioning, particularly when analyzed in today's practice and regulations. These studies were predominantly performed in young male individuals; indeed these were primarily performed on trainees that "volunteered" for the procedures. It should be noted that internal medicine residents were required to spend a year in a clinical laboratory. Perhaps driven by a mixture of inquisitiveness, selflessness, and naivety, or the desire to study scientific endeavors as part of their training and eventual careers, it is doubtful that these young subjects could foresee that they were contributing to the foundation of an entire subspecialty.

The early scientific contributions by Dr. Wood deserve a full monograph given how prolific and novel they were. A few of them deserve highlighting:

1. The definition of a "step-up" in the diagnosis of intracardiac shunts [4] – using successive O_2 saturation measurements in 26 healthy individuals, Dr. Wood described the expected blood oximetry findings and proposed cutoffs (e.g., a "step-up" of 8% from the superior vena cava to the right atrium) for the diagnosis of left-to-right shunt. Subsequently studied and validated by others, this technique is (or at least ideally should be) an integral part of every right heart catheterization procedure.

2. Pulmonary artery wedge pressure measurement as a surrogate for left atrial pressure [5] – Dr. Daniel Connolly and Dr. Wood validated the technique initially described Dr. Lewis Dexter [6], who "accidentally" advanced a catheter into the pulmonary artery wedge position while performing catheterization of renal veins. Dr. Dexter's report and the Mayo Clinic experience provided the foundation for the ubiquitous use of pulmonary artery wedge pressure in cardiac catheterization in subsequent decades, including today's practice. Importantly, they

highlighted that normally blood oxygen saturations should always exceed 95% regardless of whether central cyanosis due to ventilation-perfusion mismatch or right-to-shunt is present, a mandatory step to appropriate "wedging" that is still sometimes forgotten.

3. Use of dye-dilution curves – the so-called "green-dye" curves were introduced by Dr. Wood in our practice both for the diagnosis of intra- and extracardiac shunts [7, 8]. His work detailed the expected findings related to different arterial and venous sample sites according to each congenital lesion, also correlating these observations with blood oximetry results. Dye-dilution curves continued to be used routinely in the diagnosis of intracardiac shunts at Mayo Clinic for almost 50 years. The same principle was subsequently applied for the diagnosis of regurgitant valvular lesions [9], being instrumental in intraoperative assessment of valvular interventions prior to intraoperative transesophageal echocardiography. Lastly, "green-dye" curves for the calculation of flow (i.e., cardiac output [10]; Fig. 10.1) provided the basis for the development of the currently used thermodilution method, which now uses cold saline in lieu of indocyanine dye.

4. Description of pulmonary vein wedge pressure measurement – this subsequent observation by Drs. Connolly and Wood is of great historical value [11]. In an elegant study, they proved that discordant pressure recordings are obtained when "wedging" the pulmonary vasculature from opposite sides, namely, pressures obtained from the pulmonary artery vasculature versus the pulmonary vein. Therefore, they suggested that it would be more appropriate to describe the position in which "wedging" was performed rather than using the term "pulmonary capillary wedge pressure" (which would suggest that similar values should be obtained from both sites). Accordingly, at Mayo Clinic and several other centers, most prefer the term "pulmonary artery wedge pressure" instead of "capillary."

5. Supine exercise studies during cardiac catheterization – exercise hemodynamic studies are now routinely done in our cardiac cath lab, and Mayo Clinic has played a major role in demonstrating their invaluable role in evaluation of patients with heart failure or unexplained dyspnea. However, some might not be

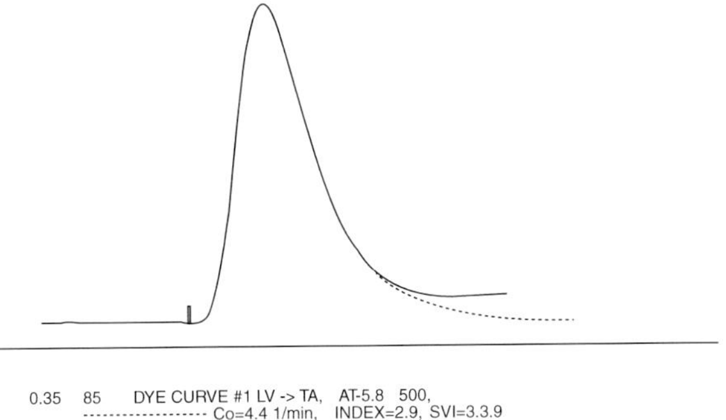

Fig. 10.1 Calculation of cardiac output.
Typical green-dye curve used for the calculation of cardiac output (4.4 l/min); in this case, dye was injected into the left ventricle and the femoral artery sampled. Note the similar appearance to the curves currently obtained by the thermodilution method

aware that supine bicycle exercise has been performed in the cardiac cath lab at our institution for more than 60 years [12]. These were initially performed in patients with congenital heart disease to study the exercise-induced changes in intracardiac and pulmonary pressures as well as flow during exercise [13]. This is even more impressive when one considers that most centers still find exercising during catheterization not feasible from a logistical standpoint.

6. Description of the catheterization findings in constrictive pericarditis [14] – one of the first descriptions of constrictive physiology during catheterization stemmed from our laboratory, highlighting the equalization of diastolic pressures and the typical contour of ventricular tracings. This work marked the beginning of a long tradition in the study of hemodynamic evaluation of constriction at Mayo Clinic.

An illustrative example of impressive work performed by Dr. Wood in the early 1950s is shown in Fig. 10.2. Dr. Wood was accompanied by another pioneer while establishing Mayo's cardiac catheterization practice – Dr. Jeremy Swan. While at Cedars-Sinai, Dr. Swan, together with Dr. William Ganz and Dr. James Forrester, developed the first balloon-tipped catheter for right heart catheterization [15]. Prior to moving to California, Dr. Swan was the head of the Mayo Clinic clinical cardiac cath lab, making numerous contributions in the field of congenital heart disease and later to the assessment of valvular disorders.

While at Mayo Clinic, Dr. Swan also mentored Dr. Shahbudin Rahimtoola, who later became a prominent cardiologist worldwide and an expert in valvular disorders. Prior to focusing on the hemodynamics in valvular disease, Dr. Rahimtoola authored important studies in congenital heart disease, including hemodynamics of single ventricle [16] and the use of the Radner procedure in patients with transposition of great vessels [17]. The Radner procedure was used for percutaneous access to the vessels and cardiac chambers, popularized in the evaluation of mitral and aortic valve diseases. A thin needle would be advanced from the base of the neck until the desired pressure measurement was obtained (frequently aortic, pulmonary, and left atrium, in this order; retrograde left ventricular access was also possible). Almost unimaginable in current practice (the method was abandoned after the introduction of transseptal and retrograde left ventricular catheterization), the Radner procedure deserves mention, as it illustrates the evolution in techniques for hemodynamic assessment.

The 1950s should also be credited for the introduction of transseptal catheterization for the measurement of the left atrial and ventricular pressures. Prior to the description of the transseptal puncture at the National Institutes of Health, in addition to the Radner procedure, two other techniques that are now of historical interest had been used to gain access to the left atrium: the posterior transthoracic (via a paravertebral puncture site) and the transbronchial approach [18]. Although transseptal catheterization was initially developed for diagnostic purposes, it provided the foundation for a number of percutaneous interventions performed in the Mayo Clinic laboratory in the 1990s and onward [19].

a

PLEASE FILE WITH HISTORY.

PHYSIOLOGY
Mayo Clinic—Rochester, Minnesota

Sheet No. _________

RESPIRATORY AND CARDIOVASCULAR LABORATORIES

DIRECT ARTERIAL PRESSURE STUDIES

No. _________ Name _________

Referred by _________

Diagnosis _ Coarctation

Simultaneous recordings were made of the intra-arterial blood pressure in the right radial artery at the wrist and the right femoral artery at Poupart's ligament   Heart rate was also recorded

The results of the tests are given in the table below. Done during catheterization.

Time of test	Heart rate	Radial pressure mm Hg		Femoral pressure mm Hg		Systolic pressure ratio femoral/radial	Pulse pressure ratio femoral/radial	Delay in onset of femoral pulse seconds	Femoral pulse build-up time seconds
		Systolic	Diastolic	Systolic	Diastolic				
Pre-operative	80	193	88	93	80	0.48	.13	.02	0.17
Post operative									
Normal subjects. Average and extreme values	64 (46 81)	130 (122 142)	68 (65 70)	127 (120 134)	64 (58 69)	0.99 (0.94 1.05)	1.02 (0.89 1.20)	0.00 (−0.01 +0.01)	0.15 (0.13-0.18)
21 patients with coarctation average and extreme values	80 (54 115)	194 (161 230)	96 (76 136)	113 (87 143)	81 (63 104)	0.59 (0.43 0.72)	0.33 (0.16 0.48)	0.03 (0.01 <0.07)	0.23 (0.17-0.30)

MC-441   (over)

b

PLEASE FILE WITH HISTORY.

PHYSIOLOGY
Mayo Clinic—Rochester, Minnesota

Sheet No. _________

CARDIOVASCULAR AND RESPIRATORY LABORTORIES

Cardiac Catheterization

No. _________ Name _________

Time	Rec. no.	Source of blood sample	Pressure (mm. Hg)	X-ray film no.	Blood sample no.	Oxygen content (vol. %)	Oxygen capacity (vol. %)	Van Slyke % sat.	Total % sat. cuvette	% art. sat. earpiece
		On air:								
9:20	3	Inferior vena cava	8/6	1	A*				75.0	96.0
9:21	4	Mid-right atrium	8/3	—	B*				77.0	96.0
9:22	7	Superior vena cava	11/6	2	C*				73.0	96.0
9:23	—	Mid-right atrium	—	—	D*				75.0	97.0
9:23	6	Inferior vena cava at diaphragm	8/5	—	E*				70.0	97.0
9:25	—	Inferior vena cava at diaphragm	—	—	F*(1)				76.0	97.0
9:26	7	Mid-right atrium	8/4	—	G*				72.0	97.0
9:27	8	Superior vena cava	8/6	—	H*				75.0	97.0
9:28	—	Right lobe hepatic wedge	—	—	I				79.0	97.0
9:30	11	Right ventricle	43/9	—	J*				71.0	97.0
9:31	12	Right atrium	7/5	—	K*				72.0	97.0
9:36	—	Coronary sinus	—	—	7.5.1	4.5	15.6	28.2	30.0	98.0
9:43	—	Right ventricular outflow	—	—	L				67.0	97.0
9:45	14	Pulmonary trunk	37/20	—	—				70.0	97.0
9:46	—	Right lower lobe wedge attempted	—	—	M				70.0	97.0
9:50	15	Right lower lobe wedge	Mean 27(2)	3	N				91.0	97.0
9:51	16	Right lower lobe wedge	(Mean 23) 30/16(1)	—	O				91.0	96.0
9:57	22	Right lower lobe (lateral) wedge	28/16(2)	—	P				99.0	96.0
9:58	23	Right pulmonary artery	37/18	—	—					
10:10	24	Radial	139/101	—	2	15.6	15.6	96.0	98.0	96.0
10:16	25	Right pulmonary artery	42/21	—	3	11.4	15.5	72.0	74.0	

MC-441   (over)

Fig. 10.2 Illustrative cardiac catheterization report from Mayo Clinic's 1950s Physiology laboratory procedural report from a cardiac catheterization performed for the investigation of coarctation of the aorta. Panel A provides values for radial and femoral artery pressures in normal individuals and summarizes the laboratory's experience in patients with coarctation. Panel B presents serial intracardiac pressure measurements and blood oximetry samples; the red asterisks mark samples drawn consecutively (without reinfusing blood or using saline flushes), a standard for a Mayo Clinic laboratory given its increased accuracy. Panel C provides the interpretation of the procedure, performed by Dr. Earl Wood. Note the comment regarding the contour of pulmonary artery wedge pressure as a marker of mitral regurgitation

c

Time	Rec. no.	Source of blood sample	Pressure (mm. Hg)	X-ray film no.	Blood sample no.	Total Oxygen content (vol. %)	Oxygen capacity (vol. %)	Van Slyke % sat.	% sat. cuvette	% art. sat. earpiece
10:21	—	100% oxygen								100.0
10:25	26	Radial)simul- taneous on O₂	184/100							
10:25	26	Right pulmonary artery)	39/19	4						
10:30	—	Dye #1 (right pulmonary artery)								
10:36	35	Left mid-lung wedge	23/10(1)						99.0	99.0
10:50	—	Dye #2 (left pulmonary artery)		5						
11:00	—	Dye #3 (pulmonary trunk)		6						
11:03	—	Pulmonary trunk			R*				76.0	
11:05	37	Right ventricular outflow	41/10		S*				76.0	
11:06	38	Mid-right atrium	10/5		T*(1)				82.0	
11:07	40	Inferior vena cava	11/7		U*				80.0	
11:08	41	Mid-right atrium	13/7		V*				77.0	
11:09	—	Superior vena cava		7	W*				75.0	
11:12	—	Dye curve #4 (superior vena cava)								
11:18	—	Radial artery			4	17.2	16.1	100.0	98.0	96.0
11:19	—	100% oxygen discontinued.								
11:23	43	Radial)simul-	202/90(2)							
11:23	43	Femoral)taneous	100/??							
11:23	43	Superior vena cava)	10/6							
11:30	53	Right radial)simultaneous	193/88							
11:30	53	Right femoral)	93/80							
		End procedure.								

$$\text{Cardiac output} = \frac{209}{15.6 - 11.4} = 5.0 \ \text{L/Min.} \qquad \text{Cardiac Index} = \frac{5.0}{1.28} = 3.9 \ \text{L/Min./M}^2$$

Metabolic studies:
Metabolic rate =
O_2 consumption = 209   cc./min-
CO_2 output = 186   cc./min.
R. Q. = 0.89
Surface area = 1.28   sq./meters

Copy to: Dr. DuShane

Dye curves: Within normal range.

* consecutive samples.

(1) Contour of wedge pressures shows prominent V-wave which is compatible with mitral insufficiency.

(2) see coarctation report (ATTACHED)

Operator: Dr. E. H. Wood

Signed _J. Leo Wright_
J. L. Wright, M.D.

Fig. 10.2 (continued)

The 1960s also demonstrated a broadening in the scope of pathologies assessed in the cardiac cath lab. The initial studies focused on typical findings of different congenital cardiac disorders, and subsequent studies reported hemodynamic determinants of surgical outcomes and mortality. In addition, a number of manuscripts reported changes in hemodynamics postoperatively. This decade also marked the beginning of a series of studies focused on mitral valve disorders. With the introduction of open mitral commissurotomy, a new therapeutic window was opened for the treatment of rheumatic mitral stenosis, a highly prevalent, debilitating, and potentially fatal disease. Similar to congenital pathologies, an accurate preoperative diagnosis was crucial, as a mistaken diagnosis of the major mitral valve lesion was of great importance as patients with dominant mitral stenosis could be well treated with commissurotomy. In contrast, a patient with predominant mitral regurgitation would not benefit from such a procedure and would have been unnecessarily exposed to one that carried significant morbidity and even mortality. The height of pulmonary artery wedge pressure v-waves as a sign of underlying mitral regurgitation was proposed to aid in the differentiation between mitral stenosis and regurgitation [20]. This simple and astute observation has survived the test of time (and echocardiography) and continues to be a useful tool in the invasive evaluation of mitral disorders and the response to percutaneous mitral valve interventions.

The 1970s: Emphasis on Ischemic Heart Disease

The introduction of selective coronary angiography in 1958 by Dr. F. Mason Sones [21] and subsequent contributions from the 1960s revolutionized the understanding of coronary artery disease and its impact on left ventricular function. Combined with the wide use of coronary artery bypassing grafting beginning in the 1960s and, particularly, the 1970s, the demographics of patients referred for cardiac catheterization dramatically changed.

Mirroring these advances, the contribution from Mayo Clinic also evolved. Under the guidance of Dr. Robert Frye, a series of studies focused on ischemic heart disease were undertaken. These ranged from acute medication-induced changes in hemodynamics (e.g., glucagon and nitroglycerin [22, 23]) to the impact of coronary artery bypass grafting on left ventricular hemodynamics and function. An invaluable contribution to literature from this period involves exercise hemodynamic studies in individuals with coronary artery disease compared to normal individuals [24, 25]. Some cardiologists and cath lab staff members might be unaware that these studies actually established the cutoffs for abnormal left ventricular filling during exercise (pulmonary artery wedge pressure ≥ 25 mmHg) that are still used in our laboratory [26] and worldwide.

In parallel to these changes in patients with acquired heart disease, the laboratory continued to be active in studying congenital heart diseases through the work of Drs. Ritter, Mair, and, later, Dr. Hagler. The publications reflected the many transformations in the care of these patients, for example, the hemodynamic assessment and midterm outcomes following the atrial switch operation for the treatment of complete transposition of the great vessels [27, 28]. This decade was also punctuated by the initial Mayo Clinic experience with the Fontan operation, a pioneering surgical endeavor that would forever change pediatric and adult congenital heart disease at the clinic [29].

Paradoxically, in the 1970s, the cardiac cath lab also gave birth to the current version of the Mayo Clinic Echocardiography Laboratory. The acquisition of a transthoracic M-mode echocardiography machine by Drs. Don Ritter, A. Jamil Tajik, and Frye to be solely used during cardiac catheterization procedures allowed echocardiography correlations with angiographic and hemodynamic data never previously performed [30, 31]. Drs. Tajik and James Seward initiated a series of landmark studies on multiple congenital pathologies that would ultimately result in the establishment of the *Mayo Clinic Echocardiography and Hemodynamic Laboratory* under their leadership. This close relationship between echocardiography and catheterization would prove to be instrumental for subsequent Doppler-catheterization studies, a hallmark of Mayo Clinic in the 1980–2000s.

The 1980–1990s: The Doppler-Cardiac Catheterization Studies

The 1980s brought the advent of Doppler echocardiography, which showed promise as a noninvasive modality to measure blood flow velocities for assessment of patients with valvular heart disease, measurement of intracardiac pressures, and evaluation of diastolic filling. However, there was initial skepticism as to the accuracy of this methodology. The Mayo Clinic Cath Lab played an essential role in evaluating the utility of Doppler echocardiography through a series of studies in which Doppler velocity curves in different disease states were obtained simultaneously with the gold standard of invasive catheterization hemodynamic pressures. This work was made possible by the combined leadership of Dr. David Holmes, chief of the Cardiac Cath Lab, and Dr. Tajik, chief of the Echocardiography Laboratory. It was through these studies that Doppler echocardiography has become well accepted as a noninvasive alternative for assessment of hemodynamics. In addition, the combined information from simultaneous Doppler-catheterization studies was then used as a powerful tool for investigating the underlying pathophysiology of various cardiac disorders.

The initial skepticism as to the accuracy of Doppler echocardiography stemmed from early studies comparing Doppler assessment of aortic valve gradients in patients with aortic stenosis to the gold standard of cardiac catheterization. These studies were retrospective nonsimultaneous studies that resulted in a gross "underestimation" of the severity of stenosis by Doppler echocardiography. However, Mayo Clinic studies subsequently showed that there was an excellent correlation between the instantaneous gradients from direct pressure measurements in the cath lab and simultaneous Doppler velocity curves. The previously described discrepancies were due to the fact that the peak aortic Doppler velocities derived from the modified Bernoulli equation measured the peak instantaneous gradient, while the standard aortic valve measurement in the cardiac catheterization was a peak-to-peak gradient – two different measurements from different times in the cardiac cycle. In addition, there were frequently different loading conditions between an outpatient examination and the cardiac catheterization examination, which directly affect the aortic valve gradient. Using simultaneous noninvasive and invasive measurements, Mayo Clinic studies clearly showed an extremely high correlation of the now widely used mean gradient between the two techniques. This excellent correlation was initially demonstrated in the animal cath lab by Drs. Mark Callahan, Alfred Bove, and A. Jamil Tajik [32], in which simultaneous Doppler echocardiography was performed and compared to direct pressure measurements with increasing severity of stenosis from a band around the ascending aorta. Subsequent simultaneous studies in the cardiac cath lab, through the work of Dr. Phil Currie and Dr. Tajik, showed an excellent correlation of the mean aortic valve gradient in patients with aortic stenosis [33]. The Doppler echocardiographic measurement of pressure gradients was shown to be accurate for patients with right ventricular outflow tract obstruction and

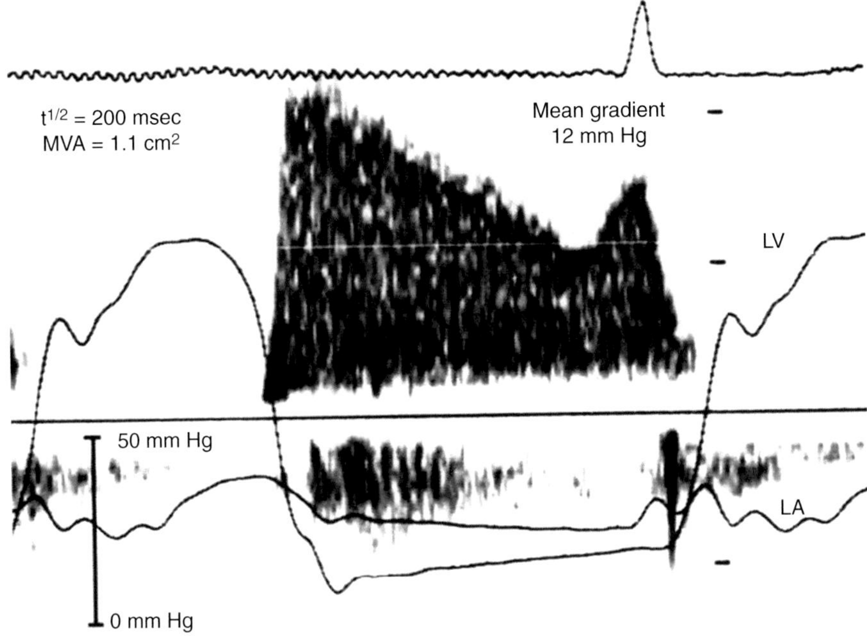

Fig. 10.3 Simultaneous Doppler and catheterization findings in mitral stenosis. Illustrative tracings show continuous-wave Doppler interrogation of the mitral valve with simultaneous left ventricular and direct left atrial pressures

those with the dynamic outflow tract obstruction of hypertrophic cardiomyopathy [34]. Gradients across prosthetic valves were shown to be similarly measured by Doppler echocardiography and cardiac catheterization [35]. Going one step further, the mean gradient and mitral stenosis measured by Doppler echocardiography (Fig. 10.3) was found to be more accurate in measuring the true left atrial to left ventricular pressure gradient than the conventional cardiac catheterization measurement using pulmonary artery wedge pressure [36].

The measurement of Doppler velocities from valve regurgitation jets was then applied for determination of intracardiac pressures. Again, simultaneous studies were performed, first examining the tricuspid regurgitation Doppler velocities (Fig. 10.4) as a method to obtain the right ventricular-right atrial pressure gradient [37]. Excellent correlations between the Doppler velocities and absolute catheterization studies were shown, resulting in a noninvasive method for determination of pulmonary artery systolic pressures. Similar correlations between the Doppler velocities and direct pressure measurements were shown with aortic regurgitation, mitral regurgitation, and pulmonary regurgitation [38], allowing determination of left ventricular end-diastolic pressures, left atrial pressures, and pulmonary artery end-diastolic pressures. The instantaneous changes in pressure gradients allowed determination of other ventricular function parameters such as positive dP/dt and

Fig. 10.4 Noninvasive estimation of right ventricular systolic pressure. Simultaneous right ventricular tracings and continuous-wave Doppler interrogation of the tricuspid regurgitation jet in a patient with normal pulmonary pressures

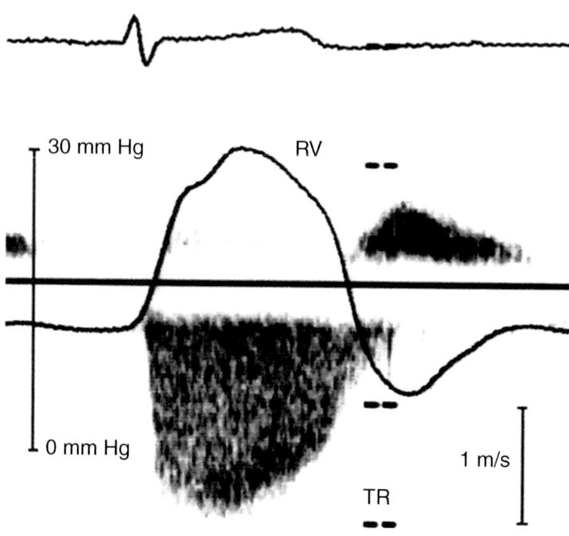

the time constant of relaxation from the mitral regurgitation and tricuspid regurgitation signals [39].

Assessment of volumetric flow, or stroke volume, was thought to be possible using pulse-wave Doppler interrogation of areas of laminar flow. Simultaneous Doppler-catheterization demonstrated the usefulness of this approach from interrogation of both the ascending aorta and left ventricular outflow tract [40]. This subsequently led to the concept of using a continuity equation to determine valve areas, in addition to the information from pressure gradients. The correlation of aortic valve areas from Doppler echocardiography compared to valve area from the Gorlin equation at catheterization was spear-headed by Dr. Jae Oh and remains a standard in all echocardiographic laboratories [41].

A major contribution to the understanding of cardiac hemodynamics that has become widely used is the analysis of diastolic filling of the heart from Doppler flow velocities across the mitral valve, compared to simultaneous high-fidelity intracardiac pressure measurements. Dr. Liv Hatle from Norway, a renowned hemodynamic investigator, spent several years on sabbatical at Mayo Clinic. Through a series of simultaneous Doppler-catheterization studies, Dr. Hatle and Mayo Clinic staff proposed a practical approach for the evaluation of diastolic filling of the left ventricle. This resulted in a noninvasive methodology for determination of left ventricular filling pressures and provided the foundation for the well-accepted four stages of diastolic function. Incremental accuracy for determination of filling pressures was provided by further studies of pulmonary vein velocities [42] and, subsequently, Doppler tissue imaging [43].

Of particular interest was the use of hemodynamics to differentiate between constrictive pericarditis and other causes of significant right heart failure. The early work in the 1960s by Connolly et al. established that early rapid filling, elevation, and end-equalization of pressures were a necessary finding to diagnose constrictive pericarditis. However, these findings could also be present in other types of abnormalities resulting in right heart failure, particularly restrictive cardiomyopathy. Through intricate simultaneous Doppler and cardiac catheterization analysis, the concept of dynamic respiratory changes found in constrictive pericarditis was evaluated (Fig. 10.5) and found to accurately differentiate constrictive pericarditis from restrictive myocardial disease [44]. Thus, using either cardiac catheterization or Doppler echocardiography, the finding of dissociation of intra-thoracic and intra-cardiac pressures combined with enhancement of ventricular interaction has become a standard by which constrictive pericarditis is now diagnosed. The incremental utility of Doppler tissue imaging (annulus reversus and annulus paradoxus), tricuspid regurgitation signals, and hepatic vein velocity curves were shown through further evaluation with simultaneous echocardiography and high-fidelity manometer-tipped catheters [45–47].

Through these simultaneous Doppler-catheterization studies, the Mayo Clinic investigators developed a powerful diagnostic methodology that combined both Doppler flow velocities and high-fidelity manometer-tipped intracardiac pressures.

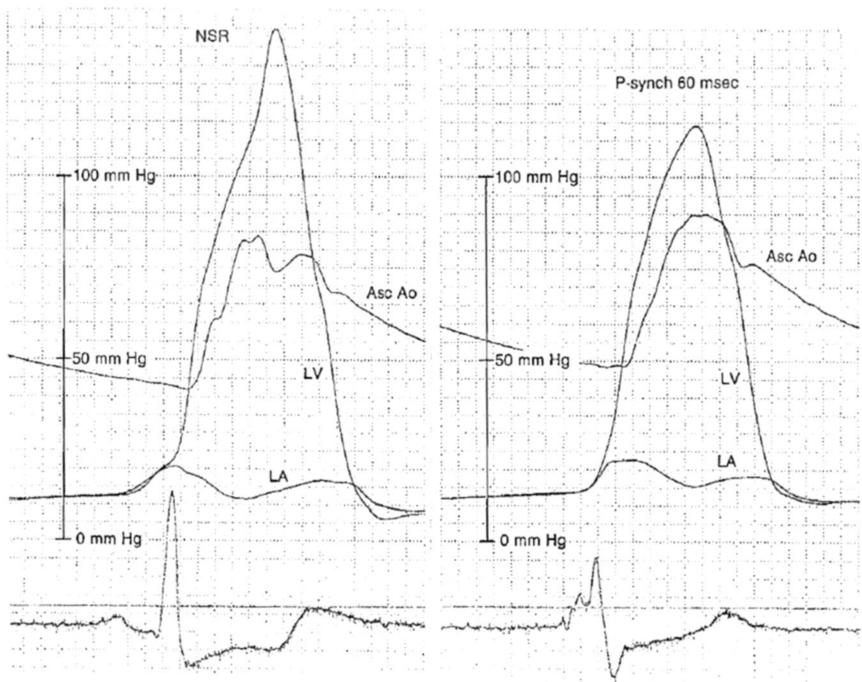

Fig. 10.5 Effects of pacing on obstructive hypertrophic cardiomyopathy.
Simultaneous left ventricular, aortic, and left atrial tracings were obtained via transseptal catheterization. The left panel demonstrates severe resting dynamic left ventricular obstruction while the patient is in sinus rhythm. After initiation of dual-chamber pacing (*right panel*), there is a marked decrease in the left ventricular outflow gradient with the typical "spike-and-dome" aortic contour no longer present

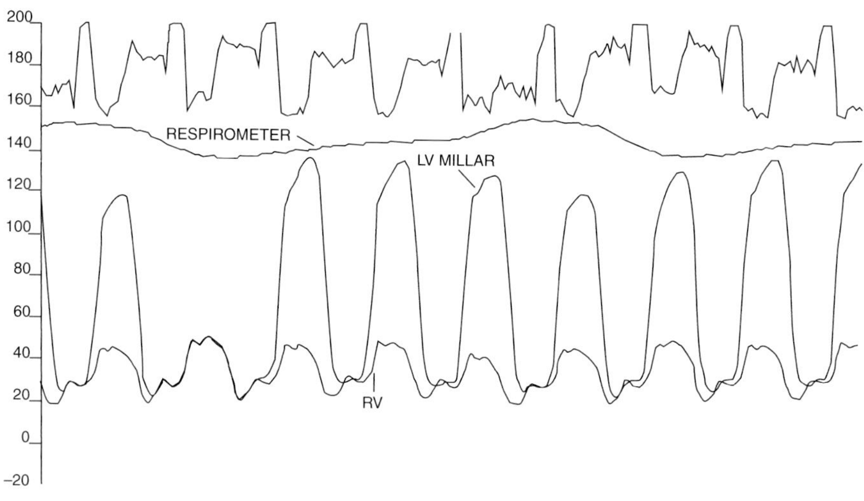

Fig. 10.6 Simultaneous right and left ventricular tracings in constrictive pericarditis
Typical findings of ventricular interdependence in a patient with constrictive pericarditis is demonstrated on simultaneous right and left ventricular tracings. At peak inspiration (sixth beat), reciprocal/discordant changes are seen in right and left ventricular peak systolic pressures and width of tracings themselves. Pulsus paradoxus is also present

Utilization of additional changes in ventricular loading and contractility by intravenous drug infusions and exercise further added to the diagnostic approach. This was and is now applied clinically for many patients presenting with complex cardiac presentations of valvular, myocardial, and pericardial disease, in whom the diagnosis cannot be made on the basis of conventional noninvasive testing. In addition, this combined Doppler-catheterization assessment of hemodynamics was used to study the underlying pathophysiologic mechanisms of different diseases and interventions. These included (1) insights into the effect of dual chamber pacing for both dilated cardiomyopathies and hypertrophic cardiomyopathies [48–50] (Fig. 10.6), (2) evaluation of patients with low flow-low gradient aortic stenosis [51], and (3) the effect of catheter-based therapies (septal ablation, balloon valvotomy) on ventricular function and outcome [52, 53].

The 2000–2010s: Further Understanding of Heart Failure and the Rise of Exercise Hemodynamics

The previous work demonstrating the role of noninvasive estimation of left filling pressures extended into different pathologies during this era. For example, our laboratory reported the limited performance of mitral E/e' as a surrogate for left ventricular mean diastolic pressure in individuals with hypertrophic cardiomyopathy [54]. In addition, it provided one of first studies evaluating the performance of noninvasive estimation of pulmonary artery wedge pressure during exercise [55]. This subject was revisited a decade later in one of the largest cohorts of patients undergoing simultaneous exercise right heart catheterization and echo-Doppler for the evaluation of dyspnea [56].

The initial description of the "dynamic criteria" for constrictive pericarditis was also refined in a subsequent publication, augmenting its performance for the recognition of ventricular interdependence [57]. Criteria for the differentiation between constrictive pericarditis and tricuspid regurgitation, a conundrum that had challenged clinician for decades, were also proposed [58]. The understanding of underlying hemodynamics in patients with severe tricuspid regurgitation was further enhanced when exercise-related hemodynamics changes were studied [59], demonstrating severe elevation in biventricular filling pressures during exertion and, thus, explaining the presence of dyspnea in some of these individuals.

The contribution from the Mayo Clinic cath lab for the invasive evaluation of valvular disorders during this time has been extensive. Accumulating data from the classic study describing the presence of left ventricular contractile reserve in low-flow, low-gradient severe aortic stenosis [51] and related prognosis/surgical outcomes to now refining the diagnosis of true low-flow, low-gradient aortic stenosis remains of great interest [60]. More recently we have characterized the low-flow variant of mitral valve stenosis [61]. Mayo Clinic has also introduced a technique for continuous left atrial pressure measurement during percutaneous mitral valve repair [62]. This technique consists of placing a 4F multipurpose catheter into the left atrium adjacent to the steerable device sheath, providing real-time hemodynamic monitoring during mitral valve interventions. Proposed by Dr. Charanjit Rihal, this approach, shown to predict outcomes, is now widely used in other centers.

Perhaps the most striking change in the way hemodynamic catheterization studies are currently performed in our laboratory is related to the use of exercise hemodynamics. Originally reported as providing incremental diagnostic information in patients with early heart failure [26], subsequent studies have confirmed its value, as nearly half of patients with heart failure will have normal resting hemodynamics [56]. The work of Dr. Barry Borlaug has transformed the practice at Mayo Clinic, and typically 5–10 exercise studies are performed in our cardiac cath lab daily. His group has also elegantly described numerous diagnostic and pathophysiologic studies in heart failure.

Similar to the work performed at our institution 60 years ago, we continue to study the impact of newly adopted interventions (now via percutaneous approach) on right and left ventricular hemodynamics in patients with valvular and congenital heart diseases [63–65]. These methodical observations remain critical for the optimal care of patients at Mayo Clinic as novel procedures are introduced into clinical practice.

The Future

As one reviews the advances in cardiology over the past 50 years, the dynamic nature of this subspecialty is made clear. Driven by the introduction of new percutaneous and surgical interventions, the field is constantly evolving. In addition, as the population ages, diseases themselves change. This is reflected in the current challenges in the management of degenerative mitral and aortic disorders and tricuspid regurgitation. As very successful therapies for congenital heart disease have been applied at younger ages, and the population continues to grow older, a new specialty of adult congenital heart disease has developed with unique features and issues. This group will continue to grow. Other groups of patients and diseases continue to be explored. Despite the major advances in the treatment of heart failure with reduced ejection fraction, therapy for those with preserved ejection fraction remains incipient. In these patients there will be interest in cell therapeutics for strategies of care. As we embark on a new decade, our mission remains to continue the legacy of the Mayo Clinic hemodynamic laboratory in supporting the demands of clinical care with meticulous, high-quality hemodynamic data, advancing the field from a research and innovation standpoint, and, similar to Drs. Wood, Swan, and others, educating the hemodynamic experts of the future.

References

1. Cournand A, Riley RL, Breed ES, Baldwin ED, Richards DW, Lester MS, et al. Measurement of cardiac output in man using the technique of catheterization of the right auricle or ventricle. J Clin Invest. 1945;24(1):106–16.
2. Wood EH. Normal oxygen saturation of arterial blood during inhalation of air and oxygen. J Appl Physiol. 1949;1(8):567–74.
3. Barratt-Boyes BG, Wood EH. Cardiac output and related measurements and pressure values in the right heart and associated vessels, together with an analysis of the hemo-dynamic response to the inhalation of high oxygen mixtures in healthy subjects. J Lab Clin Med. 1958;51(1):72–90.
4. Barratt-Boyes BG, Wood EH. The oxygen saturation of blood in the venae cavae, right-heart chambers, and pulmonary vessels of healthy subjects. J Lab Clin Med. 1957;50(1):93–106.
5. Connolly DC, Kirklin JW, Wood EH. The relationship between pulmonary artery wedge pressure and left atrial pressure in man. Circ Res. 1954;2(5):434–40.
6. Hellems HK, Haynes FW, Dexter L. Pulmonary capillary pressure in man. J Appl Physiol. 1949;2(1):24–9.
7. Swan HJ, Zapata-Diaz J, Wood EH. Dye dilution curves in cyanotic congenital heart disease. Circulation. 1953;8(1):70–81.
8. Broadbent JC, Wood EH. Indicator-dilution curves in acyanotic congenital heart disease. Circulation. 1954;9(6):890–902.
9. Woodward E Jr, Swan HJ, Wood EH. Evaluation of a method for detection of mitral regurgitation from indicator-dilution curves recorded from the left atrium. Proc Staff Meet Mayo Clin. 1957;32(19):525–35.
10. Hetzel P, Swan HJ, Ramirez De Arellano AA, Wood EH. Estimation of cardiac output from first part of arterial dye-dilution curves. J Appl Physiol. 1958;13(1):92–6.

11. Connolly DC, Wood EH. The pulmonary vein wedge pressure in man. Circ Res. 1955;3(1):7–13.
12. Barratt-Boyes BG, Wood EH. Hemodynamic response of healthy subjects to exercise in the supine position while breathing oxygen. J Appl Physiol. 1957;11(1):129–35.
13. Swan HJ, Marshall HW, Wood EH. The effect of exercise in the supine position on pulmonary vascular dynamics in patients with left-to-right shunts. J Clin Invest. 1958;37(2):202–13.
14. Connolly DC, Wood EH. Cardiac catheterization in heart failure and cardiac constriction. Trans Am Coll Cardiol. 1957;7:191–201.
15. Thakkar AB, Desai SP. Swan, Ganz, and their catheter: its evolution over the past half century. Ann Intern Med. 2018;169(9):636–42.
16. Rahimtoola SH, Ongley PA, Swan HJ. The hemodynamics of common (or single) ventricle. Circulation. 1966;34(1):14–23.
17. Rahimtoola SH, Ongley PA, Swan HJ. Percutaneous suprasternal puncture (Radner technique) of the pulmonary artery in transposition of the great vessels. Circulation. 1966;33(2):242–8.
18. Ross J Jr. Transseptal left heart catheterization a 50-year odyssey. J Am Coll Cardiol. 2008;51(22):2107–15.
19. Holmes DR Jr, Hildner FJ. Transseptal catheterization 1992: it is here to stay. Catheter Cardiovasc Diagn. 1992;26(4):264–5.
20. Connolly DC, Wood EH. Hemodynamic data during rest and exercise in patients with mitral valve disease in relation to the differentiation of stenosis and insufficiency from the pulmonary artery wedge pressure pulse. J Lab Clin Med. 1957;49(4):526–44.
21. Sones FM Jr, Shirey EK. Cine coronary arteriography. Mod Concepts Cardiovasc Dis. 1962;31:735–8.
22. Campion BC, Frye RL, Zitnik RS. Effects of nitroglycerin on capacitance vessels: a mechanism for reduction of left ventricular end-diastolic pressure. Mayo Clin Proc. 1970;45(8):573–8.
23. Greenberg BH, McCallister BD, Frye RL. Effects of glucagon on resting and exercise haemodynamics in patients with coronary heart disease. Br Heart J. 1972;34(9):924–9.
24. Saltups A, McCallister BD, Hallermann FJ, Wallace RB, Smith RE, Frye RL. Left ventricular hemodynamics in patients with coronary artery disease and in normal subjects. Correlations with the extent of coronary artery lesions and the electrocardiogram. Am J Med. 1971;50(1):8–19.
25. Rutherford BD, Gau GT, Danielson GK, Pluth JR, Davis GD, Wallace RB, et al. Left ventricular haemodynamics before and soon after saphenous vein bypass graft operation for angina pectoris. Br Heart J. 1972;34(11):1156–62.
26. Borlaug BA, Nishimura RA, Sorajja P, Lam CS, Redfield MM. Exercise hemodynamics enhance diagnosis of early heart failure with preserved ejection fraction. Circ Heart Fail. 2010;3(5):588–95.
27. Hagler DJ, Ritter DG, Mair DD, Davis GD, McGoon DC. Clinical, angiographic, and hemodynamic assessment of late results after mustard operation. Circulation. 1978;57(6):1214–20.
28. Hagler DJ, Ritter DG, Mair DD, Tajik AJ, Seward JB, Fulton RE, et al. Right and left ventricular function after the mustard procedure in transposition of the great arteries. Am J Cardiol. 1979;44(2):276–83.
29. Gale AW, Danielson GK, McGoon DC, Mair DD. Modified Fontan operation for univentricular heart and complicated congenital lesions. J Thorac Cardiovasc Surg. 1979;78(6):831–8.
30. Ritter DG, Seward JB, Moodie D, Danielson GK. Univentricular heart (common ventricle): preoperative diagnosis. Hemodynamic, angiocardiographic and echocardiographic features. Herz. 1979;4(2):198–205.
31. Wilcox WD, Seward JB, Hagler DJ, Mair DD, Tajik AJ. Discrete subaortic stenosis: two-dimensional echocardiographic features with angiographic and surgical correlation. Mayo Clin Proc. 1980;55(7):425–33.
32. Callahan MJ, Tajik AJ, Su-Fan Q, Bove AA. Validation of instantaneous pressure gradients measured by continuous-wave Doppler in experimentally induced aortic stenosis. Am J Cardiol. 1985;56(15):989–93.

33. Currie PJ, Seward JB, Reeder GS, Vlietstra RE, Bresnahan DR, Bresnahan JF, et al. Continuous-wave Doppler echocardiographic assessment of severity of calcific aortic stenosis: a simultaneous Doppler-catheter correlative study in 100 adult patients. Circulation. 1985;71(6):1162–9.
34. Currie PJ, Hagler DJ, Seward JB, Reeder GS, Fyfe DA, Bove AA, et al. Instantaneous pressure gradient: a simultaneous Doppler and dual catheter correlative study. J Am Coll Cardiol. 1986;7(4):800–6.
35. Burstow DJ, Nishimura RA, Bailey KR, Reeder GS, Holmes DR Jr, Seward JB, et al. Continuous wave Doppler echocardiographic measurement of prosthetic valve gradients. A simultaneous Doppler-catheter correlative study. Circulation. 1989;80(3):504–14.
36. Nishimura RA, Rihal CS, Tajik AJ, Holmes DR Jr. Accurate measurement of the transmitral gradient in patients with mitral stenosis: a simultaneous catheterization and Doppler echocardiographic study. J Am Coll Cardiol. 1994;24(1):152–8.
37. Currie PJ, Seward JB, Chan KL, Fyfe DA, Hagler DJ, Mair DD, et al. Continuous wave Doppler determination of right ventricular pressure: a simultaneous Doppler-catheterization study in 127 patients. J Am Coll Cardiol. 1985;6(4):750–6.
38. Nishimura RA, Tajik AJ. Determination of left-sided pressure gradients by utilizing Doppler aortic and mitral regurgitant signals: validation by simultaneous dual catheter and Doppler studies. J Am Coll Cardiol. 1988;11(2):317–21.
39. Chung N, Nishimura RA, Holmes DR Jr, Tajik AJ. Measurement of left ventricular dp/dt by simultaneous Doppler echocardiography and cardiac catheterization. J Am Soc Echocardiogr. 1992;5(2):147–52.
40. Nishimura RA, Callahan MJ, Schaff HV, Ilstrup DM, Miller FA, Tajik AJ. Noninvasive measurement of cardiac output by continuous-wave Doppler echocardiography: initial experience and review of the literature. Mayo Clin Proc. 1984;59(7):484–9.
41. Oh JK, Taliercio CP, Holmes DR Jr, Reeder GS, Bailey KR, Seward JB, et al. Prediction of the severity of aortic stenosis by Doppler aortic valve area determination: prospective Doppler-catheterization correlation in 100 patients. J Am Coll Cardiol. 1988;11(6):1227–34.
42. Nishimura RA, Abel MD, Hatle LK, Tajik AJ. Relation of pulmonary vein to mitral flow velocities by transesophageal Doppler echocardiography. Effect of different loading conditions. Circulation. 1990;81(5):1488–97.
43. Ommen SR, Nishimura RA, Appleton CP, Miller FA, Oh JK, Redfield MM, et al. Clinical utility of Doppler echocardiography and tissue Doppler imaging in the estimation of left ventricular filling pressures: a comparative simultaneous Doppler-catheterization study. Circulation. 2000;102(15):1788–94.
44. Hurrell DG, Nishimura RA, Higano ST, Appleton CP, Danielson GK, Holmes DR Jr, et al. Value of dynamic respiratory changes in left and right ventricular pressures for the diagnosis of constrictive pericarditis. Circulation. 1996;93(11):2007–13.
45. Ha JW, Oh JK, Ling LH, Nishimura RA, Seward JB, Tajik AJ. Annulus paradoxus: transmitral flow velocity to mitral annular velocity ratio is inversely proportional to pulmonary capillary wedge pressure in patients with constrictive pericarditis. Circulation. 2001;104(9):976–8.
46. Klodas E, Nishimura RA, Appleton CP, Redfield MM, Oh JK. Doppler evaluation of patients with constrictive pericarditis: use of tricuspid regurgitation velocity curves to determine enhanced ventricular interaction. J Am Coll Cardiol. 1996;28(3):652–7.
47. Reuss CS, Wilansky SM, Lester SJ, Lusk JL, Grill DE, Oh JK, et al. Using mitral 'annulus reversus' to diagnose constrictive pericarditis. Eur J Echocardiogr. 2009;10(3):372–5.
48. Nishimura RA, Hayes DL, Holmes DR Jr, Tajik AJ. Mechanism of hemodynamic improvement by dual-chamber pacing for severe left ventricular dysfunction: an acute Doppler and catheterization hemodynamic study. J Am Coll Cardiol. 1995;25(2):281–8.
49. Nishimura RA, Hayes DL, Ilstrup DM, Holmes DR Jr, Tajik AJ. Effect of dual-chamber pacing on systolic and diastolic function in patients with hypertrophic cardiomyopathy. Acute Doppler echocardiographic and catheterization hemodynamic study. J Am Coll Cardiol. 1996;27(2):421–30.

50. Nishimura RA, Trusty JM, Hayes DL, Ilstrup DM, Larson DR, Hayes SN, et al. Dual-chamber pacing for hypertrophic cardiomyopathy: a randomized, double-blind, crossover trial. J Am Coll Cardiol. 1997;29(2):435–41.
51. Nishimura RA, Grantham JA, Connolly HM, Schaff HV, Higano ST, Holmes DR Jr. Low-output, low-gradient aortic stenosis in patients with depressed left ventricular systolic function: the clinical utility of the dobutamine challenge in the catheterization laboratory. Circulation. 2002;106(7):809–13.
52. Klarich KW, Rihal CS, Nishimura RA. Variability between methods of calculating mitral valve area: simultaneous Doppler echocardiographic and cardiac catheterization studies conducted before and after percutaneous mitral valvuloplasty. J Am Soc Echocardiogr. 1996;9(5):684–90.
53. Nishimura RA, Holmes DR Jr, Reeder GS, Tajik AJ, Hatle LK. Doppler echocardiographic observations during percutaneous aortic balloon valvuloplasty. J Am Coll Cardiol. 1988;11(6):1219–26.
54. Geske JB, Sorajja P, Nishimura RA, Ommen SR. Evaluation of left ventricular filling pressures by Doppler echocardiography in patients with hypertrophic cardiomyopathy: correlation with direct left atrial pressure measurement at cardiac catheterization. Circulation. 2007;116(23):2702–8.
55. Talreja DR, Nishimura RA, Oh JK. Estimation of left ventricular filling pressure with exercise by Doppler echocardiography in patients with normal systolic function: a simultaneous echocardiographic-cardiac catheterization study. J Am Soc Echocardiogr. 2007;20(5):477–9.
56. Obokata M, Kane GC, Reddy YN, Olson TP, Melenovsky V, Borlaug BA. Role of diastolic stress testing in the evaluation for heart failure with preserved ejection fraction: a simultaneous invasive-echocardiographic study. Circulation. 2017;135(9):825–38.
57. Talreja DR, Nishimura RA, Oh JK, Holmes DR. Constrictive pericarditis in the modern era: novel criteria for diagnosis in the cardiac catheterization laboratory. J Am Coll Cardiol. 2008;51(3):315–9.
58. Jaber WA, Sorajja P, Borlaug BA, Nishimura RA. Differentiation of tricuspid regurgitation from constrictive pericarditis: novel criteria for diagnosis in the cardiac catheterisation laboratory. Heart. 2009;95(17):1449–54.
59. Andersen MJ, Nishimura RA, Borlaug BA. The hemodynamic basis of exercise intolerance in tricuspid regurgitation. Circ Heart Fail. 2014;7(6):911–7.
60. Lloyd JW, Nishimura RA, Borlaug BA, Eleid MF. Hemodynamic response to nitroprusside in patients with low-gradient severe aortic stenosis and preserved ejection fraction. J Am Coll Cardiol. 2017;70(11):1339–48.
61. El Sabbagh A, Reddy YNV, Barros-Gomes S, Borlaug BA, Miranda WR, Pislaru SV, et al. Low-gradient severe mitral stenosis: hemodynamic profiles, clinical characteristics, and outcomes. J Am Heart Assoc. 2019;8(5):e010736.
62. Eleid MF, Sanon S, Reeder GS, Suri RM, Rihal CS. Continuous left atrial pressure monitoring during MitraClip: assessing the immediate hemodynamic response. JACC Cardiovasc Interv. 2015;8(7):e117–9.
63. Eleid MF, Padang R, Pislaru SV, Greason KL, Crestanello J, Nkomo VT, et al. Effect of transcatheter aortic valve replacement on right ventricular-pulmonary artery coupling. JACC Cardiovasc Interv. 2019;12(21):2145–54.
64. Miranda WR, Hagler DJ, Reeder GS, Warnes CA, Connolly HM, Egbe AC, et al. Temporary balloon occlusion of atrial septal defects in suspected or documented left ventricular diastolic dysfunction: hemodynamic and clinical findings. Catheter Cardiovasc Interv. 2019;93(6):1069–75.
65. Misumida N, Guerrero M, Pislaru SV, Alkhouli M, Rihal CS, Eleid MF. Hemodynamic response to transseptal transcatheter mitral valve replacement in patients with severe mitral stenosis due to severe mitral annular calcification. Catheter Cardiovasc Interv. 2021;97(7):E992–E1001.

Chapter 11
New Insights into Heart Failure: From the Beginning to Now

Barry A. Borlaug

Introduction

In 1929, Werner Forssmann performed the first-known cardiac catheterization in a human being, on himself. Dr. Forssmann advanced a urinary catheter from his antecubital vein into the right atrium, then walked down to the radiology suite to document the event, publishing the results of his self-experiment in 1931. Twelve years later at the Bellevue Hospital in New York, Andre Cournand and Dickinson Richards read his paper and began brainstorming new ideas, opening the door to a new era of cardiac catheterization in clinical cardiology. For the next 40 years, hemodynamic right and left heart catheterizations were performed on a routine basis to define pathophysiology and guide treatment decisions for a wide range of cardiovascular disorders ranging from congenital to structural heart diseases to heart failure (HF).

The late 1980s brought a shift in the United States and Europe coupled with decreased utilization of invasive hemodynamic assessment in clinical cardiology. This shift was related to two key developments occurring around this time. The first was related to rapid advances in the use of echocardiography to noninvasively evaluate cardiac function and estimate hemodynamics, and the second relates to a shift in the catheterization practice from being a diagnostic to a therapeutic laboratory, with the rapidly expanding field of percutaneous coronary intervention. After two decades of decreased utilization, the early 2000s marked the beginning of a new renaissance in the use of invasive hemodynamic assessment in the evaluation and treatment for people with heart failure, which has risen to become even more widespread than ever before.

B. A. Borlaug (✉)
The Department of Cardiovascular Medicine, Mayo Clinic, Rochester, MN, USA
e-mail: borlaug.barry@mayo.edu

© Mayo Foundation for Medical Education and Research,
under exclusive license to Springer Nature Switzerland AG 2021
D. R. Holmes Jr., R. L. Frye (eds.), *The Mayo Clinic Cardiac Catheterization Laboratory*, https://doi.org/10.1007/978-3-030-79329-6_11

The Emergence of a New Gold Standard Test

HF represents the final common symptomatic expression for a wide array of cardio-vascular disorders spanning from ischemic heart disease to hypertensive, congenital, and valvular heart diseases. Heart failure was historically defined clinically, based exclusively upon the impressions of the providing physician from history, physical examination, and radiography [1]. This definition, while useful, is highly subjective, poorly reproducible, and, as we later learned, insufficiently sensitive. In 1971, McKee and colleagues from the Framingham group proposed a new set of diagnostic criteria for HF based upon signs and symptoms and chest X-ray findings, adopting the approach that had previously been applied by Jones for diagnosis of acute rheumatic fever [2]. These criteria were informed by time-honored clinical observations dating back centuries but were not based upon objective quantitative data or a priori definitions of cardiac failure.

Thirty years later, echocardiography was becoming widely used in the evaluation of patients with dyspnea. The demonstration of a reduced ejection fraction (EF) by echocardiography in a patient with dyspnea was taken as strong evidence that left ventricular (LV) systolic dysfunction was present, making the diagnosis of HF and reduced EF (HFrEF) secure. However, around this time it was becoming increasingly evident that roughly half of patients with the clinical syndrome of HF in fact had a normal EF [3]. These patients were initially referred to as having "diastolic HF" because systolic function (estimated crudely by the EF) was normal or near normal. Subsequent studies identified subtle but important deficits in systolic function that are present despite a normal EF, as well as other nondiastolic mechanisms, leading to the use of the term HF with preserved EF (HFpEF) to describe this condition [3].

Since those early descriptions, there has been a steady increase in the incidence and prevalence of HFpEF [4], while incidence of HFrEF has been decreasing, likely related to improved treatments for ischemic heart disease [5]. HFpEF is mechanistically tied to comorbid conditions that have become highly prevalent in Western societies in the modern era, in particular, obesity, hypertension, and diabetes, making this the most common form of HF among older adults in the United States [6]. The Framingham criteria described above can certainly be applied to make the diagnosis of HFpEF, just as they can for HFrEF, but an important limitation is that the Framingham criteria reflect congestion that is present at the time of evaluation, at rest, and that also rely heavily on the presence of right-sided HF. Thus the Framingham criteria refer mostly to patients with acutely decompensated HF, often requiring hospitalization. Echocardiography had been relied upon to estimate filling pressures, but a number of studies had raised questions regarding the accuracy of noninvasive estimates for cardiac filling pressures as compared to direct invasive measures [7, 8]. Unlike HFrEF, we could not simply look at the EF to determine whether a patient has HF.

Thus with this burgeoning epidemic there was a critical unmet need for a method to diagnose (or exclude) HFpEF among ambulatory patients who were not volume-overloaded at the time of assessment in the clinic and therefore did not meet the Framingham criteria. Ideally, HF should not be defined subjectively but conceptually and using objective, measurable quantities that reflect this conceptual definition. The hemodynamic definition of HF is an inability of the heart to pump blood to the body at a rate commensurate with its needs at normal diastolic filling pressures [9–11]. Therefore, a patient with typical symptoms (e.g., dyspnea and fatigue) meeting these criteria with normal EF ($\geq$50%) should be properly diagnosed as having HFpEF.

This definition is very important because it includes variables that can be directly and quantitatively measured in the catheterization laboratory (filling pressures, cardiac output). Importantly, this definition of HFpEF does not simply refer to rest, as it also encompasses the ability of the heart to fulfill its duties during stress. The most common stress encountered in everyday life is physical exercise, and this is where patients with HFpEF experience symptoms. Thus, to adequately address the question as to whether a patient has HFpEF, we reasoned that it was necessary to perform hemodynamic measurements both at rest and then again during the stress of exercise. Exercise taxes the heart due to marked increases in venous return along with changes in heart rate, contractility, and loading conditions. Most patients with HF are not symptomatic at rest, but they are symptomatic during exercise. Why then would we conclude that they do not have HF based upon the observation of normal resting hemodynamics? To do so would be analogous to reassuring a patient with exertional angina and severe stenosis in the left anterior descending artery that they do not have coronary disease based upon a normal resting ECG or perfusion scan. It is the application of stress that is critical to reach the correct diagnosis.

Thus, around 2006 we began to perform right heart catheterization at rest and during supine exercise in the Mayo Clinic Cath Lab in the diagnostic evaluation of HFpEF. The first studies were performed variably using arm weights or isometric handgrip devices, as vascular access was often performed through the femoral artery and vein. However, we soon appreciated that the degree of hemodynamic duress that could be recreated with upper body exercise alone was not sufficient. Blood pressure and arterial afterload may increase dramatically with upper arm exercise, but changes in heart rate and venous return are much less dramatic as compared with dynamic lower extremity exercise, leading us to switch to supine cycle ergometry. Using jugular and radial artery access, we were able to free up the legs for exercise, and we soon appreciated the incredible diagnostic power of this new testing modality.

Following the first 6 invasive exercise tests performed to evaluate for HFpEF in 2006, we observed a steady increase in referrals for evaluation, such that just one decade later the Mayo Clinic Cath Lab was performing over 400 invasive hemodynamic exercise tests per year. We published our initial experience with invasive exercise testing in 2010, showing for the first time that despite normal clinical findings at rest, just over half of patients referred to the lab showed conclusive hemodynamic evidence of HF when evaluated during the stress of exercise, defined as an increase in pulmonary capillary wedge pressure (PCWP) to 25 mmHg or higher during exertion [11]. At the time it was believed that echocardiographic abnormalities or elevation in plasma natriuretic peptide levels were necessary for diagnosis of HFpEF, and this paper demonstrated that was not the case, pointing to the importance of exercise assessment. Less than a decade later in 2019, expert consensus guidelines from the European Society of Cardiology emphasized invasive hemodynamic exercise testing as the gold standard to diagnose HFpEF [12], and today this test is performed yearly in over 400 Mayo Clinic patients with unexplained dyspnea.

New Insights from Exercise Testing

Performance of invasive exercise testing in the evaluation of HF led to a number of new pathophysiologic observations that have just begun to reshape how we conceptualize and treat HFpEF. One observation of clinical importance is the great challenge of how to treat an abnormality (elevation in LV filling pressures) that develops only during exercise. Prescribing a patient a diuretic or vasodilator when pressures are normal at rest could be hazardous, as it may precipitate hypotension or azotemia, especially among older patients who may be more vulnerable. What was needed was a "magic bullet" that would be more effective to reduce LV filling pressures selectively during exercise, without causing excessive preload reduction at rest [11].

Around 2009 we began performing echocardiography simultaneously with invasive exercise testing to learn more about diastolic compliance properties in the pathophysiology of HFpEF. Recent studies had raised questions with the primary role of diastolic dysfunction in this disorder, something that had not been questioned for years [13]. Pressure can be measured with exquisite precision and accuracy using high-fidelity micromanometers in the catheterization lab, but assessment of LV volumes is more challenging, particularly during exercise. Integrating LV volume during exercise based upon transmitral Doppler flow profiles, we were able to generate single beat LV end-diastolic pressure volume relationships (EDPVR) at rest and during exercise [14]. We observed that the EDPVR in HFpEF was indeed shifted upward and to the left, in keeping with increased diastolic stiffness, but during exercise, the EDPVR shifted upward in parallel, an effect that could be caused by an increase in external restraint on the heart, mediated by the pericardium. It was known from prior studies that pericardial restraint and right heart compression across the septum account for ~40% of measured LV diastolic pressure [15], and in older animal studies where the pericardium is removed, the EDPVR shifts to the right (less stiff, lower pressure relative to volume) and peak aerobic capacity improves [16, 17]. This led to the birth of a new idea: could an intervention to remove pericardial restraint lower filling pressures and therefore improve symptoms in patients with HFpEF?

We then set out to test this hypothesis, first in bench studies, then in beating heart experiments performed in normal dogs, and then in a porcine model of HFpEF using the Mayo animal catheterization laboratory in the Stabile building. However, even if this technique were to be effective, uptake could be limited. Patients with HFpEF are often elderly and frail, with multiple comorbidities. This makes a conventional surgical pericardiectomy less palatable. However, we suspected that simply opening the anterolateral pericardium over the LV might produce similar results, and if this could be accomplished percutaneously, the eligible patient population would be greatly expanded. In the first set of experiments, we showed that while LV end-diastolic pressure (LVEDP) at rest was not affected by pericardiectomy, the increase in LVEDP in response to saline loading (as a surrogate for exercise) was substantially attenuated, an effect that would be expected to reduce lung congestion and dyspnea [18]. Remarkably, the benefit was just as great with percutaneous anterior pericardiotomy performed with the chest intact as it was with full pericardiectomy. We then went on to show that pericardiotomy produced similar hemodynamic benefits in humans evaluated at the time of cardiac surgery [19] and that the effects were sustained chronically in the animal model of HFpEF. This series of work finally culminated in the first human study conducted at Mayo Clinic in collaboration with Dr. Phillip Rowse and Dr. Hartzell Schaff, where we have performed surgical anterior pericardiotomy in four women suffering with severe, recalcitrant HFpEF. All of the patients have reported improvement, and three of four have reported major improvements in activity tolerance and quality of life. We are currently in the process of further developing this approach as a novel treatment for patients with HFpEF.

In addition to surgical or device-based interventions, there could also be pharmacologic treatments that preferentially target the increase in LVEDP that occurs during exercise in people with HFpEF. Inorganic nitrite (NO_2) is one such molecule. Nitrite was formerly considered to be an inert byproduct of nitric oxide (NO) metabolism, but a number of seminal studies conducted at the NIH showed that nitrite in fact serves as a novel NO donor that is activated during exercise as venous pH and O_2 content decrease, essentially a hypoxia-sensitive vasodilator [20, 21]. This led us to hypothesize that nitrite could mitigate the rise in LVEDP that occurs during exercise (where venous hypoxia and acidosis occur) in patients with HFpEF. To test this hypothesis, we conducted an acute, single-dose randomized clinical trial in the Mayo Clinic Cath Lab enrolling patients who had been referred clinically for exercise catheterization [22]. We observed that, as compared to placebo, patients treated with nitrite had much less increase in pulmonary capillary wedge pressure (PCWP) and pulmonary artery (PA) pressure with exercise, with an improvement in cardiac output. We went on to replicate this finding using an inhaled form of nitrite [23]. This served as the basis for a multicenter trial of inhaled nitrite in HFpEF [24]. While this trial proved neutral, a number of ongoing studies from our group and others are currently testing oral formulations of nitrite, which are hoped to be effective to improve hemodynamics and clinical status in HFpEF.

Other studies have also targeted exercise-induced elevations in PCWP in patients with HF since these earlier experiences, including studies testing a novel device that creates an interatrial shunt to reduce left atrial pressure in HFpEF [25] and other studies using alternative pharmacologic approaches including phosphodiesterase 5 inhibitors, sodium glucose protein transport inhibitors, and calcium sensitizers [26, 27]. New studies on the horizon at Mayo Clinic will test the effects of other novel approaches in the catheterization laboratory on hemodynamic endpoints, including pharmacologic weight loss strategies for patients with obesity, transvascular splanchnic nerve ablation, and an implantable PA balloon device to improve vascular compliance.

One consistent observation from invasive hemodynamic testing independent of diastolic dysfunction is that many patients with HFpEF display abnormal pulmonary vascular dilatation during exercise, even when resting vascular function appears relatively normal [28]. In an earlier study we had shown that patients with HFpEF display marked pulmonary vasodilation in response to the beta-adrenergic agonist dobutamine, significantly greater than the amount of vasodilation seen in people without HF [29]. While dobutamine is a parenteral drug that is not suitable for chronic use, we extended this observation to suggest a new hypothesis: that albuterol, a commonly used inhaled beta-agonist, might improve pulmonary vascular reserve with exercise in HFpEF. To test this hypothesis, we conducted a randomized double-blind placebo-controlled trial in the laboratory, again evaluating patients with HFpEF who had been referred for clinical testing, where it was found that albuterol improves dynamic pulmonary vasodilation during exercise to enhance right heart function and left heart filling [30]. A larger, longer duration follow-up trial is currently in the planning stages.

The invasive hemodynamic practice has afforded an incredible opportunity to make other observations to help gain a richer understanding of HF. Notable observations in this regard include a direct comparison of saline loading and exercise [31], an evaluation of the effects of high PCWP on breathing mechanics and pulmonary reserve [32], exploration of the hemodynamic determinants of lung congestion during exercise [33], evaluations on the role of cardiac ischemia and injury on cardiac function and hemodynamics [34], effects of neurohormonal activation [35], the impact of obesity and visceral fat [36, 37], effects of therapeutic left-to-right shunt on the pulmonary vasculature [38], and unique hemodynamic signatures of patients with HFpEF and severe pulmonary hypertension [39]. None of this would have been possible without a world-class dedicated catheterization laboratory staffed with expert, highly committed team members and, most importantly, patients who were willing to give of their time and body to participate in clinical research in order to advance the science and help others, even when they had little to gain themselves.

Memorable and Instructive Cases

While research is richly rewarding in itself, the greatest satisfaction in academic medicine comes from playing a role to help arrive at the correct diagnosis and administer treatments that help people to feel better. The culture at Mayo Clinic dating back to the very beginning emphasizes the needs of the patient, and this culture has promoted an uncompromising and often aggressive diagnostic workup that is pursued to reach the correct diagnosis. Many times these "n of one" series can incubate new ideas that are translated to other diagnostic and treatment modalities. While there are too many instructive cases to review here, there are a few that stick out as being particularly notable.

One was the case of a 76-year-old man with HFpEF and a history of atrial fibrillation found to have elevated pulmonary artery pressures by echocardiography. His primary complaint was of exercise-induced syncope. He had formerly been very active but had withdrawn from athletics due to concern for falls. He came to the catheterization laboratory where we observed elevated PCWP (30 mmHg), moderate pulmonary hypertension (mean PA 41 mmHg), and normal cardiac index at rest (2.4 l/min*m^2). But like most patients with HFpEF, his main concerns were not of symptoms at rest, but rather with exercise. During supine cycle ergometry at 30 watts, he became dizzy and nearly lost consciousness. At this time his mean PA pressure had increased to 50 mmHg, but his systolic blood pressure dropped from 140 mmHg to 85 mmHg, with reduction in cardiac index to 1.8 l/min*m^2. With cessation of exercise his systemic pressure rose just as his PA pressure returned closer to baseline and cardiac index increased. We reasoned that the exercise-induced pulmonary hypertension had caused acute right heart dilatation, with bowing of the septum toward the LV, leading to LV underfilling and reduction in cardiac output due to Frank Starling failure. Within days of starting a new prescription of low-dose sildenafil (a pulmonary vasodilator), he had no recurrent dizziness and was again playing doubles tennis. His peak oxygen consumption (VO$_2$) during cardiopulmonary exercise testing increased from 10.9 to 14.5 ml/kg/min, with an increase in exercise blood pressure from 72 to 110 mmHg. This case was rewarding in that it led to the correct diagnosis for this man, but this "n of one" observation also inspired a larger series of studies in patients with HFpEF and pulmonary hypertension, showing that the pathophysiology, while extreme in this gentleman, was not peculiar to him but common to others [39].

Another remarkable case was that of a 55-year-old man with idiopathic dilated cardiomyopathy [40]. Prior to the onset of LV dysfunction, he had been a marathon runner, and he continued to be an avid exerciser despite his cardiac failure. His EF was 20% with a dilated LV. At rest his PCWP was 20 mmHg and mean PA pressure 35, with a cardiac output of 4.0 l/min. Strikingly, despite his severe LV dysfunction, he was able to exercise to a peak exercise workload of 120 watts (VO$_2$ 1388 mL/min). Because of his cardiomyopathy, he could only increase cardiac output modestly, to a peak value of 7.9 l/min, which would normally be insufficient to reach this load. However, as dictated by the Fick principle, VO$_2$ is equivalent to the product of cardiac output and arterial-venous O$_2$ content difference (AVO$_2$D). During exercise, whole-body VO$_2$ increases due to combined effects of increases in cardiac output and AVO$_2$D. Because systemic arterial O$_2$ content cannot increase to significant extent (arterial saturation is 94%–100% at rest), AVO$_2$D is augmented predominantly by increased extraction of O$_2$ in the tissues, which reduces mixed venous (PA) O$_2$ content. Two groups of humans have the greatest ability to augment O$_2$ extraction in the tissues: patients with severe HF (an adaptation to chronic hypoperfusion from low output), and elite athletes (who condition skeletal muscle and mitochondria to adapt to very high workloads). This gentleman ticked both boxes and was remarkably able to lower his PA saturation to 6% at peak exercise, the lowest value ever reported in humans [40].

Over the years, the author has repeatedly noted that other extremely active patients seem to be minimally symptomatic with exertion and retain robust functional capacity despite severe impairments in cardiac function. Another example was a 65-year-old man with severe amyloid cardiomyopathy. Resting PCWP was 22 mmHg with a severely depressed cardiac output of 2.7 l/min at rest. During low-level exercise (20 W), his cardiac output increased to 5.1 l/min, but there was no further increase beyond this, even as he continued to exercise through the 40 W, 60 W, 80 W, and 100 W workloads, at which time he was able to reduce his PA saturation to 12%. It was very striking that despite such profound impairment in cardiac output and elevation in filling pressures, he remained minimally symptomatic during submaximal exercise, presumably due to compensations in skeletal muscle involving the afferent pathways that normally communicate metabolic duress to the brain (so-called metaboreceptors). These latter two cases emphasize the remarkable ability of the periphery, including vasculature, endothelium, and skeletal muscle, to compensate for what the heart cannot do in heart failure. This emphasizes the benefits of exercise training, which is one of the few interventions tested to date that has been shown to improve clinical status in patients with HFpEF and one that we continue to test as part of ongoing trials at Mayo Clinic.

Conclusions

Cardiac catheterization was responsible for many of the crucial pathophysiologic observations leading to advances in the field of heart failure since its advent in the 1940s, and after a brief hiatus in the 1990s, its importance is greater now more than ever before. The Mayo Clinic Catheterization Laboratory has been in the center of this renaissance in invasive assessment of HF, and with the rapid expansion of novel, innovative, catheter-based diagnostics and treatments, the coming years are expected to hold even greater promise to make new strides to improve the lives of the patients we care for.

Acknowledgment BAB is supported by R01 HL128526.

References

1. Klainer LM, Gibson TC, White KL. The epidemiology of cardiac failure. J Chronic Dis. 1965;18(8):797–814.
2. McKee PA, Castelli WP, McNamara PM, Kannel WB. The natural history of congestive heart failure: the Framingham study. N Engl J Med. 1971;285(26):1441–6.
3. Pfeffer MA, Shah AM, Borlaug BA. Heart failure with preserved ejection fraction in perspective. Circ Res. 2019;124(11):1598–617.

4. Owan TE, Hodge DO, Herges RM, Jacobsen SJ, Roger VL, Redfield MM. Trends in prevalence and outcome of heart failure with preserved ejection fraction. N Engl J Med. 2006;355(3):251–9.
5. Tsao CW, Lyass A, Enserro D, Larson MG, Ho JE, Kizer JR, et al. Temporal trends in the incidence of and mortality associated with heart failure with preserved and reduced ejection fraction. JACC Heart Fail. 2018;6(8):678–85.
6. Shah AM, Claggett B, Loehr LR, Chang PP, Matsushita K, Kitzman D, et al. Heart failure stages among older adults in the community: the atherosclerosis risk in communities study. Circulation. 2017;135(3):224–40.
7. Mullens W, Borowski AG, Curtin RJ, Thomas JD, Tang WH. Tissue Doppler imaging in the estimation of intracardiac filling pressure in decompensated patients with advanced systolic heart failure. Circulation. 2009;119(1):62–70.
8. Maeder MT, Thompson BR, Brunner-La Rocca HP, Kaye DM. Hemodynamic basis of exercise limitation in patients with heart failure and normal ejection fraction. J Am Coll Cardiol. 2010;56(11):855–63.
9. Obokata M, Kane GC, Reddy YN, Olson TP, Melenovsky V, Borlaug BA. Role of diastolic stress testing in the evaluation for heart failure with preserved ejection fraction: a simultaneous invasive-echocardiographic study. Circulation. 2017;135(9):825–38.
10. Abudiab MM, Redfield MM, Melenovsky V, Olson TP, Kass DA, Johnson BD, et al. Cardiac output response to exercise in relation to metabolic demand in heart failure with preserved ejection fraction. Eur J Heart Fail. 2013;15(7):776–85.
11. Borlaug BA, Nishimura RA, Sorajja P, Lam CS, Redfield MM. Exercise hemodynamics enhance diagnosis of early heart failure with preserved ejection fraction. Circ Heart Fail. 2010;3(5):588–95.
12. Pieske B, Tschope C, de Boer RA, Fraser AG, Anker SD, Donal E, et al. How to diagnose heart failure with preserved ejection fraction: the HFA-PEFF diagnostic algorithm: a consensus recommendation from the Heart Failure Association (HFA) of the European Society of Cardiology (ESC). Eur Heart J. 2019;40(40):3297–317.
13. Kawaguchi M, Hay I, Fetics B, Kass DA. Combined ventricular systolic and arterial stiffening in patients with heart failure and preserved ejection fraction: implications for systolic and diastolic reserve limitations. Circulation. 2003;107(5):714–20.
14. Borlaug BA, Jaber WA, Ommen SR, Lam CS, Redfield MM, Nishimura RA. Diastolic relaxation and compliance reserve during dynamic exercise in heart failure with preserved ejection fraction. Heart. 2011;97(12):964–9.
15. Dauterman K, Pak PH, Maughan WL, Nussbacher A, Arie S, Liu CP, et al. Contribution of external forces to left ventricular diastolic pressure. Implications for the clinical use of the starling law. Ann Intern Med. 1995;122(10):737–42.
16. Hammond HK, White FC, Bhargava V, Shabetai R. Heart size and maximal cardiac output are limited by the pericardium. Am J Phys. 1992;263(6 Pt 2):H1675–81.
17. Stray-Gundersen J, Musch TI, Haidet GC, Swain DP, Ordway GA, Mitchell JH. The effect of pericardiectomy on maximal oxygen consumption and maximal cardiac output in untrained dogs. Circ Res. 1986;58(4):523–30.
18. Borlaug BA, Carter RE, Melenovsky V, DeSimone CV, Gaba P, Killu A, et al. Percutaneous pericardial resection: a novel potential treatment for heart failure with preserved ejection fraction. Circ Heart Fail. 2017;10(4):e003612.
19. Borlaug BA, Schaff HV, Pochettino A, Pedrotty DM, Asirvatham SJ, Abel MD, et al. Pericardiotomy enhances left ventricular diastolic reserve with volume loading in humans. Circulation. 2018;138(20):2295–7.
20. Cosby K, Partovi KS, Crawford JH, Patel RP, Reiter CD, Martyr S, et al. Nitrite reduction to nitric oxide by deoxyhemoglobin vasodilates the human circulation. Nat Med. 2003;9(12):1498–505.
21. Gladwin MT, Shelhamer JH, Schechter AN, Pease-Fye ME, Waclawiw MA, Panza JA, et al. Role of circulating nitrite and S-nitrosohemoglobin in the regulation of regional blood flow in humans. Proc Natl Acad Sci U S A. 2000;97(21):11482–7.

22. Borlaug BA, Koepp KE, Melenovsky V. Sodium nitrite improves exercise hemodynamics and ventricular performance in heart failure with preserved ejection fraction. J Am Coll Cardiol. 2015;66(15):1672–82.
23. Borlaug BA, Melenovsky V, Koepp KE. Inhaled sodium nitrite improves rest and exercise hemodynamics in heart failure with preserved ejection fraction. Circ Res. 2016;119(7):880–6.
24. Borlaug BA, Anstrom KJ, Lewis GD, Shah SJ, Levine JA, Koepp GA, et al. Effect of inorganic nitrite vs placebo on exercise capacity among patients with heart failure with preserved ejection fraction: the INDIE-HFpEF randomized clinical trial. JAMA. 2018;320(17):1764–73.
25. Feldman T, Mauri L, Kahwash R, Litwin S, Ricciardi MJ, van der Harst P, et al. Transcatheter interatrial shunt device for the treatment of heart failure with preserved ejection fraction (REDUCE LAP-HF I [Reduce Elevated Left Atrial Pressure in Patients With Heart Failure]): a phase 2, randomized, sham-controlled trial. Circulation. 2018;137(4):364–75.
26. Andersen MJ, Ersboll M, Axelsson A, Gustafsson F, Hassager C, Kober L, et al. Sildenafil and diastolic dysfunction after acute myocardial infarction in patients with preserved ejection fraction: the Sildenafil and Diastolic Dysfunction After Acute Myocardial Infarction (SIDAMI) trial. Circulation. 2013;127(11):1200–8.
27. Omar M, Jensen J, Frederiksen PH, Kistorp C, Videbaek L, Poulsen MK, et al. Effect of empagliflozin on hemodynamics in patients with heart failure and reduced ejection fraction. J Am Coll Cardiol. 2020;76(23):2740–51.
28. Borlaug BA, Kane GC, Melenovsky V, Olson TP. Abnormal right ventricular-pulmonary artery coupling with exercise in heart failure with preserved ejection fraction. Eur Heart J. 2016;37(43):3293–302.
29. Andersen MJ, Hwang SJ, Kane GC, Melenovsky V, Olson TP, Fetterly K, et al. Enhanced pulmonary vasodilator reserve and abnormal right ventricular: pulmonary artery coupling in heart failure with preserved ejection fraction. Circ Heart Fail. 2015;8(3):542–50.
30. Reddy YNV, Obokata M, Koepp KE, Egbe AC, Wiley B, Borlaug BA. The beta-adrenergic agonist albuterol improves pulmonary vascular reserve in heart failure with preserved ejection fraction. Circ Res. 2019;124(2):306–14.
31. Andersen MJ, Olson TP, Melenovsky V, Kane GC, Borlaug BA. Differential hemodynamic effects of exercise and volume expansion in people with and without heart failure. Circ Heart Fail. 2015;8(1):41–8.
32. Obokata M, Olson TP, Reddy YNV, Melenovsky V, Kane GC, Borlaug BA. Haemodynamics, dyspnoea, and pulmonary reserve in heart failure with preserved ejection fraction. Eur Heart J. 2018;39(30):2810–21.
33. Reddy YNV, Obokata M, Wiley B, Koepp KE, Jorgenson CC, Egbe A, et al. The haemodynamic basis of lung congestion during exercise in heart failure with preserved ejection fraction. Eur Heart J. 2019;40(45):3721–30.
34. Obokata M, Reddy YNV, Melenovsky V, Kane GC, Olson TP, Jarolim P, et al. Myocardial injury and cardiac reserve in patients with heart failure and preserved ejection fraction. J Am Coll Cardiol. 2018;72(1):29–40.
35. Obokata M, Kane GC, Reddy YNV, Melenovsky V, Olson TP, Jarolim P, et al. The neurohormonal basis of pulmonary hypertension in heart failure with preserved ejection fraction. Eur Heart J. 2019;40(45):3707–17.
36. Obokata M, Reddy YN, Pislaru SV, Melenovsky V, Borlaug BA. Evidence supporting the existence of a distinct obese phenotype of heart failure with preserved ejection fraction. Circulation. 2017;136(1):6–19.
37. Sorimachi H, Obokata M, Takahashi N, Reddy YNV, Jain CC, Verbugge FH, et al. Pathophysiologic importance of visceral fat in women with heart failure and preserved ejection fraction. Eur Heart J. 2021;42(16):1595–605.
38. Obokata M, Reddy YNV, Shah SJ, Kaye DM, Gustafsson F, Hasenfubeta G, et al. Effects of interatrial shunt on pulmonary vascular function in heart failure with preserved ejection fraction. J Am Coll Cardiol. 2019;74(21):2539–50.

39. Gorter TM, Obokata M, Reddy YNV, Melenovsky V, Borlaug BA. Exercise unmasks distinct pathophysiologic features in heart failure with preserved ejection fraction and pulmonary vascular disease. Eur Heart J. 2018;39(30):2825–35.
40. Reddy YNV, Obokata M, Haykowsky MJ, Borlaug BA. Skeletal muscle compensation for cardiac muscle insufficiency in heart failure and reduced ejection fraction. Circ Heart Fail. 2018;11(1):e004714.

Chapter 12
Congenital Cardiac Catheterization Lab

Donald J. Hagler, Umberto Squarcia, and Paul R. Julsrud

In the early 1950s, the leadership at the Mayo Clinic worked to establish an effective program for congenital heart disease. Drs. James W. DuShane, Howard B. Burchell, Earl H. Wood, and John W. Kirklin (Fig. 12.1 through Fig. 12.3) were instrumental in this effort. Dr. DuShane was appointed a Mayo Clinic consultant in pediatrics in 1946 and was head of the sections of pediatrics (1957–1969) and pediatric cardiology (1969–1973). He was a member of Mayo Clinic's Board of Governors (1961–1973) and Board of Trustees (1967–1973). It was through the efforts of Drs. DuShane and Kirklin that they were able to achieve in 1955 the first successful closure of a ventricular septal defect at the Mayo Clinic utilizing the Mayo-Gibbon heart-lung machine in a 5-year-old girl. With the advent of cardiopulmonary bypass and open heart surgery at Mayo Clinic, they realized that more accurate diagnosis for potential surgical patients was required.

Dr. Earl Wood, a career investigator of the American Heart Association, established a clinical cardiac catheterization laboratory in the medical sciences building and was the director of that laboratory. From 1955 to 1960, this laboratory carried out diagnostic procedures utilizing pressure measurements, oximetric data, and indocyanine green dye curves with instrumentation often developed in Dr. Wood's research laboratory. The catheterization studies were complex and thorough while improving our knowledge of the physiology of congenital heart disease.

D. J. Hagler (✉)
Department of Cardiovascular Diseases, Mayo Clinic, Rochester, MN, USA
e-mail: Hagler.donald@mayo.edu

U. Squarcia
University of Parma, Italy, Parma, Italy

P. R. Julsrud
Mayo College of Medicine, Mayo Clinic, Rochester, MN, USA
e-mail: Julsrud.paul@mayo.edu

© Mayo Foundation for Medical Education and Research,
under exclusive license to Springer Nature Switzerland AG 2021
D. R. Holmes Jr., R. L. Frye (eds.), *The Mayo Clinic Cardiac Catheterization Laboratory*, https://doi.org/10.1007/978-3-030-79329-6_12

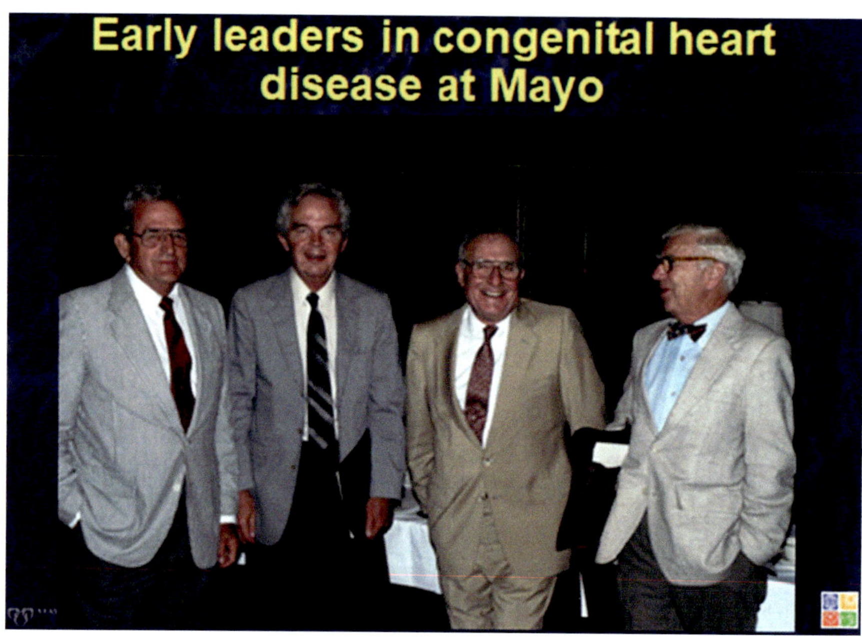

Fig. 12.1 Early leaders in the development of congenital cardiovascular medicine and surgery L–R – James W. DuShane (pediatric cardiology), Dwight C. McGoon (cardiovascular surgery), Jessie E. Edwards (cardiac pathology), and Howard B. Burchell (adult cardiology)

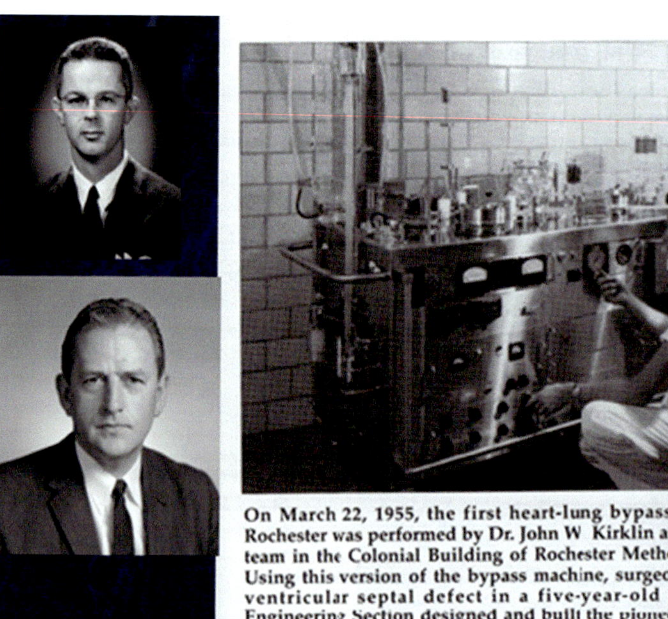

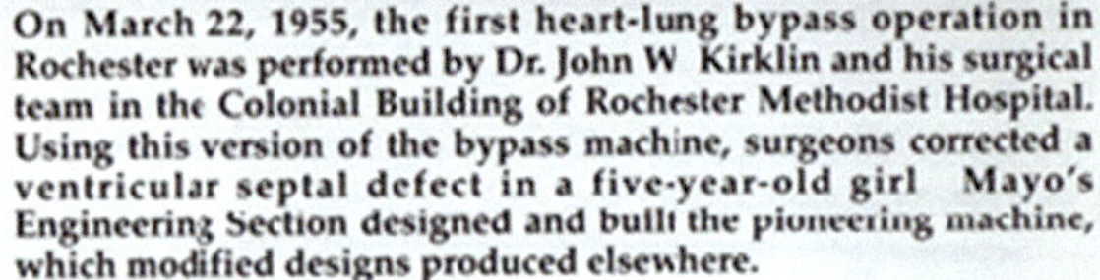
On March 22, 1955, the first heart-lung bypass operation in Rochester was performed by Dr. John W Kirklin and his surgical team in the Colonial Building of Rochester Methodist Hospital. Using this version of the bypass machine, surgeons corrected a ventricular septal defect in a five-year-old girl Mayo's Engineering Section designed and built the pioneering machine, which modified designs produced elsewhere.

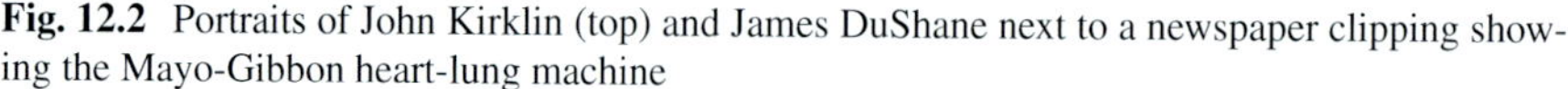

Fig. 12.2 Portraits of John Kirklin (top) and James DuShane next to a newspaper clipping showing the Mayo-Gibbon heart-lung machine

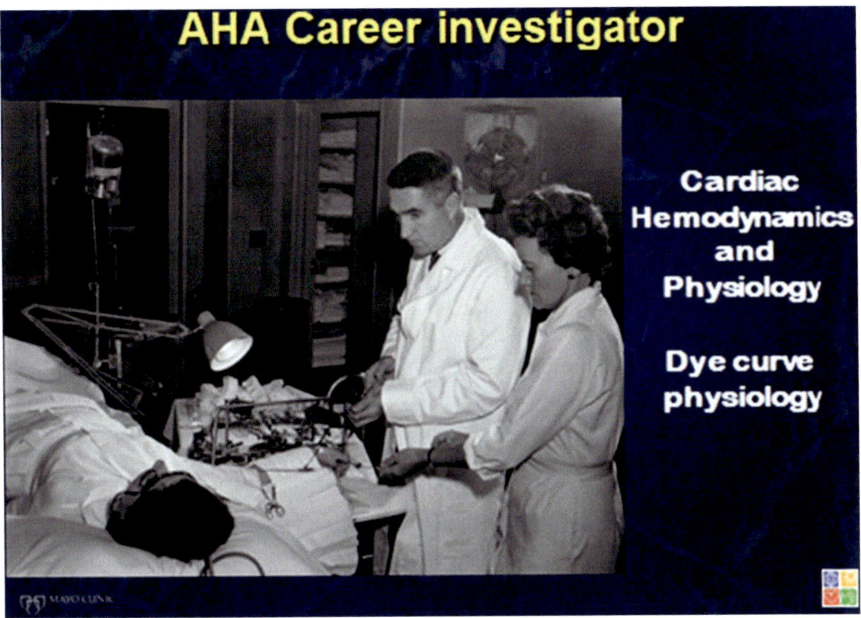

Fig. 12.3 Dr. Earl Wood performing early catheter diagnostic studies in the medical science cardiac catheterization laboratory

Mayo Clinic's open heart surgery program moved from Methodist Hospital to St. Mary's Hospital in September 1956. In the late 1950s, because of increasingly complex congenital heart disease, it became apparent that high-quality angiographic images would be necessary to achieve successful surgical repair. There were also concerns then for the risks associated with transferring sick children back and forth from St. Mary's Hospital to the Medical Science building [1] (p. 247). To achieve these goals, it was necessary to establish a clinical cardiac catheterization laboratory at St. Mary's Hospital. Dr. Jeremy Swan, a research fellow in Dr. Wood's research laboratory, was selected by the Mayo Clinic Board of Governors as the director of the St. Mary's Hospital cardiac catheterization laboratory in 1958. Dr. Swan determined that the location and design of the new clinical laboratory would permit collaboration between cardiologists and radiologists in the use of angiography to image the heart in congenital heart disease. Dr. Wood remained focused in physiology research at the Medical Sciences cath lab. Shortly thereafter, Dr. Shahbudin Rahimtoola, who had previously worked in physiology with Dr. Swan, also joined the staff in the new clinical laboratory. Dr. Owings W. Kincaid and Dr. George Davis, Mayo Clinic staff radiologists, who had already performed angiography at St. Mary's Hospital, were selected to help develop and maintain cardiac angiocardiography in the cardiac catheterization laboratory. In 1964, Dr. Donald G. Ritter completed his pediatric cardiology residency and was invited to join the Mayo Clinic staff to work in the laboratory. In 1965, Dr. Robert Feldt also joined the staff with his duties also involving work in the catheterization laboratory. Dr. Feldt subsequently became the medical director of the infant intensive care unit and left the cardiac laboratory in 1974.

Dr. Swan left Mayo Clinic in 1965, and Dr. Rahimtoola returned to England. This resulted in new leadership for the laboratory at St. Mary's Hospital with establishment in 1966 of four codirectors to provide leadership for the laboratory in their various areas of expertise (Fig. 12.4): Dr. Donald G. Ritter, as the director for congenital heart disease; Dr. Robert L. Frye, adult cardiovascular disease; Dr. Robert A. Devloo, anesthesiology; and Dr. Owings W. Kincaid, radiology. Dr. George Davis soon replaced Dr. Kincaid as the radiology director. Drs. Davis and Ritter rapidly developed an internationally recognized expertise in angiographic study of complex congenital heart disease primarily utilizing the large roll film format of the Elema-Schonander film changer (Fig. 12.5). This system allowed the high spatial resolution needed for complex congenital heart disease but only allowed a maximum of 12 frames per second. This was therefore complimented with cineangiography for better time resolution. Figure 12.6 [2] details a combined pathologic and angiographic study by Dr. Somkid Sridaromont in 72 patients with double outlet right ventricle.

Dr. Ritter served as a director of the cardiac laboratory from 1965 to 1974 and became chair of the Division of Pediatric Cardiology from 1973 to 1984. It was significant that he was the laboratory director of congenital heart disease which also included many adults with congenital heart disease. This was an unusual clinical arrangement but a unique trademark of the Mayo Clinic cardiac laboratory which has persisted to today. Interventional procedures in congenital heart disease became

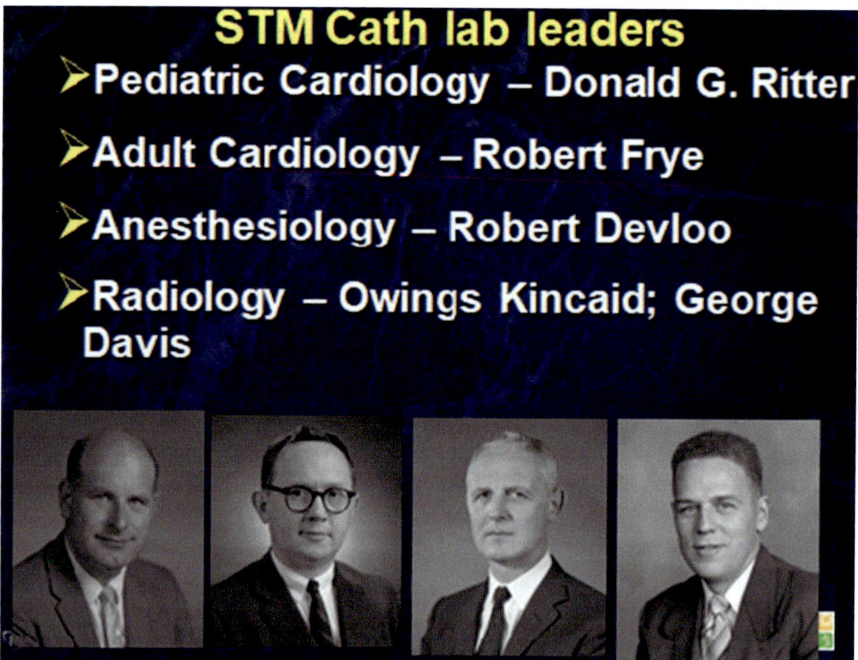

Fig. 12.4 New cardiac cath lab leaders in 1966

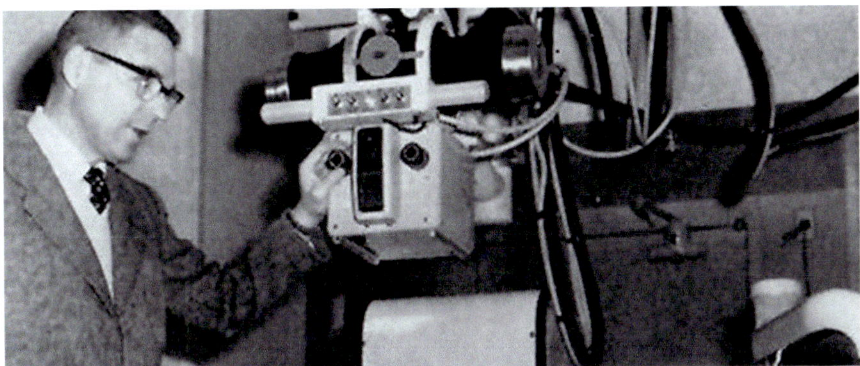

Fig. 12.5 Dr. George Davis adjusting the collimator for a large film angiography with the Elema-Schonander film changer

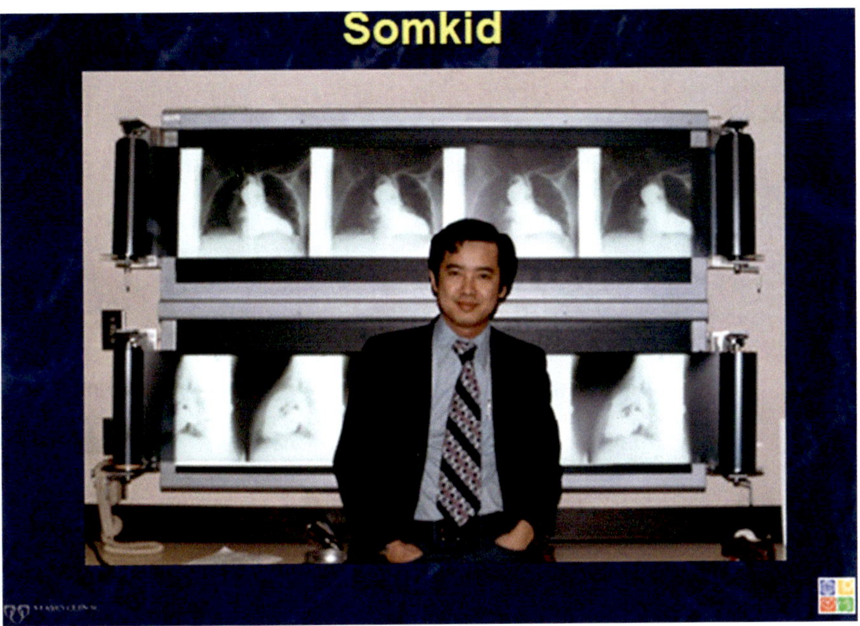

Fig. 12.6 Dr. Somkid Sridaromont, as a 1973 Mayo Clinic pediatric cardiology fellow standing in front of typical roll film study of one of his favorite topics "double outlet right ventricle"

standard practice in the congenital laboratory in 1969, first with adaptation of the balloon atrial septostomy procedure developed by William Rashkind for palliation of complete transposition of the great arteries. The high international profile of the congenital laboratory in conjunction with highly successful cardiovascular surgical interventions achieved by Drs. John Kirklin, Dwight McGoon, Robert Wallace, and Gordon Danielson attracted many interested physicians who would train at Mayo as fellows in congenital heart disease. These early fellows such as Fergus Macartney,

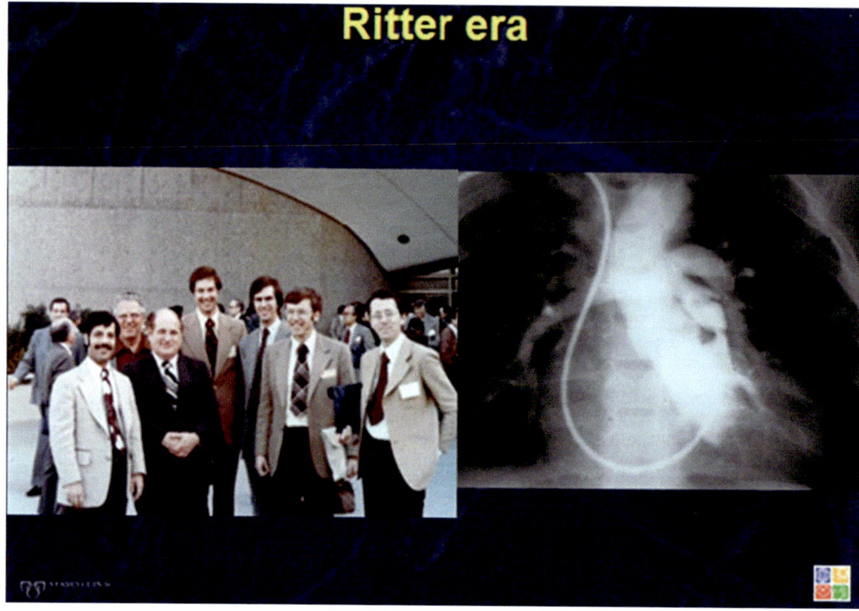

Fig. 12.7 Left: Photo of Dr. Ritter, Tajik, Seward, Squarcia, and participating fellows at an AHA meeting in the 1970s. On the right: A frame from a film study of a patient with tetralogy of Fallot shows typical catheter placement from the right ax

Umberto Squarcia, and Boonchob Pongpanich subsequently became pediatric cardiology leaders at their home institutions (Fig. 12.7).

Here are some remembrances from Umberto Squarcia:

The Cardiac Laboratories of the Mayo Clinic was my first "docking" when I started my fellowship in Pediatric Cardiology at May. And the main reason was that I had a very good knowledge of all English medical terminology, but not so good of the spoken English. So I began in the Cardiac Lab where I soon started learning the jokes of Dr. Donald Ritter, but besides the English of the jokes I learned from his skillful and masterly teaching the "art" of doing the cardiac catheterization in newborn, babies and children. And I learned from him all the secrets of the complex congenital heart diseases.

The single episode which remain more vivid in my memory of the time I spent in the Cardiac Lab is when one afternoon Gian Rastelli came in the small office of the residents , coming from the OR that was one floor below us, and started telling me that Dr. Robert Wallace had just finished to operate on a child with TGA VSD and PS using with the same technique that Gian had envisioned and experimented successfully in dogs in laboratory. He made a schematic drawing while explaining the various steps of the procedure. The surgical procedure went well and was followed by countless operations with the same technique that since then will be called the Rastelli procedure [3].

It was the 26th of July 1968.

Gian had been my mentor in my last year of Medical School at the University of Parma. He was assistant professor at that University and soon he would leave Italy and Parma to come to the United States, to the Mayo Clinic. I followed him some years later and on 1st of July 1968 I started my fellowship in Pediatric Cardiology at the Mayo Clinic. We had many things in common, the first of them was the dream of coming back together to Italy and start the work of Pediatric Cardiology and Pediatric Cardiac Surgery, so badly needed at that time in our country. That afternoon of 26th of July 1968 in the Cardiac Lab we were enjoying together for the early success of the first surgical procedure of TGA, VSD, PS that Gian had experimented. I would love to still have with me that schematic drawing made by Gian showing all the details of the Rastelli procedure.

Dr. Douglas Mair completed his pediatric cardiology training in 1970 and joined the Mayo Clinic staff to spend most of his time in the congenital catheterization laboratory. When Dr. Ritter left the cardiac laboratory in 1974, Dr. Mair replaced him as a codirector of the cardiac lab and as director of the congenital lab. Dr. Frye was named the chairman of adult cardiology, and Dr. Hugh Smith who was also a fellow in Earl Wood's lab was then appointed as director of the adult cardiac laboratory. Drs. Mair and Smith then functioned as the codirectors of the catheterization laboratory.

In the 1960s most of the catheterization procedures, even in infants, were performed by surgical cutdown technique from the femoral or axillary approach. However, in the 1970s this was easily replaced by the now standard percutaneous Seldinger techniques. Also, new video angiographic recordings and videodensitometric techniques began to replace the large roll film and cineangiographic filming. Videodensitometry also was a benefit of the continued research efforts in Dr. Wood's medical science laboratory. These techniques applied to clinical ventriculography for the first time allowed accurate assessment of ventricular function even in complex congenital heart disease such as after Mustard or Senning operations for repair of complete transposition of the great arteries [4]. Thus, we were able to make accurate determinations of right and left ventricular systolic function and ejection fraction in these patients for the first time. This information was particularly helpful to direct clinical and surgical efforts in the repair of complete transposition of the great arteries utilizing the arterial switch procedure to allow the left ventricle to function as the systemic ventricle.

Also during the 1970s, Dr. Ritter encouraged the training of several adult cardiology fellows in congenital cardiac catheterization techniques. In 1974, Dr. Jamil Tajik completed his adult cardiology fellowship and joined the Mayo Clinic staff while continuing his participation in the work of the congenital catheterization laboratory. Dr. Tajik recognized the importance of application of ultrasound techniques in the study of congenital heart disease and began efforts to develop the application of M-mode echocardiography to congenital heart disease with the continued support and assistance from Dr. Ritter. Dr. Donald Hagler joined the Mayo Clinic staff in 1974 as an associate consultant and also utilized M-mode echocardiographic techniques on infants and children with congenital heart disease [5]. The application of these echocardiographic techniques continued to expand but remained primarily utilized during cardiac catheterization procedures. It was with the significant support both financially and personally that Dr. Ritter helped to establish echocardiography as an adjunct imaging tool in the assessment of congenital heart disease in the catheterization laboratory. With his investment in the latest ultrasound equipment for the laboratory, Dr. Ritter provided the opportunity for enterprising new staff, Drs. Tajik, Hagler, and James Seward, to recognize and publish concepts of contrast echocardiography, straddling atrioventricular valves, and single ventricle morphology. Dr. James Seward completed his Mayo cardiology training and joined the staff in 1976. He also had great interest in congenital heart disease and was also assigned to work in the congenital cardiac laboratory. He was actively involved in many of the morphologic publications which originated from the cardiac laboratory.

Having established the utility of echocardiography in the catheterization laboratory, it was a natural development in 1976 to advance these techniques with the purchase of the first Mayo Clinic 2-dimensional echocardiograph – the Varian phased array sector scanner. This was recognized by all of us who clearly saw that this new technology suddenly provided a whole new dimension to echocardiography and cardiac imaging. This instrument not only provided a new imaging modality for adult and pediatric cardiology patients throughout the hospital, but it also spurred efforts in the catheterization laboratory to expand and publish our morphologic understanding of very complex forms of congenital heart disease [6]. Figure 12.8a, b illustrates the use of one of the early 2-dimensional and Doppler echocardiographs which was routinely utilized during procedures in the catheterization laboratory. They also show the door to the small dark room in the back which housed the Elema-Schonander roll film changer. During this time frame, the use of Doppler echocardiography became an important tool to better understand the physiology of congenital cardiac defects [7]. Dr. Phillip Currie came to Mayo Clinic from Australia to compliment his cardiology training and was intimately involved in many of the studies to demonstrate the utility of continuous wave Doppler echocardiography in congenital cardiac defects. The simultaneous catheter-measured valve gradients with continuous wave Doppler studies defined the methodology and the accuracy of clinical application of these Doppler techniques [8]. This methodology was particularly important in recognizing and defining the role of pressure recovery in lesions such as aortic valve stenosis. As a natural extension of the application of Doppler technique in echocardiography, color flow imaging became an integral part of echocardiographic imaging in the cardiac laboratory in the early 1980s [9].

Dr. Davis retired from the Mayo Clinic in 1977, and Dr. Paul R. Julsrud became the director of cardiac radiology in 1983 (Fig. 12.9). During these years, the cardiac laboratory benefited from collaboration with IBM to develop computerization of the data recording and to develop a complete cardiac catheterization report. The computerization of input data allowed substantial improvements in reporting accuracy and development of new, easier calculations of hemodynamic parameters.

The Early Days: The Radiological Perspective

Dr. Paul Julsrud provided some memories of the early years of the cath lab.

In 1958 Dr. John Kirklin, head of cardiac surgery at Mayo Clinic, and Dr. James DuShane, head of pediatric cardiology at Mayo Clinic, led the initiative for the establishment of a

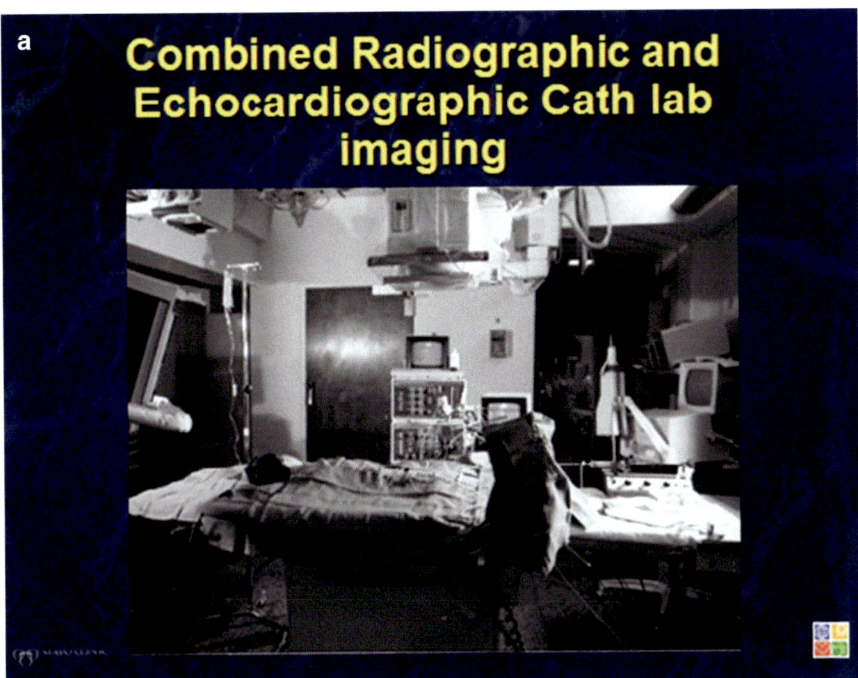

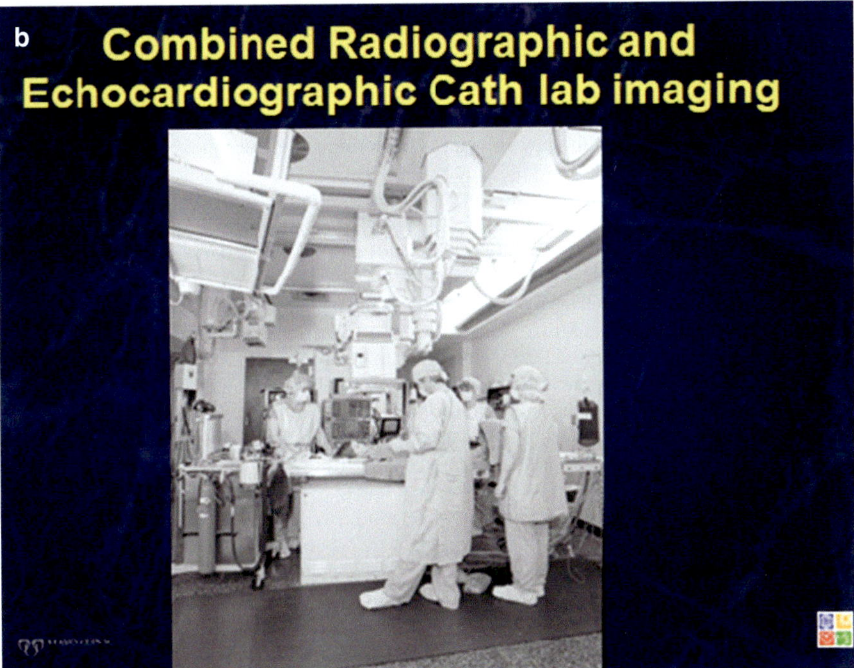

Fig. 12.8 (**a**) Photograph shows the combined echocardiographic imaging and radiography in the early St. Mary's cardiac laboratory. The wood door in the background is the entrance to the dark room for the Elema-Schonander roll film changer. (**b**) Photograph shows a simulated catheterization procedure with cardiologist, anesthesia, and tech support in the room. Separate X-ray tubes are noted above for the roll film images

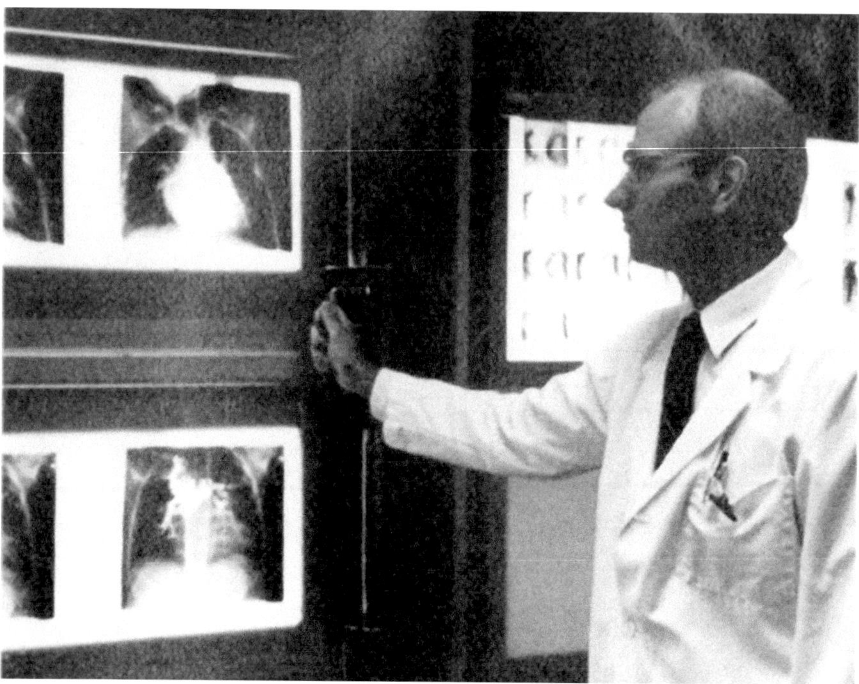

Fig. 12.9 Dr. Paul R. Julsrud, cardiac radiologist, became director of cardiac radiology in the cardiac catheterization laboratory in 1980

cardiac catheterization laboratory at St. Mary's Hospital. This would accomplish two important goals: bringing the physiological monitoring techniques pioneered in Dr. Earl Wood's laboratory into the hospital setting and also developing a much-needed angiographic capability. The later task was felt to be critically important in order to establish the exact anatomic nature of the abnormality of the congenital heart defects being investigated at the time. Dr. Kirklin was well aware of recent advances in medical imaging since he was the son of the chair of roentgenology at Mayo Clinic, Dr. Byrl R. Kirklin. Dr. Byrl Kirklin was the first Mayo Clinic chair of roentgenology from 1930 to 1951. He had established the first angiographic facility at Mayo Clinic in the hospital setting in the old Colonial Building in 1949. Dr. Byrl Kirklin hired Dr. George Davis to be in charge of this angiographic facility. Dr. Owings Kincaid joined the radiology staff in 1952, and together Drs. Davis and Kincaid were charged with the responsibility for imaging in the newly created St. Mary's Hospital laboratory, while Dr. Jeremy Swan was responsible for its physiologic aspects.

In 1959, Drs. Davis and Kincaid were sent on a trip to various US academic centers including Boston (Harvard), while Dr. Swan was sent to Sweden to study at the Karolinska Institute. In January 1960, Dr. Davis also traveled to Sweden and was convinced that the role film capabilities at the Karolinska Institute were superior to the cut film format which was initially installed in the cardiac catheterization laboratory (Figs. 12.5, and 12.6). The initial filming capabilities in the cath lab were with the large cut film format at six frames per second alternating between AP and lateral and a 16 mm cine capability at 60 frames per second. The cut film capability was soon felt to be insufficient, and in 1962 the roll film capability was installed which had simultaneous AP and lateral filming rates up to 12 frames per second.

In 1960, the cardiac catheterization laboratory became functional with the first angiogram of an aortic coarctation obtained in March of 1960. Dr. Kincaid did the first angiogram employing the Seldinger technique at Mayo Clinic in 1961. In 1970 Dr. Kincaid left the cardiac cath lab due to health reasons. In the same year Dr. James Stewart and Dr. Franz Hallermann made contributions to the radiologic activities in the cath lab but later left Mayo Clinic for private practice. Dr. Davis retired in 1977. Prior to Dr. Davis's retirement, Dr. Richard Fulton had become Dr. Davis' coworker in the cardiac catheterization laboratory (cardiac radiology). He then directed cardiac radiology when Dr. Davis retired. Dr. Anthony Stanson supported the radiology efforts in the catheterization laboratory after Dr. Fulton left Mayo Clinic in 1979.

During 1979–1980, I was a Mayo Foundation Scholar. The first 6 months from July to end of December 1979 was spent at the Boston Children's Hospital, part of the Harvard Medical establishment. There I was under the mentorship of pediatric radiologist Dr. Kenneth Fellows who taught me a great deal, particularly about the new angulated views of the heart for angiographic assessment of congenital heart diseases which I helped introduce in the pediatric cardiac cath lab on returning to Mayo Clinic [10].

In addition to Dr. Fellows, I spent as much time as possible with Dr. Richard Van Praagh. Dr. Van Praagh was a world expert cardiac pathologist who specialized in the cardiac malformations encountered in patients with congenital heart disease. I learned a great deal about the anatomy of congenital heart diseases and also how important it was to know the embryology behind these lesions which not only helped understand these malformations better but aided in the ability to diagnose them.

Dr. Enge was my principal mentor while studying in Norway from January to July 1980. In addition to his sage advice and angiographic knowledge, he was instrumental in introducing me to individuals who would play an important role in my activities once I got back to the pediatric cardiac catheterization laboratory at Mayo Clinic. A prime example was becoming aware of the revolutionary work in low osmolar contrast agents being developed by a small Norwegian company, Nyegaard. They had recently formed a partnership with Dr. Torsten Almen, a Swedish radiologist, who invented the first low osmolar, nonionic, contrast agent (metrizamide) and at the time I met him had recently introduced the second generation of nonionics (iohexol). This eventually played a part in my role as principal investigator in 1994 for a Phase III, randomized, blinded comparison of iodixanol and iohexol in pediatric patients requiring angiocardiography, performed in the pediatric cardiac catheterization laboratory.

Another example of how my time as a Mayo Foundation Scholar influenced working in the pediatric cardiac catheterization laboratory is illustrated by the following. During my 6 months in Oslo, Norway, I worked primarily under the guidance of a gifted pediatric radiologist, Professor Gunnar Stake, at the Rikshospitalet (Norway's nation hospital). He and his cardiac surgical colleagues had recently published a paper describing the first successful balloon angioplasty of a stenotic pulmonary valve using an inflated angiographic balloon catheter to rupture the valve employing a "pull through" technique [11]. During my training at Mayo Clinic, I had seen our vascular radiologists using the percutaneous transluminal angioplasty technique first described by radiologists, Dr. Charles Dotter and Dr. Melvin Judkins, in patients with arteriosclerotic obstructive disease [12]. It seemed to me that using this technique would provide a more controlled radial force at the stenotic valve level and might be advantageous in attempting a "controlled" rupture of the valve.

On January 13, 1981, a 6-year-old boy came to the pediatric cardiac catheterization laboratory for a measurement of the gradient of his presumed pulmonary valve stenosis. Dr.

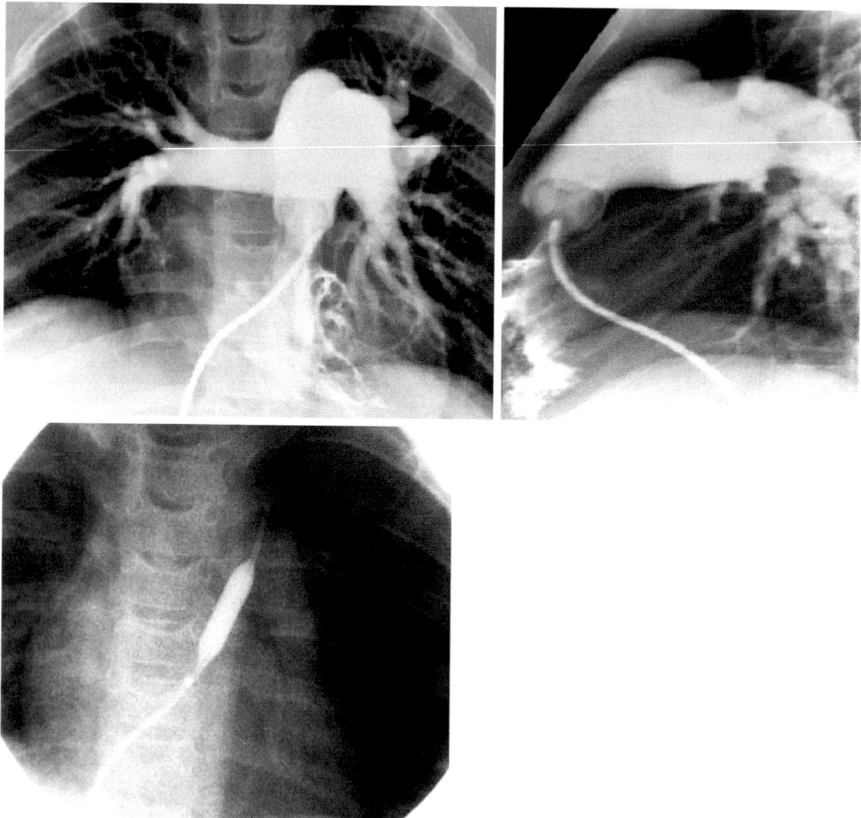

Fig. 12.10 Top figures illustrate large roll film right ventricular angiogram demonstrating severe pulmonary valvular and infundibular stenosis in a 12-year-old boy. The image balloon was obtained with cineangiography, while Dr. Julsrud inflated a balloon catheter across the valve in an attempt to dilate the valvular stenosis

James Seward was the cardiologist in the laboratory that day, and after measuring a 60 mmHg gradient at the pulmonary valve level, we discussed the possibility of attempting a balloon angioplasty. I secured one of the larger inflatable angioplasty balloons from vascular radiology and after consulting with the appropriate parties elected to proceed. I performed multiple balloon inflations at the valve level (Fig. 12.10), but no change in the gradient was achieved. A surgical valvectomy 2 days later was successful in relieving the obstruction to right ventricular outflow. The attempted balloon dilatation taught us that the patient tolerated the transient super-systemic pressure experienced by the right ventricle during balloon inflation which totally occluded right ventricular outflow and, also, that larger and stronger balloons would be desirable.

In May 1981, radiologist Dr. Robert White, who had trained with Dr. Kurt Amplatz at the University of Minnesota from July 1, 1970, to June 30, 1971, along with pediatric cardiologist Dr. Jean Kan, successfully dilated a stenotic pulmonary valve using the percutaneous balloon angioplasty technique which they reported in the *New England Journal of Medicine*, August 26, 1982 [13, 14].

Another activity related to any radiographic practice is the constant attention that needs to be taken in order to reduce radiation exposure as much as possible to the patient. This is especially important in the pediatric population due to the fact that children are more sensitive than adults to the induction of cancers, and they frequently require multiple cardiac catheterizations during their childhood. These catheterizations employ both fluoroscopic and cineangiographic type radiation and result in radiation exposures as much as ten times as most other radiographic type examinations. By implementing simple steps such as increasing X-ray tube filtration, removing the antiscatter grid during fluoroscopy, and decreasing frame rates for appropriate cineangiographic studies, as well as implementing more sophisticated pulsed progressive fluoroscopic techniques introduced by our video engineer, Mr. Merrill Wondrow, we were able to decrease the fluoroscopic exposure by as much as five times and reduce the cineangiographic exposure rates by as much as three times [15, 16].

The application of advanced technology to deliver long distance care was an important component of cath lab practice. Merrill Wondrow had previously worked on implementing our pulsed progressive fluoroscopic system and was instrumental in initiating our collaboration with the Defense Advanced Research Projects Agency (DARPA) to utilize satellite communication capability. Drs. Jerome Breen and Julsrud evaluated the feasibility of telemedical consultation for patients with complex congenital heart diseases, which was undertaken with the Phoenix Children's Hospital. Such strategies of care would become increasingly important in the years to come [17].

I am ending my recollection of the pediatric catheterization laboratory by referencing an article written by the cardiac surgeons in 1993. In this article describing surgical techniques that were devised for modification of the so-called Fontan procedure in patients with anomalous venous connections, Dr. Gordon Danielson refers to one of the procedures as the Julsrud procedure. I point this out not to suggest any personal accomplishment on my part but rather to draw attention to his generosity of spirit and to illustrate the high level of mutual respect and admiration the individual team members of the congenital heart team had for each other [18].

Dr. Julsrud has reported the role of radiology in the development of the angiographic and interventional capabilities of the cardiac catheterization laboratory. In that arena, interventional cardiac catheterization, which started in the laboratory as balloon atrial septostomy, developed spontaneously as an effort to provide relief of pulmonary valve stenosis without surgical intervention. He pointed out their first efforts for balloon pulmonary valvotomy which mimicked similar, later efforts by other pediatric cardiologists. With development of new balloons and stents for vascular dilation, the interventional efforts in the catheterization laboratory expanded rapidly in the 1980s to include conduits, tissue valve prostheses, pulmonary, venous and aortic stents, and coil embolization of collateral vessels [19].

Dr. Erik Ritman had been Dr. Earl Wood's protégé in physiology research in medical sciences. One of Dr. Woods's last uncompleted projects prior to his retirement was taken up by Dr. Ritman and by the mid-1980s had developed a clinical model, and parenthetically for our history, some congenital heart patients returned to the medical science facility to undergo angiographic assessment for their complex congenital heart disease using the dynamic spatial reconstructor. This amazing device became our first efforts to obtain 4-dimensional reconstructions of congenital heart defects [20]. These important efforts evolved into the subsequent development of clinical utility with cardiac CT imaging. These important early efforts clearly illustrate the close association and affiliation of the Mayo Clinic cardiac catheterization laboratory with the ongoing physiology research in medical sciences. One clear illustration of this relationship is the current designation of our cardiac laboratory at St. Mary's Hospital as the Earl Wood Cardiac Catheterization Laboratory.

Dr. Smith had accepted the chairmanship of adult cardiology, and Dr. David Holmes was appointed as a cardiac lab codirector and director of the adult catheterization lab in 1984. Dr. Mair stepped down as director of the congenital cardiac catheterization laboratory, and Dr. Donald Hagler assumed that responsibility as a codirector of the laboratory in 1992. Dr. Mair retired from Mayo Clinic in 2002.

In 1993, Dr. Seward left the cardiac catheterization laboratory to become the director of the echocardiographic laboratory which was now located in the Plummer building. Because of his physiologic background from the catheterization laboratory, he emphasized in the echocardiographic lab the physiologic capabilities of echocardiography, including both its imaging and Doppler capabilities. During his tenure in the echo laboratory, he also expanded the echocardiographic imaging to include transesophageal echocardiography and published several premier manuscripts illustrating the techniques and anatomic correlations for biplanar and multiplane TEE [21]. Very soon after this, the TEE imaging became available for the pediatric population and became the Mayo Clinic standard practice for all congenital cardiac surgery [22].

The patient population in the congenital catheterization laboratory continued to expand in interventional procedure and including many adult patients with adult congenital heart disease. By 1997, the congenital laboratory began participation in the first US trial for use of the Amplatz atrial septal occluder for percutaneous device closure of secundum atrial septal defects. Dr. Hagler was the PI for Mayo Clinic's participation in this trial. Because of a large population of adult patients who had experienced a cryptogenic stroke and recognized as having a patent foramen ovale, the same device was frequently utilized to close PFO in such patients [23]. With the implementation of ASD closure, we also led in the utilization of intracardiac echocardiographic techniques to assist in the device ASD closures [24]. ICE imaging remains the mainstay for intracardiac imaging in the catheterization laboratory.

Dr. Kurt Amplatz from the University of MN was a genius and inventor who rapidly developed other new closure devices which we rapidly applied for and participated in studies for implantation of the Amplatz patent ductus arteriosus occluder (ADO I), the muscular VSD occluder, post-infarction VSD occluder, and a variety of vascular plug such as the Amplatz vascular plugs (AVP I-IV) (Fig. 12.11) [25]. Dr. Hagler also participated as the Mayo Clinic PI for the national trials of these devices. The AVP II became a popular device in our efforts for closure of paravalvular leaks. Unfortunately, between 2002 and 2011, there were over 100 instances of Amplatz atrial septal occluder wall erosions which produced acute

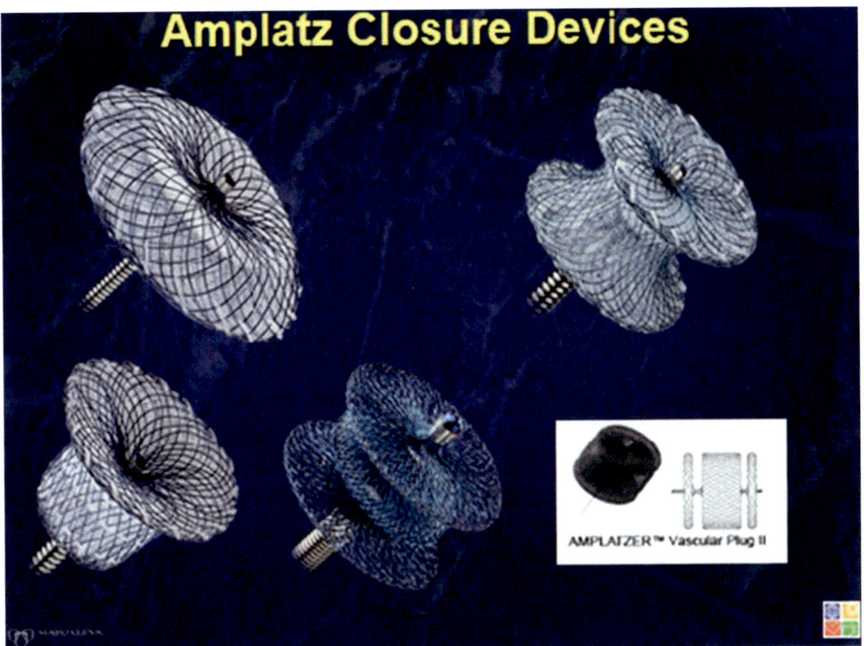

Fig. 12.11 Amplatz Closure devices: Top row left Amplatz ASD device; right Amplatz muscular VSD occluder. Bottom row: left Amplatz ADO I ductal occluder; middle Amplatz Piccolo ductal occluder; right Amplatz AVP II occluder

cardiac tamponade secondary to development of progressive accumulation of bloody pericardial effusion [26]. This unfortunate development dramatically changed Mayo Clinic cardiac catheterization laboratory practice for ASD and PFO device closure. On the other hand, it prompted the progressive development of newer device which were less metallic and softer which have not had any history of wall erosion. Mayo Clinic cardiac laboratory was asked to participate in the Gore Cardioform Atrial Septal Occluder "Assured" trial and was taken on by Dr. Hagler as PI. Following FDA approval of this device in 2019, device closure of secundum ASDs as large as 35 mm in diameter was again possible. New studies are now in preparation for Gore Cardioform Septal Occluder closure of PFO in patients with debilitating migraine (Fig. 12.12). The Cardioform Septal Occluder is a similar but smaller device which we now routinely use for device closure of PFO in patients who unfortunately have experienced stroke secondary to embolic event through the PFO.

Dr. Allison Cabalka completed her training in pediatric cardiology at Texas Children's Hospital in 1992 and after working for 7 years in private practice at the Children's Heart clinic in Minneapolis joined the Mayo Clinic staff in 1999. Dr.

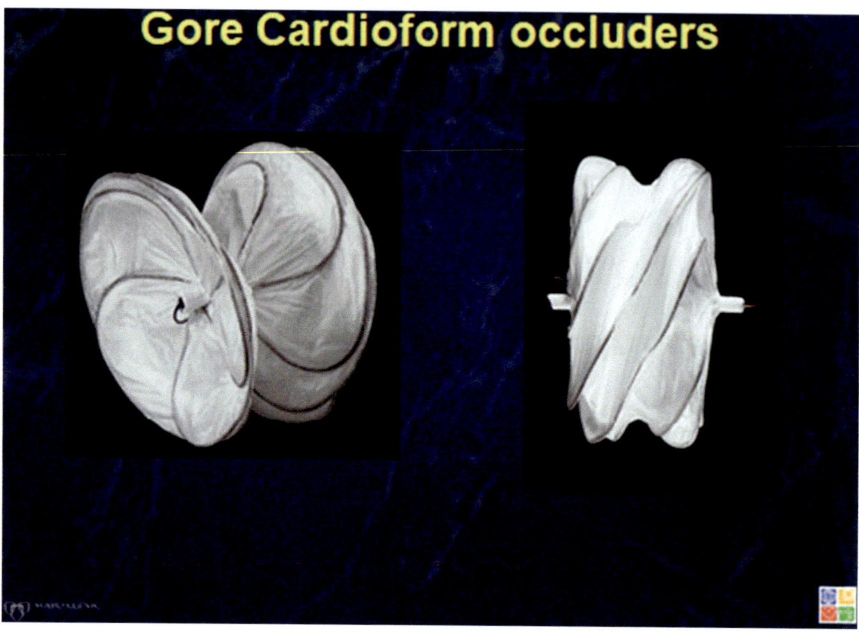

Fig. 12.12 Gore Cardioform occluders. Left – Cardioform septal occluder; Right – Cardioform atrial septal occluder

Cabalka had maintained her primary interest in interventional catheterization and readily continued to work in the cardiac catheterization laboratory. Dr. Cabalka was also heavily involved in international mission work and subsequently participated in interventional cardiac catheterization missions in multiple countries. Dr. Cabalka became an American College of Cardiology IMPACT steering committee member from 2014 to 2018.

Dr. Frank Cetta completed his Mayo Clinic training in pediatric cardiology in 1995. He initially worked at Loyola University Hospital in Chicago but returned to Mayo Clinic as the chair of the Division of Pediatric Cardiology in 2004. He also continued to pursue his interest in interventional cardiology in the catheterization laboratory and in particular was an important addition because of his commitment to adult congenital heart disease with boards in pediatric cardiology and adult internal medicine.

Intravascular stents, although originally designed for peripheral vascular and biliary use, rapidly became part of the congenital catheterization laboratory armamentarium because of the limited success achieved with simply balloon dilation. Similar to the success noted with coronary artery stenting, pulmonary artery stents allow successful noninvasive palliation of pulmonary artery branch stenosis often encountered after otherwise successful surgical repair. In 2008 we reported the use of pulmonary artery stents as a hybrid intraoperative procedure for congenital heart disease [27]. Because of these successes, intravascular stenting soon was adapted to coarctation of the aorta, and the Mayo Clinic laboratory participated in several multi-institutional studies to assess its safety and effectiveness [28]. With Dr. Cabalka as the PI, Mayo Clinic participated in the first FDA-approved clinical trial of intravascular stents for treatment of coarctation of the aorta, which eventually resulted in FDA approval of the bare metal and covered versions of the NuMed Platinum stent. This was the first intravascular stent officially approved in 2016 by the FDA for clinical use in congenital heart disease [29]. In addition, the same stent was given approval by the FDA for use in right ventricular outflow tract conduits in 2017. The application of stent therapy now encompasses venous and postoperative conduits allowing successful resolution of conduit and pulmonary artery obstruction without surgical intervention [30].

Dr. Nathaniel W. Taggart completed his Mayo Clinic training in pediatric cardiology in 2011 and as a Mayo Clinic Scholar procured additional interventional catheterization training at UC San Francisco. He returned to Mayo Clinic in 2012 and rapidly developed his participation in the cardiac catheterization laboratory. He has been active in the Society of Cardiovascular Angiography and Interventions and served as the president of the Society of Cardiac Angiography and Interventions PICECS group from 2016 to 2018. Similarly, Dr. Jason H. Anderson completed pediatric cardiology training at Mayo Clinic in 2017 and subsequently had cardiac interventional catheterization training as a Mayo Clinic Scholar at UC San Francisco in 2018.

Upon returning to Mayo Clinic, both congenital interventionalists have started new practice efforts directed to infants and premature patients. Mayo Clinic congenital catheterization lab now has developed experience in techniques for device closure of patent ductus arteriosus in premature infants weighing as little as 500 grams with the Amplatzer Piccolo Ductal Occluder or ADO II AS. In addition, they have expanded cardiac catheterization laboratory efforts to create shunts in the newborn with limited pulmonary blood flow, such as pulmonary atresia. This primarily has been achieved with patent ductus arteriosus stent placement with coronary artery size stents. Additionally new efforts have been directed to create aortopulmonary communications with radiofrequency wire perforation and subsequent placement of small covered stents. These efforts in fact have been encourage by the CV surgical group who have recognized the difficulty of safely and effectively creating such communications.

Philipp Bonhoeffer reported the first percutaneous replacement of a pulmonary valve in a dysfunctional conduit in 2000 in a 12-year-old boy. This valve was eventually manufactured by Medtronic as the Melody Valve (Fig. 12.13) and subsequently developed into one of the most highly utilized interventional practices for congenital heart disease both in children and adults. Because of the large number of congenital heart patients at Mayo who had a conduit placed to repair defects such as tetralogy of Fallot, pulmonary atresia, truncus arteriosus, and pulmonary autograft procedures for aortic stenosis, this procedure offered the

Fig. 12.13 Illustration of the Medtronic Melody valve and delivery system

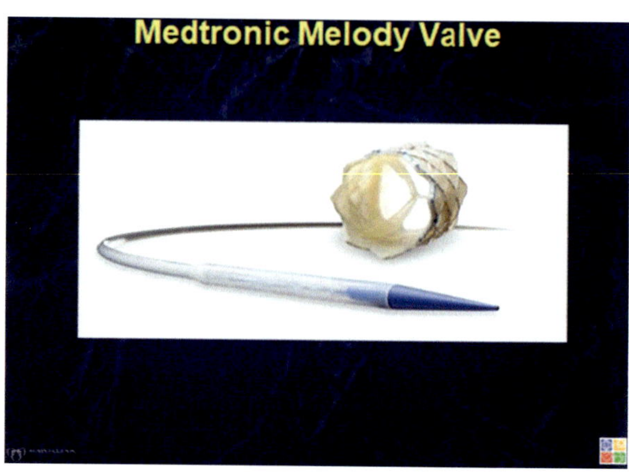

opportunity to save these patients one or more surgical sternotomy procedures for pulmonary valve replacement. Dr. Cabalka accepted the role of PI for Mayo's participation in the Melody US post-approval study after successfully approved by the FDA in 2010. Dr. Cabalka also was the national PI for the Melody Transcatheter Pulmonary Valve (TPV) study in patients with dysfunctional bioprosthetic valve in the pulmonary position. This was approved by the FDA in 2017 for use in bioprosthetic valves. In 2015, the FDA approved the use of the Edwards Sapien valve which was developed for percutaneous aortic valve replacement in adults. The Sapien valve then became available for pulmonary valve replacement in larger conduits up to 29 mm in size. These valves also have been part of the cardiac lab armamentarium for tricuspid valve-in-valve replacement in patients who have had a previous surgical bioprosthetic tricuspid valve replacement most often for Ebstein's anomaly [31].

In all of the years of progress and advancement of congenital cardiac interventions at our Earl Wood cardiac catheterization laboratory, one striking feature was persistent in all of the active staff catheterization lab members which is unusual for catheterization laboratories. Figure 12.14 illustrates the current cardiologists working in the Mayo Clinic congenital cardiac laboratory. All of the participating pediatric cardiology staff members have continued to maintain both expertise in angiography and catheter interventions as well as in all forms of cardiac ultrasonography. This has persisted as a direct result of Donald Ritter's vision and support of the combined roles of radiographic and ultrasound imaging techniques for the best diagnostic capabilities in congenital heart disease.

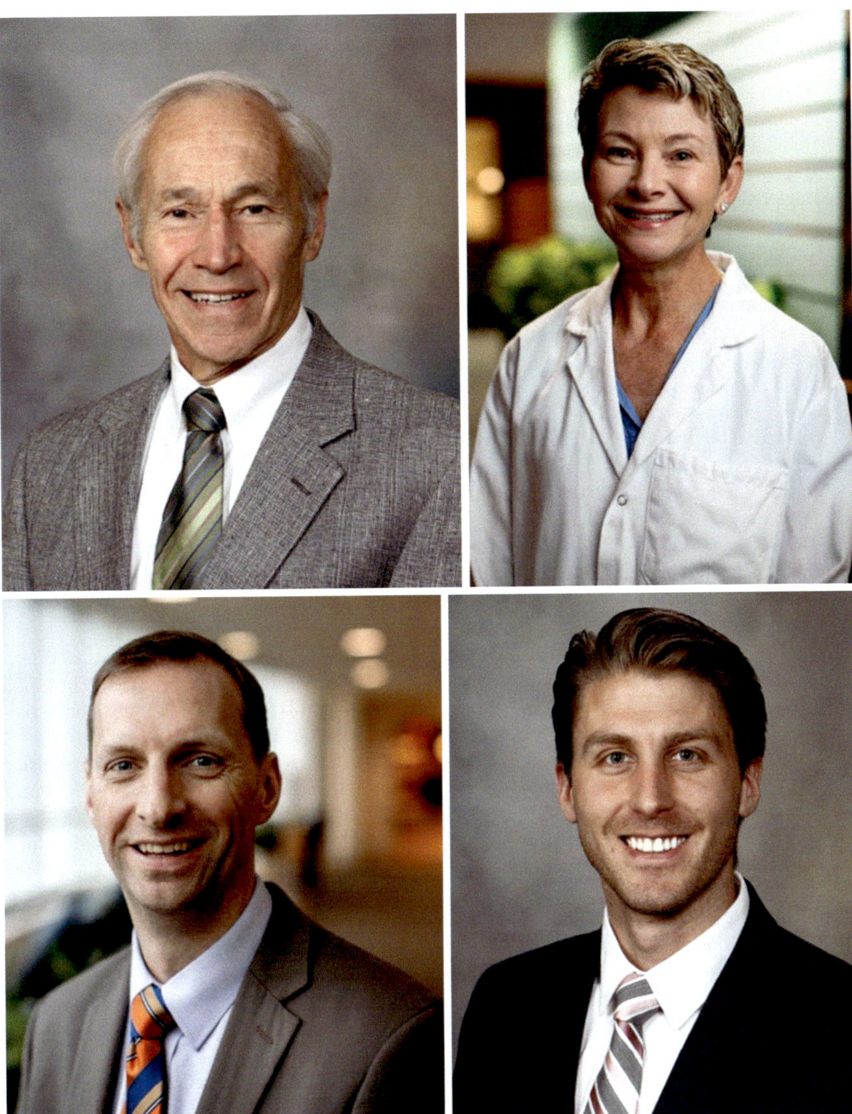

Fig. 12.14 Current photographs illustrate the current pediatric cardiologists working in the Mayo Clinic congenital cardiac catheterization laboratory. From left to right Upper panel: Dr. Donald Hagler; Dr. Alison Cabalka; Lower panel: Dr. Nathaniel Taggart, Dr. Jason Anderson

References

1. Fye W. Caring for the heart, vol. 672. New York: Oxford University Press; 2015.
2. Sridaromont S, Ritter DG, Feldt RH, Davis GD, Edwards JE. Double-outlet right ventricle. Anatomic and angiocardiographic correlations. Mayo Clin Proc. 1978;53(9):555–77.
3. Rastelli GC. A new approach to "anatomic" repair of transposition of the great arteries. Mayo Clin Proc. 1969;44(1):1–12.

4. Hagler DJ, Ritter DG, Mair DD, Davis GD, McGoon DC. Clinical, angiographic, and hemodynamic assessment of late results after mustard operation. Circulation. 1978;57(6):1214–20.
5. Hagler DJ. The utilization of echocardiography in the differential diagnosis of cyanosis in the neonate. Mayo Clin Proc. 1976;51(3):143–54.
6. Huhta JC, Hagler DJ, Seward JB, Tajik AJ, Julsrud PR, Ritter DG. Two-dimensional echocardiographic assessment of dextrocardia: a segmental approach. Am J Cardiol. 1982;50(6):1351–60.
7. Hagler DJ, Seward JB, Tajik AJ, Ritter DG. Functional assessment of the Fontan operation: combined M-mode, two-dimensional and Doppler echocardiographic studies. J Am Coll Cardiol. 1984;4(4):756–64.
8. Currie PJ, Seward JB, Reeder GS, Vlietstra RE, Bresnahan DR, Bresnahan JF, et al. Continuous-wave Doppler echocardiographic assessment of severity of calcific aortic stenosis: a simultaneous Doppler-catheter correlative study in 100 adult patients. Circulation. 1985;71(6):1162–9.
9. Reeder GS, Currie PJ, Hagler DJ, Tajik AJ, Seward JB. Use of Doppler techniques (continuous-wave, pulsed-wave, and color flow imaging) in the noninvasive hemodynamic assessment of congenital heart disease. Mayo Clin Proc. 1986;61(9):725–44.
10. Fellows KE, Keane JF, Freed MD. Angled views in cineangiocardiography of congenital heart disease. Circulation. 1977;56(3):485–90.
11. Semb BK, Tjönneland S, Stake G, Aabyholm G. "Balloon valvulotomy" of congenital pulmonary valve stenosis with tricuspid valve insufficiency. Cardiovasc Radiol. 1979;2(4):239–41.
12. Dotter CT, Judkins MP. Transluminal treatment of arteriosclerotic obstruction. Description of a new technic and a preliminary report of its application. 1964. Radiology. 1989;172(3 Pt 2):904–20.
13. Kan JS, White RI Jr, Mitchell SE, Gardner TJ. Percutaneous balloon valvuloplasty: a new method for treating congenital pulmonary-valve stenosis. N Engl J Med. 1982;307(9):540–2.
14. Kan JS, White RI Jr, Mitchell SE, Anderson JH, Gardner TJ. Percutaneous transluminal balloon valvuloplasty for pulmonary valve stenosis. Circulation. 1984;69(3):554–60.
15. Schueler BA, Julsrud PR, Gray JE, Stears JG, Wu KY. Radiation exposure and efficacy of exposure-reduction techniques during cardiac catheterization in children. AJR Am J Roentgenol. 1994;162(1):173–7.
16. Wondrow MA, Bove AA, Holmes DR Jr, Gray JE, Julsrud PR. Technical consideration for a new X-ray video progressive scanning system for cardiac catheterization. Catheter Cardiovasc Diagn. 1988;14(2):126–34.
17. Julsrud PR, Breen JF, Jedeikin R, Peoples W, Wondrow MA, Bailey KR. Telemedicine consultations in congenital heart disease: assessment of advanced technical capabilities. Mayo Clin Proc. 1999;74(8):758–63.
18. Michielon G, Gharagozloo F, Julsrud PR, Danielson GK, Puga FJ. Modified Fontan operation in the presence of anomalies of systemic and pulmonary venous connection. Circulation. 1993;88(5 Pt 2):Ii141–8.
19. Ensing GJ, Hagler DJ, Seward JB, Julsrud PR, Mair DD. Caveats of balloon dilation of conduits and conduit valves. J Am Coll Cardiol. 1989;14(2):397–400.
20. Liu YH, Mair DD, Hagler DJ, Seward JB, Julsrud PR, Ritman EL. Angiography for delineation of systemic-to-pulmonary shunts in congenital pulmonary atresia: evaluation with the dynamic spatial reconstructor. Mayo Clin Proc. 1986;61(12):932–41.
21. Seward JB, Khandheria BK, Freeman WK, Oh JK, Enriquez-Sarano M, Miller FA, et al. Multiplane transesophageal echocardiography: image orientation, examination technique, anatomic correlations, and clinical applications. Mayo Clin Proc. 1993;68(6):523–51.
22. Randolph GR, Hagler DJ, Connolly HM, Dearani JA, Puga FJ, Danielson GK, et al. Intraoperative transesophageal echocardiography during surgery for congenital heart defects. J Thorac Cardiovasc Surg. 2002;124(6):1176–82.
23. Khositseth A, Cabalka AK, Sweeney JP, Fortuin FD, Reeder GS, Connolly HM, et al. Transcatheter Amplatzer device closure of atrial septal defect and patent foramen ovale in patients with presumed paradoxical embolism. Mayo Clin Proc. 2004;79(1):35–41.

24. Earing MG, Cabalka AK, Seward JB, Bruce CJ, Reeder GS, Hagler DJ. Intracardiac echocardiographic guidance during transcatheter device closure of atrial septal defect and patent foramen ovale. Mayo Clin Proc. 2004;79(1):24–34.
25. Martinez MW, Mookadam F, Sun Y, Hagler DJ. Transcatheter closure of ischemic and post-traumatic ventricular septal ruptures. Catheter Cardiovasc Interv. 2007;69(3):403–7.
26. Taggart NW, Dearani JA, Hagler DJ. Late erosion of an Amplatzer septal occluder device 6 years after placement. J Thorac Cardiovasc Surg. 2011;142(1):221–2.
27. Menon SC, Cetta F, Dearani JA, Burkhart HA, Cabalka AK, Hagler DJ. Hybrid intraoperative pulmonary artery stent placement for congenital heart disease. Am J Cardiol. 2008;102(12):1737–41.
28. Forbes TJ, Moore P, Pedra CA, Zahn EM, Nykanen D, Amin Z, et al. Intermediate follow-up following intravascular stenting for treatment of coarctation of the aorta. Catheter Cardiovasc Interv. 2007;70(4):569–77.
29. Taggart NW, Minahan M, Cabalka AK, Cetta F, Usmani K, Ringel RE. Immediate outcomes of covered stent placement for treatment or prevention of aortic wall injury associated with coarctation of the aorta (COAST II). JACC Cardiovasc Interv. 2016;9(5):484–93.
30. Hagler DJ, Miranda WR, Haggerty BJ, Anderson JH, Johnson JN, Cetta F, et al. Fate of the Fontan connection: mechanisms of stenosis and management. Congenit Heart Dis. 2019;14(4):571–81.
31. Cullen MW, Cabalka AK, Alli OO, Pislaru SV, Sorajja P, Nkomo VT, et al. Transvenous, antegrade melody valve-in-valve implantation for bioprosthetic mitral and tricuspid valve dysfunction: a case series in children and adults. JACC Cardiovasc Interv. 2013;6(6):598–605.

Chapter 13
1980s: EP and Pacing

David R. Holmes Jr. and Stephen C. Hammill

Mayo Clinic's Department of Cardiovascular Diseases has a long history of interest in and experience with electrocardiography, cardiac pacemakers, and electrophysiology. Henry Plummer had been an initial pioneer at Mayo Clinic; an internist with special interest in cardiovascular disease, he had established an ECG laboratory in 1914. This was only 5 years after the first ECG machine in the United States had been installed. Mayo Clinic's interest expanded with the addition of Fredrick Willius who came to join Mayo Clinic in 1915 and became a key member of the staff. He would become one of the first "academic cardiologists" who directed not only the ECG laboratory but also the cardiology section. During his long and very prolific career, he published extensively on atrial flutter, paroxysmal ventricular tachycardia, complete heart block, atrial fibrillation, and chronic bradycardia. In addition, he published books complete with 368 illustrations on "Clinical Electrocardiograms: Their Interpretation and Significance" (Philadelphia: WB Saunders Co, 1929) [1] (Fig. 13.1). The long list of subsequent productive investigations on cardiac rhythms included fundamentally important papers such as that of Howard Burchell on supernormal conduction, among many others [2]. Fast forward to the early and mid-1970s, when both pacing and invasive electrophysiology procedures were an increasingly important part of clinical cardiovascular practice. During that time, records of pacing were kept both for patient indications and procedural performance. "His bundle" procedures, as they were known, were introduced in the practice with increasing expertise focusing on evaluating conduction defects requiring evaluation for cardiac pacing. In addition, early studies in patients presenting with tachycardia found tachycardia mechanisms that were a component of

D. R. Holmes Jr. (✉)
Department of Cardiovascular Diseases, Mayo Clinic, Rochester, MN, USA
e-mail: Holmes.david@mayo.edu

S. C. Hammill
Department of Cardiovascular Diseases (retired), Mayo Clinic, Rochester, MN, USA

D. R. Holmes Jr., R. L. Frye (eds.), *The Mayo Clinic Cardiac Catheterization Laboratory*, https://doi.org/10.1007/978-3-030-79329-6_13

Fig. 13.1 Book cover

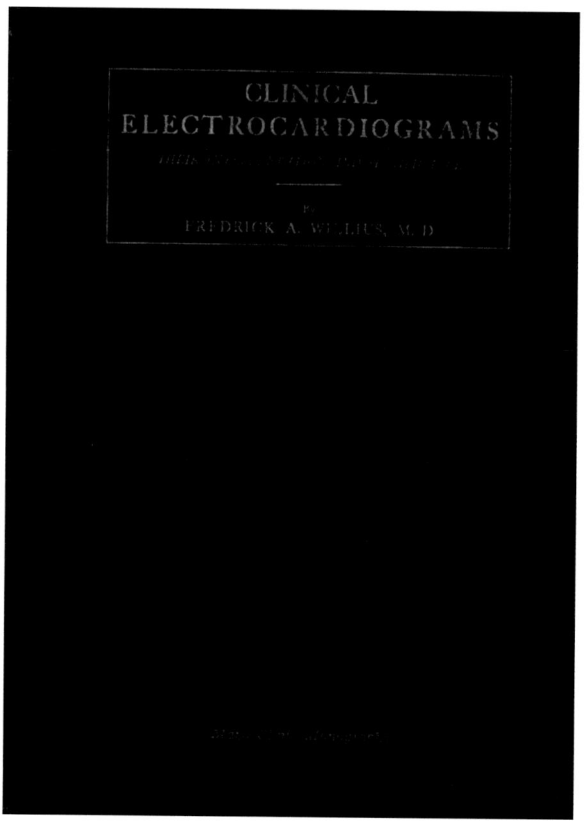

Wolff-Parkinson-White (WPW) syndrome as well as other SVT mechanisms, such as AV nodal reentry. These earlier studies were all analyzed and measured by hand with calibrated rulers and recorded in handwritten notes.

They formed the crucial basis of scientific information and conjecture for the 1980s during which there was a virtual electrical explosion (Figs. 13.2, 13.3, and 13.4). Early on the studies were performed by Dr. James Maloney, an established cardiologist/"electrophysiologist" physician and who was joined by Dr. Geoff Hartzler and later Dr. David Holmes, both of whom worked in cardiac pacing, electrophysiology, and invasive/interventional cardiology. Dr. Ron Vlietstra, who worked in pacing and invasive/interventional cardiology, also joined.

Two decades of permanent pacing from 1961 to 1981 were reviewed and published by Drs. Peter Hanley, Vlietstra, Merideth, Holmes, Broadbent, Osborn, McGoon, and Connolly [3]. Of importance, the authors included multiple stakeholders – invasive interventional cardiology, clinical EP, clinical cardiology, and cardiovascular surgery. Published in 1984, it included information on changes in trends and practice, the tremendous numerical growth of procedures, changing indications for permanent pacing, technology alternatives available with new modes of pacing, and changes in implantation strategies (Table 13.1). As noted in that

Fig. 13.2 Handwritten records were essential for categorization of clinical practice, evaluation of results, selection of patient subsets for more intensive scientific investigation, and development of quality practice initiatives. Books such as these were filled out on each patients – identifying diagnosis, date of procedure, and operator

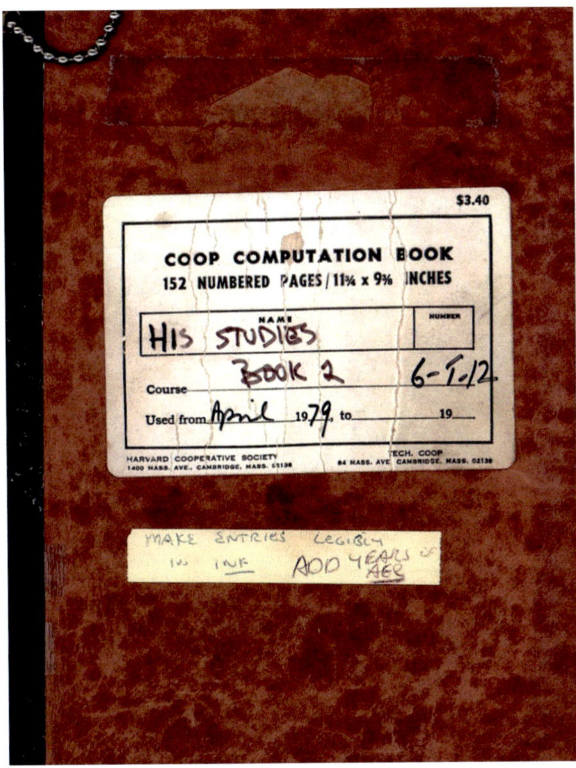

publication, in 1961 12 patients had undergone permanent pacing, all of whom had epicardial leads placed by surgeons during thoracotomy. These numbers increased greatly such that by 1971 there were 138 patients who underwent 170 procedures, all of which were still performed by surgeons. By 1981, this number increased even further to 262 patients undergoing 295 procedures. During these two decades, indications for pacing changed as did the specific pacing mode used (Table 13.2). An even more significant change occurred in the specialty of the implanting physicians; in 1971 all pacing systems were inserted by surgeons, while in 1981 only 4.4% were inserted by surgeons with the remainder being placed by invasive cardiologists. This was the result of a dramatic change in practice that had been implemented in 1978 when cardiologists assumed the dominant role. This transition required a shift from the location of implantation in the surgical operating theater to the cardiac catheterization laboratory in an angiographic suite. Since that time, the location of permanent pacemaker implantation has continued to be in the cath lab. However, even in the late 1970s through 1981, when procedures were performed in the cardiac cath lab, both specialties were involved. The cardiovascular surgeon, typically a surgical fellow, would make the incision, develop the pocket, and cannulate the cephalic vein and, soon thereafter, the subclavian vein. After cannulation, the transvenous lead/leads were placed by the cardiologist using fluoroscopic guidance. During

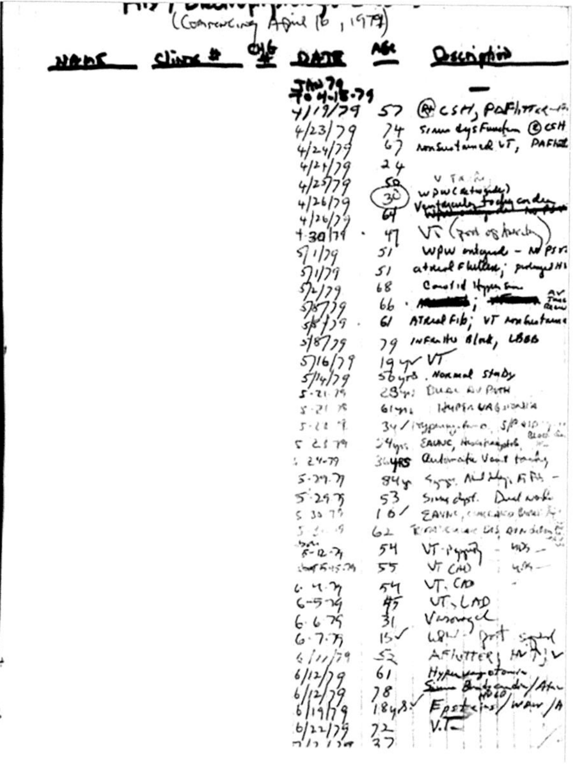

Fig. 13.3 A more detailed description of the types of cases being performed can be seen ranging from VT to hypervagotonia to conduction defects and enhanced AV nodal conduction. The specific handwriting of the entries provided a table of the specific operators involved; their handwriting remain easily identifiable over the lens of the past

cannulation of the subclavian vein, contrast was injected by anesthesia into a vein in the ipsilateral hand so that cannulation could be directed when the contrast was transiting the subclavian vein, thus avoiding inadvertent subclavian artery entry as well as pneumothorax. During this time, peel-away sheaths were introduced in the practice, making the procedure more efficient as both leads could be placed without problem through the same entry port. After thresholds and satisfactory pacemaker function were documented, the lead/leads were sutured in place, and the pocket was then closed by the waiting surgeon. Gradually the procedure evolved, and the cardiologists were trained in surgical skills for developing and then closing the pocket, making it not only secure but cosmetically very acceptable, at which time the entire procedural performance passed to the cardiologists. The decade of the 1980s would continue to show marked expansion in the practice of both cardiac pacing and electrophysiology; the future would evolve into further subspecialization with specific focus on either field by itself or both.

Upon his return to the Mayo Clinic staff from the Navy, Holmes was identified as a participant in the pacing and electrophysiology group along with James D. Maloney and John Merideth. To this group would be added Vlietstra, Wood, Osborn, Gersh, Broadbent, and David Hayes as well as Jane Trusty, the nurse coordinator, who was essential for scheduling, follow-up of patients, processes of care, and compilation of

Fig. 13.4 The more complete list of categories can be seen. Each procedure was indexed with this scheme and allowed for compilation of cases clustered by diagnosis which facilitated analysis

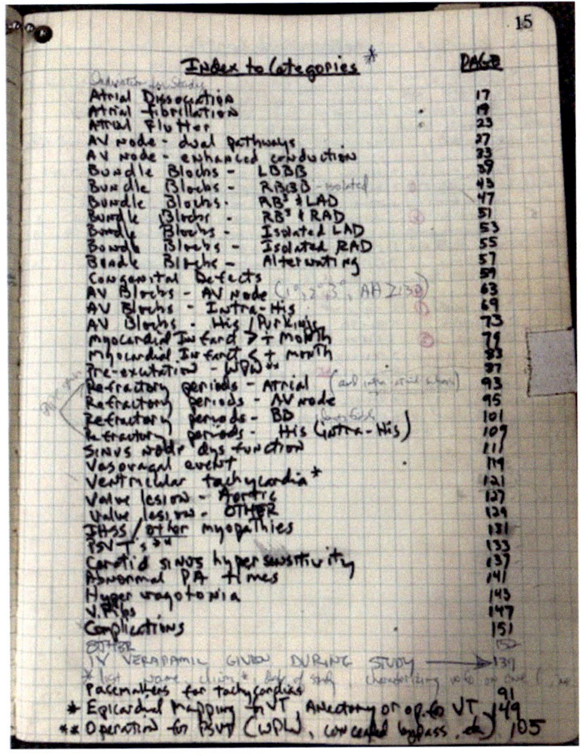

Table 13.1 Hanley et al. reviewed two decades of pacing beginning in 1961. During that interval, the number of patients increased markedly from 12 to 262, as striking were the operators. In 1961, surgeons performed all the procedures via thoracotomy. By 1981, cardiologists became the dominant implanters

Summary of data and analysis by patient and procedure subgroups				
	1961	1971	1981	Absolute change (%), 1971–1981
Patient groups				
All patients	12	138	262	Increased 90
No previous pacemaker	10	72	210	Increased 192
Previous pacemaker(s)	2	66	52	Decreased 21
Pacemaker placement	10	134	253	Increased 89
Postinfarction	0	0	7	…
Surgical bradycardia	1	4	11	Increased 175
Pacemaker syndrome	0	0	5	…
Procedures: 1 only	11	116	234	Increased 102
2	1	22	28	Increased 27
3	0	9	5	Decreased 44
4	0	3	0	Decreased 100

(continued)

Table 13.1 (continued)

Summary of data and analysis by patient and procedure subgroups

	1961	1971	1981	Absolute change (%), 1971–1981
Procedure groups				
All procedures	13	172	295	Increased 72
No previous pacemaker	11	92	236	Increased 157
Previous pacemaker(s)	2	80	59	Decreased 26
No pacemaker implant	0	4	9	Increased 125
Pacemaker placement	11	141	258	Increased 83
Operator				
Surgeon	13	172	13	Decreased 92
Cardiologist	0	0	282	…
Procedure duration (min)	…	92	78	Decreased 15
Male patients (%)	67	63	66	Increased 5
Mean age (yr)	49.8	66.7	66.2	Decreased 0.7

From Hanley et al. [3]; used with permission

Table 13.2 During the two decades of pacing analyzed by Hanley et al., there were also marked changes in pacing mode from VOO to VUI. Further changes in mode were seen in subsequent decades with dual chamber pacemakers becoming dominant

Pacing mode used (no previous pacemaker group)

Mode	1961 (%)	1971 (%)	1981 (%)
VOO	100	0	0
VVI	0	100	75
AAI	0	0	1
DVI	0	0	21
DDD	0	0	2
VDD	0	0	1

The first letter designates the chamber paced (A = atrium, V = ventricle, D = dual); the second, the chamber sensed (A = atrium, V = ventricle, D = dual, O = none); and the third, the response to sensing (I = inhibited, T = triggered, D = dual [atrial triggered and ventricular inhibited], O = none). From Hanely et al [3]; used with permission

data which resulted in multiple scientific manuscripts and presentations. Hayes joined the pacing group after participating in the Mayo Clinic Scholars Program spending his first 6 months of pacemaker training in New York City with Dr. Seymour Furman where they published the first paper on pacemaker-mediated tachycardia [4]. In addition to the science, Hayes had the chance to network and create close connections with others in the field both in the United States and Europe. After his first 6 months as part of this Mayo Clinic Scholars Program, he spent 3 months just outside of Paris during the spring working with Professor Jacques Mugica. The practice there was incredibly busy working with surgical colleagues doing many procedures per day often with multiple cephalic vein access approaches in contrast to the Mayo Clinic practice. Out of that experience, similar to that in

Table 13.3 Books published

Furman S, Hayes DL, Holmes DR Jr.: *A Practice of Cardiac Pacing*; Futura Publishing Company, Mount Kisco NY, 1986
Furman S, Hayes DL, Holmes DR Jr.: *A Practice of Cardiac Pacing, Second Revised and Enlarged Edition*; Future Publishing Company, Mount Kisco NY, 1989
Furman S, Hayes DL, Holmes DR Jr.: *A Practice of Cardiac Pacing, third Edition*, Future Publishing Co., Inc., New York, 1993

New York City, many connections were made throughout pacing centers in Europe. From these connections there were multiple visits to Nice, France, to explore the beaches and enjoy the spectacular but sometimes somewhat scant beautiful scenery but more importantly to evaluate the convention facilities as Hayes became the codirector of the international Cardiostim meeting held in Nice every 2 years. This meeting was a showcase for new technologies from around the world with leading experts and wide industry exposure as well as the latest data and strategies of care. In addition, during that time, he had the opportunity to develop strategies for analysis of large data sets of patients undergoing permanent pacing. With the strategies of efficiencies and practice patterns learned, the pacing service grew greatly in procedural volume, assessment of the science, and working with collaborators from other institutions and industry to bring to Mayo Clinic patients the most advanced developments for optimizing outcome. This growth resulted in three complete books on cardiac pacing by Furman, Hayes, and Holmes (Table 13.3) during the decade. Hayes subsequently went on to a prominent rise becoming director of the Mayo Clinic pacing service and president of the North American Society of Pacing and Electrophysiology (NASPE) which later evolved to the Heart Rhythm Society (HRS). Close collaborators included the prominent Seymour Furman, the first editor of the journal PACE, and colleague Doris Escher. These books documented what was being performed as well as led the way toward future approaches as the technology rapidly evolved; they continue to influence practice to the current time.

Close interaction with industry colleagues including Medtronic and CPI was essential with bidirectional input in the field. The close relationship was formalized by the establishment of the Visiting Scientist Program that allowed engineers and research scientists in industry to spend 3-month rotations at Mayo Clinic observing clinical procedures and participating in conferences. This collaboration allowed Mayo Clinic clinicians to work closely with industry scientists on the development of new pacing techniques such as those used to treat and prevent atrial fibrillation.

Early on, admittance to the pacing and electrophysiology group required attendance and active participation at a classic course devoted to electrocardiography held in Chicago at Michael Reese Hospital. The course featured and was directed by the legendary figures of Drs. Alfred Pick and Richard Langendorf, who had established our understanding of concealed conduction, the rule of bigeminy, and the basis for WPW syndrome, among many other seminal observations. The auditorium at Michael Reese Hospital held eager but very nervous participants; in theater style, they were seated before a dais immediately behind which was a large screen upon which exceedingly complex 12-lead electrocardiograms, vector cardiograms, and rhythm strips were projected to the whole auditorium. On the dais, there was a blackboard for Pick and Langendorf which was ideal for diagramming concepts and impulse conduction wave fronts. With each new ECG, vectorcardiogram, or rhythm strip, one of the course participants would be asked to identify themselves, the institution they were from, and then were invited to come forward in front of the entire audience. The participant would be given a large, foot-long pair of wooden calipers, and then Pick and Langendorf would ask that individual to work through the electrocardiograms and rhythms on the screen to make the diagnosis and discuss the relevant issues both known and unknown. Occasionally, the participant would be given one-half of a rhythm strip on a slide and then asked to diagram on the blackboard what the second half of the rhythm strip would need to show to make the diagnosis of what was happening, such as concealed conduction. During the course, every participant was asked to participate in this rich, emotional experience. As terrifying as you might imagine, lessons and strategies learned became imprinted for life.

The decade of the 1980s was one of extraordinary growth in pacing driven by improving programmable pacemakers with greater functionality, marked changes in implantation techniques with peel-away sheaths, fixation leads to minimize the chance of dislodgement, identifying optimal strategies for treatment of pacemaker infections, broadening of patient selection criteria, placement of the automatic implantable cardioverter defibrillator (AICD), and combining the lessons learned from electrophysiology. During that decade, pacing and electrophysiology formed a single group. The whole atmosphere was "electrified" by physicians who had come from around the world to become leaders at Mayo Clinic such as Bernard Gersh in 1978 who continued with an active pacing career before branching out into ischemic and structural heart disease. In addition, people came to train in Rochester, Minnesota, as well as those in the Mayo Clinic training program such as Dr. Rob Brandenburg. The international flavor, intellectual excitement, and pertinent probing questions asked were typified by Dr. Declan Sugrue from Ireland, Dr. Chris McLaren from Brisbane, Australia, and Dr. Maurice Choo from Singapore, among many others. Teaching, conferencing, questioning, and problem-solving were eclectic, far-ranging, and included input from the physician and nurse attendees and industry representatives. At that time, industry technical experts were able to be present in the procedure room for discussion of optimal programming and troubleshooting and were an invaluable asset.

Particularly prominent and popular were the late afternoon sessions which were open to all and quite well attended. At approximately 5:00 pm, we gathered in a specific nearby restaurant which had an adjacent room for liquid bread (aka beer) and free popcorn. During these sessions, topics ranged from who was writing up a series of patients, to clinical questions, to review of complex rhythm strips, to issues about MRI interference with pacemaker function and even other important issues such as Australian rules of football or cricket. These were special times of interaction and learning reminiscent of past meetings in Atlantic City where the doyen of basic electrophysiology, Dr. Gordon Moe, would invite fellows to a room in the evening at the end of a full day of science to discuss fundamentals of EP.

Out of those meetings in Atlantic City, which at times lasted several hours, as well as the meetings in Rochester, Minnesota, came robust scientific observations, several books on cardiac pacing, multiple publications including first in-human use applications, initial experiences, and large series. It also provided the opportunity to network with investigators from around the world including such luminaries as Furman, Escher, John Fischer, H.J.J. Wellens, Doug Zipes, Jacques Mugica, and others. This collaboration also included two individuals from Duke, Drs. Stephen Hammill and Douglas Packer, who would be enticed to join the staff and each of whom played extremely important roles after joining the Mayo Clinic cardiovascular group in EP and pacing. Both went on to play fundamentally important roles as national presidents of the Heart Rhythm Society.

Multiple areas of cardiac pacing were the subject of considerable interest and formed the basis of multiple investigations and publications.

Evaluation of Pacemaker/Lead Function

Lead function and durability had been a major issue in the earlier days of cardiac pacing highlighted by Hanley et al. [3]. Innovations in lead design had allowed more reliable function with implementation and widespread use of lead fixation using either passive leads, specifically bipolar tined polyurethane leads and/or screw-in active fixation leads. Lead design changes had also focused on late lead failure by changing to multifilament helical construction. By 1981, Mayo Clinic had evaluated long-term stimulation thresholds by measuring chronic strength duration curves, which led to important emphasis on measurement of these thresholds at the time of implantation for projecting longer-term outcome. An important topic of discussion centered around the advantages and disadvantages of bipolar versus unipolar systems.

During the decade, MRI units came into more frequent clinical use. One of the earliest Mayo Clinic experiences evaluated the effect of MRI studies on external and implantable pacemakers. Studies were made on discrete pulse generator components as well as single- and dual-chamber external pulse generators. In addition, the effect of MRI was studied in an anesthetized in vivo animal model study conducted after hours in radiology at St. Mary's Hospital after all clinical radiology procedures had been completed. All pulse generator reed switches closed in response to the magnetic field. The external pulse generators reverted from the demand mode to the asynchronous mode or exhibited total inhibition. In the in vivo experiments, changes in the stimulation rate analogous to the RF field pulse rate were seen, with the pacemaker acting as a potential antennae (Figs. 13.5 and 13.6). The in vivo test results depended on the mode and lead configuration. In a single-chamber pulse generator, the VVI mode reverted to an asynchronous mode which was related to reed switch closure. In another system, the pacing generator was found to act as an antenna and could be stimulated, and the heart could potentially be stimulated at the RF pulse period (Figs. 13.5 and 13.6). This work, among others, led to the development of hazard warnings for this interaction and spurred the eventual development of MRI-safe pacemakers [5].

An important part of evaluation of longer-term pacemaker function related to the issue of pacemaker infections. These had been seen since the initial days of

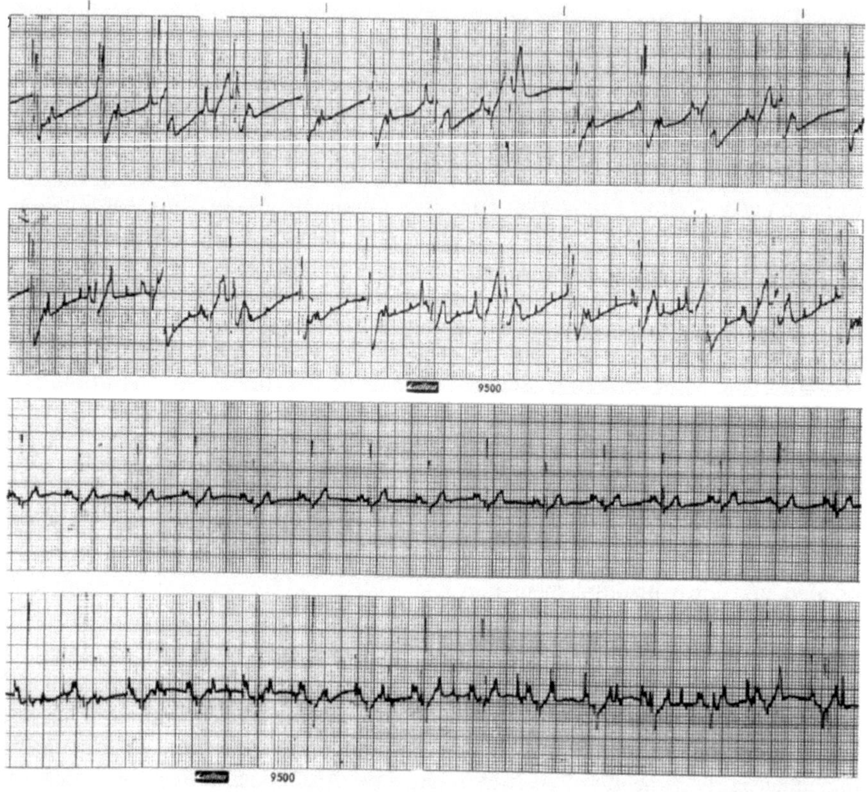

Figs. 13.5 and 13.6 The in vivo experiments with both single- and dual-chamber pacemakers documenting that with RF energy, pacing function changed from VVI a DDD to VOO or DOO. This occurred even when pacing rate was not affected by the RF field. (From Fetter, J., et al. Pacing Clin Electrophysiol 7 (4):720–727, 1984; used with permission)

pacemakers, but more complete knowledge of characterization and management was needed to optimize care. Early treatment approaches varied and included chronic suppressive antibiotic therapy, partial device removal, or the need for complete extraction of the pacing system including the leads. The approaches coming out of Mayo Clinic investigations during that time, in particular, the findings and conclusions made by cardiology fellow Choo, dramatically changed the field by focusing emphasis on the need for complete extraction of infected systems to optimize outcome and prevent recurrent infection. Such approaches became and remain standard.

Changes in Pacemaker Technology

Pacemakers in the 1980s and beyond became increasingly complex and included multi-programmable dual chamber devices with physiologic adaptability using a number of different sensors, transcutaneous interrogation telemetry, and anti-tachycardia pacing. Such extensive changes raised questions about utility, applicability, longer-term durability, outcome, and cost-effectiveness. The importance of industry collaboration was essential in keeping Mayo practice at the forefront.

At the end of the 1970s and then more frequently in the 1980s, Mayo Clinic was involved in application of patient-activated transvenous cardiac stimulation for both the treatment of supraventricular and ventricular arrhythmias. One of the earlier experiences published by Hartzler reported on two patients with drug-resistant chronic and recurrent ventricular tachycardia, each of whom was successfully treated with an implantable patient-activated unit [6, 7]. These cases were always extremely important as well as interesting from the standpoint that the specific pacing sequence selected needed to be reliably successful for terminating the arrhythmia, but which would not entrain the rhythm and result in clinically dangerous acceleration of either the supraventricular or, more importantly, the ventricular arrhythmia. Units were implanted, and for those with ventricular arrhythmias, patients were in the CCU for earliest testing (Fig. 13.7). Once the device was implanted, the arrhythmia was induced either by delivering programmed ventricular or supraventricular stimuli at the bedside using the previously placed temporary pacing lead. It was always of considerable interest to watch the entire medical and nursing team gathered around the patient as they activated the unit and then were so satisfied when it terminated the event. Many of these patients had excellent, clinical

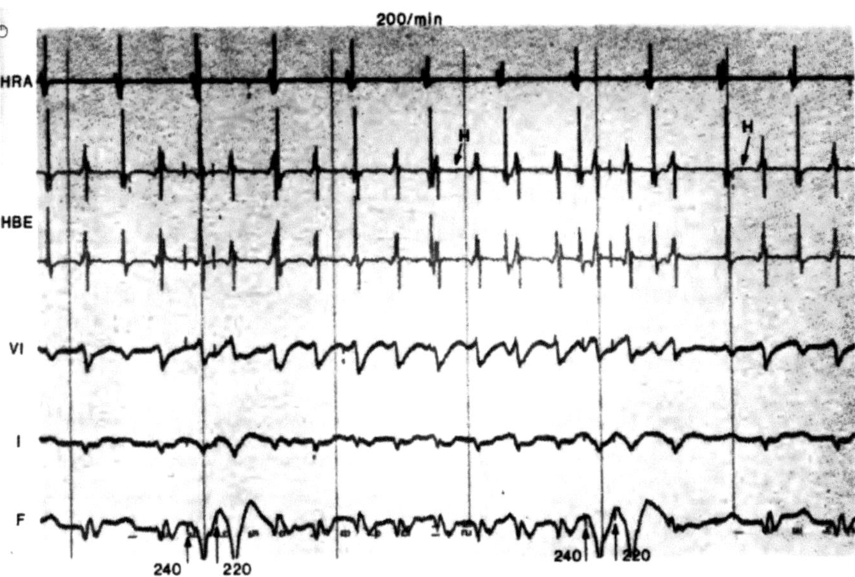

Fig. 13.7 A 21-year-old patient seen in 1978 with an IVC and non-obstruction hypertrophic cardiomyopathy had a history of recurrent ventricular tachycardia which had been resistant to multiple medications. During repeat EP studies, HIS Bundle reentrant tachycardia could be induced and terminated by paired ventricular stimuli at 240 and 220 msec. Subsequent to this, a patient-activated unit was implanted

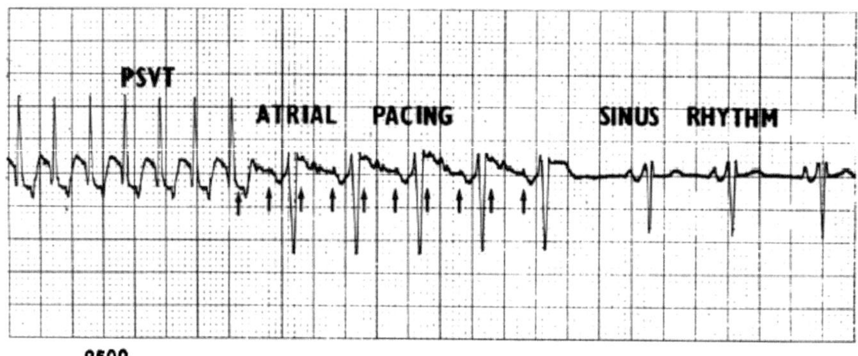

Fig. 3 (case 2). Surface electrocardiogram (lead V₁), showing restoration of sinus rhythm with overdrive pacing at 220 beats/min. PSVT = paroxysmal supraventricular tachycardia.

Fig. 13.8 Spontaneous PSVT – terminated by overdrive pacing at 220 beats/minute. (Sugrue, D.D. Mayo Clin Proc 60 (3):169–172, 1985; used with permission of Mayo Foundation)

longer-term successes and sometimes avoided the need for chronic medications. Evaluation of temporary antitachycardia pacing for supraventricular tachycardia was also the focus of considerable interest, particularly in very young children in hospital settings [8] (Fig. 13.8). These efforts continued throughout the decade and formed some of the basis and science needed in the development and now widespread use of the current advanced devices which include both antitachycardia algorithms and capabilities for cardioversion and defibrillation.

Significant attention throughout the decade focused on initial and early followup of the clinical efficacy of the multiparameter programmable generators and universal DDD pacing devices, the results of which were excellent and set the stage for more widespread acceptance of the use of these devices and expanded the indications.

Other important data were accumulated on the hemodynamics and systematic consequences of ventricular pacing, particularly the importance of ventriculoatrial conduction [9, 10] (Fig. 13.9). This specific study paved the way for the transition of what had been more frequent use of single-chamber VVI pacing to more physiologic approaches which have become standard. Related observations dealt with dual-chamber pacing for pacemaker syndrome (Table 13.4).

Other investigations included analysis of transvenous pacemakers in young children. An early case of an 18-month-old child raised important questions of how much lead redundancy to insert so that the child's growth could be accommodated without having to place new leads as the child grew. Other considerations related to the fact that the device was relatively large and modifications were often needed for development of a suitable pacemaker pocket.

Mayo Clinic had had a long history of involvement with what had become the vibrant field of electrophysiology. The field of more basic electrophysiology was one of particular growth. Supernormal conduction had been puzzling but of great interest. Howard Burchell had made observations on this in 1942 [2]. The term

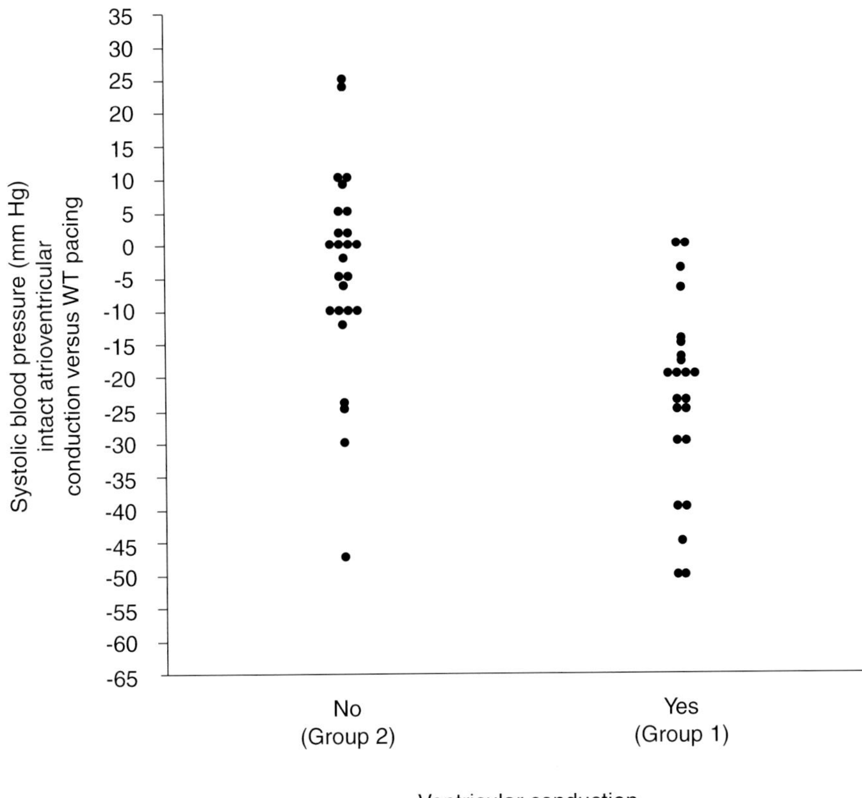

Fig. 13.9 Patients undergoing hemodynamic evaluation for chronic pacing, patients with intact ventriculoatrial conduction, and patients with ventricular pacing had significant decrease in arterial pressure. (From Nishimura et al. PACE, Vol. 5, 1982; used with permission)

"supernormal conduction" was confusing, as it did not refer to conduction which was faster than normal. Instead it referred to conduction which was better than anticipated under the circumstances. Multiple case examples and experiments identified what had been felt to represent this phenomenon. In an iconic article, the basic principles of "supernormal A-V conduction" had been published by John Merideth, a pioneer at Mayo Clinic working at the Masonic Medical Research Laboratory in Utica, New York, with Drs. Moe and Mendez [11]. This article discussed and evaluated multiple examples that had been attributed to the phenomenon but in which the authors were able to identify alternative explanations. In their summary, they identified three major categories that had been attributed to "supernormal conduction" including (1) occult 2:1 AV block in which an idioventricular beat "retracts" an otherwise refractory AV nodal barrier, (2) vagal depression of nodal conductivity, and (3) alternation between dissociated intranodal pathways. Such conceptual work remained a focus of interest as it was applied clinically to interpret complex

Table 13.4 Evaluation of the outcome of dual chamber pacing for the pacemaker syndrome. As seen, in patients with intact AV conduction, with VVI pacing there is a reduction in blood pressure. Programming the mode in the patients to DDD or DVI restored blood pressure to that seen when the patient was in normal sinus rhythm

Blood pressure responses to VVI pacing

Case	Ventriculoatrial conduction	Blood pressure (mm Hg)[a]				
		NSR	VVI	DDD or DVI	CSM	Δ (NSR to VVI)
1	+	144/82	120/76	140/70	80/...	24
2	+	150/90	100/90	164/80	100/90	50
3	+	168/80	90/80	160/80	90/...	78
4	+	120/80	96/80	134/80	76/80	24
5	−	94/54	84/50	90/50	85/48	10
6	+	140/80	98/60	135/65	98/...	42
7	+	120/80	66/...	130/80	66/...	54
8	+	120/80	90/60	110/80	90/60	30
9	+	190/90	140/85	180/80	90/...	50

[a]*NSR* normal sinus rhythm, *VVI* ventricular paced, ventricular inhibited, *DDD* atrial and ventricular sensing and pacing, *DVI* atrioventricular sequential pacing, *CSM* carotid sinus massage, Δ change

arrhythmias and then concluded that "the alternatives we have proposed should be considered before any complex arrhythmia is accepted as evidence of supernormal conduction."

Along with interest in basic electrophysiology, there was a rapidly evolving experience with clinical conditions.

Some of the earliest experience evaluated patients with atrioventricular and ventriculoatrial preexcitation in WPW syndrome. Mayo Clinic had been interested in this syndrome and had performed "His bundle" procedures in patients with this syndrome. In August of 1966, a 43-year-old man was seen at Mayo Clinic with the main complaint of episodes of "rapid heart action" which had been present for approximately 20 years but had become increasingly frequent up to several times a month. At the time of his evaluation, the electrocardiogram (Fig. 13.10a, b) documented a classic pattern of WPW type B, and the vectorcardiogram documented that the initial (delta) vector was oriented to the left, anterior, and superior. The analysis suggested that the early excitation of the right ventricle was a "bundle" (accessory muscular connection) at the right lateral border of the heart (Fig. 13.11). There had been a case report of the "histologic demonstration of accessory muscular connections between the auricle and ventricle in a case of short P-R interval and prolonged QRS complex" in 1943 and another report earlier that year in 1967. The Mayo Clinic authors, with this information, a "Heart Team" of three cardiologists and one cardiac surgeon (Drs. Frye, Anderson, and McGoon) led by Dr. Howard Burchell, designed a strategy which presaged the field of surgical interruption of these "bundles of Kent." It included exploration of the right ventricle below the A-V groove to determine the time of earliest activation (Fig. 13.11). Pressure on that point of earliest activation terminated the frequent short paroxysms of tachycardia

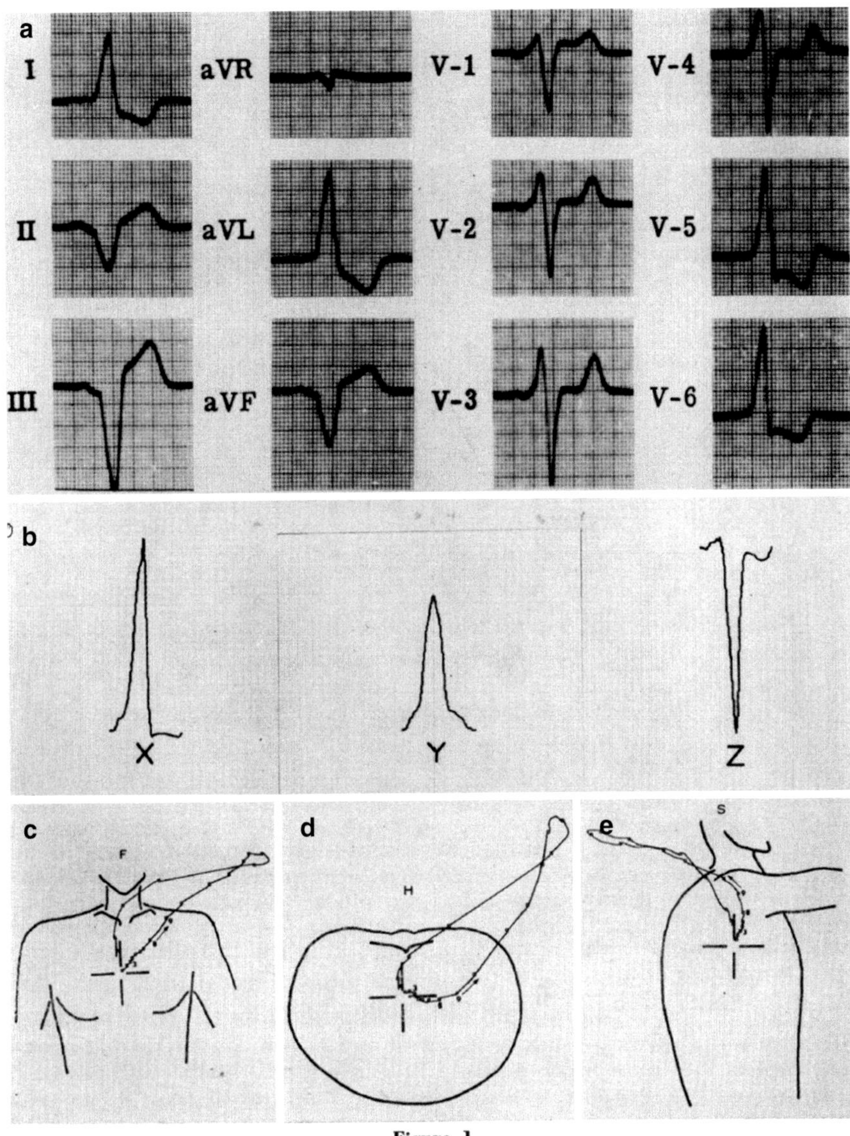

Figure 1

(A) Routine electrocardiogram. Recording speed 50 mm/sec. (B) X, Y, and Z leads. (C, D, and E) Vectorcardiogram as computer plotted from X, Y, and Z modified Frank system (Mayo).

Fig. 13.10 (**a** and **b**) Baseline electrocardiogram and vector cardiogram on a 43-year-old man with frequent episodes of STT document and what was then called type B with initial delta vector oriented to the left and anterior and superior. (From Burchell, H.B., et al. Circulation 36 (5):663–672, 1967; used with permission)

Fig. 13.11 Mapping at the time of surgery documented earliest activation at the points seen and was consistent with the vector of the impulse. (From Burchell, H.B., et al. Circulation 36 (5):663–672, 1967; used with permission)

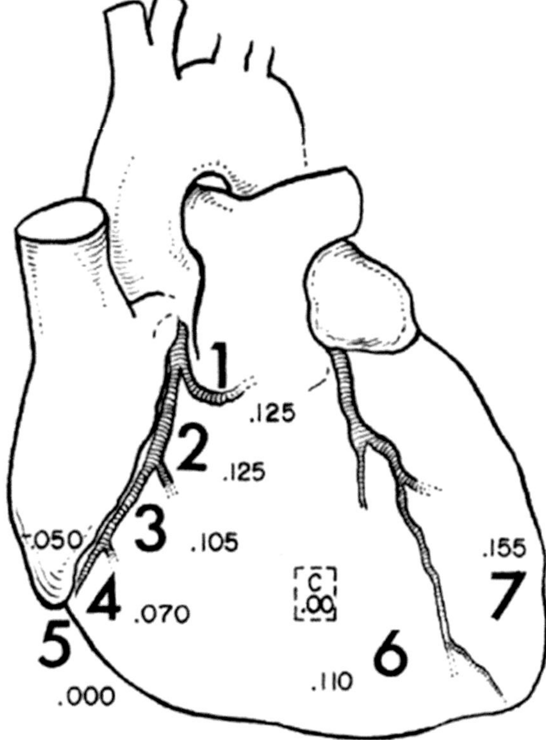

Figure 2

Diagram, as utilized in operating theater, for identification of points of exploration by unipolar electrode. Values for excitation are given in reference to earliest intrinsic deflection (marked .000) on right border of right ventricle near groove. Measurements are between sites on base-line intercept by sharp intrinsic deflection. The rectangle enclosing CO refers to excitation deflection at zero time within the right ventricular cavity.

during the surgical procedure which had been initiated by a premature atrial contraction. The authors then injected procaine at the right ventricular muscle site of earliest activation which resulted in disappearance of the preexcitation of the right ventricle. Dr. McGoon then made a transverse 1-cm-long incision on the inside of the right atrium close to and parallel to the AV ring, and then the intracardiac repair of the ASD was completed during which time the P-R interval was normal, without evidence of ventricular preexcitation. However, at the end of the procedure, preexcitation had returned. In the discussion, the authors stated "in retrospect the incision…seems unduly timid but may be defended because the patient was not disabled by his episodes and one could neither jeopardize the results of the operation recommended for cure of the ASD or risk the remote chances of complete heart block." They also planned subsequent surgical approaches which were implemented in the years to come.

Working closely with the cardiac surgeons, specifically Gordon Danielson, the surgical treatment of accessory atrioventricular pathways became more frequently applied [12]. The use of cryoablation for treating AV nodal and focal atrial tachycardias during cardiac surgery became common and improved the efficacy and safety of selected surgical procedures. An example of the innovative surgical approaches taking place during this time period involved the surgical treatment of a patient with atrial tachycardia refractory to medications. Sinus tachycardia at the time of surgery suppressed the atrial focus preventing mapping. Temporary suppression of the sinus node by cooling allowed the atrial focus to become active, facilitating successful mapping and cryoablation [13]. Along with surgery was the introduction and then wider use of percutaneous ablation strategies for treatment of tachycardia in a variety of clinical circumstances, including the use of DC ablation for the production of AV nodal block in patients with atrial fibrillation resistant to all pharmacologic agents [14].

These observations spurred interest over the 1980s in the Mayo Clinic laboratory in the study of concealed retrograde bypass tracts, enhanced AV nodal conduction, and clinical and electrophysiologic characteristics of patients with accelerated atrioventricular nodal conduction. Initial studies were often performed under the direction of Hartzler who had developed superb experience in the field. A written logbook was initiated in which we recorded each "His study" (Figs. 13.2, 13.3, and 13.4). Before the days of computer records, the His records were manually reviewed and intervals painstakingly measured on roll records with calipers. This logbook formed a valuable resource for development of new approaches to a variety of patient groups including patients with tachycardia-induced cardiomyopathy, symptomatic bundle branch block, syncope of unknown etiology, and out-of-hospital cardiac arrest in patients without clinically significant coronary artery disease.

An important group of patients were those presenting with loss of consciousness (syncope) of unknown etiology. Multiple issues in these patients included the need for prolonged monitoring in the hospital or electrophysiologic studies to assess conduction. Brandenburg, an advanced cardiology trainee, analyzed the largest group of these patients that had been recorded and reported the results at a national meeting. Skeptics of the study results in these patients and the actual clinical need for study in this group abounded. However, subsequent investigations in the field confirmed the initial Mayo Clinic experience and validated the need for careful evaluation including tilt table testing [15]. It also stimulated the introduction of tilt-table testing as an integral component of evaluation of patients with a variety of clinical symptoms to evaluate the mechanisms of cardioinhibitory and vasodepressor syncope [16]. Hammill, now a staff member from Duke and subsequent director of pacing/electrophysiology, developed the Mayo Clinic protocol for tilt-table testing in a small procedure room that had been developed for barium UGI swallows in which the patient lies supine initially and then the table could be brought to a vertical position where measurements of blood pressure and heart rate could be analyzed along with patient symptomatology to help define the etiology of the clinical events. Along with this, the tilt table could be used after catheters had been placed to evaluate the effect of position on rhythm disturbances. Hammill et al. evaluated this application in 104 patients, of whom 59 had supraventricular tachycardia, 6 had vasovagal syncope, and 39 had carotid sinus hypersensitivity. In this group, 23 (22%) had significant abnormalities when upright that were not present when supine. In one of the patients (Fig. 13.12a–c), SVT with sinus node reentry could be induced while supine and was well tolerated, but on assuming the upright position on the tilt table had acceleration and near syncope, reproducing the patient's symptoms. Other important related observations were focused on the natural history and results of treatment of symptomatic "isolated carotid sinus hypersensitivity" with anticholinergic drugs or pacemakers and evaluation and treatment of "hypervagatonia" as a cause of syncope.

The Mayo Clinic group was one of the first to report on patients with tachycardia-induced cardiomyopathy and that the abnormal depressed ventricular function in such patients had the potential to improve after control of their tachycardia [17, 18].

An important component of the practice during this time was the interaction with other physicians in the state. Drs. Holmes and Benditt, from the University of Minnesota, initiated a regularly scheduled meeting, open to all physicians in the state that was case-based and very interactive. Some of the earliest ideas about etiology and treatment of syncope originated from this collaboration.

In addition to syncope, supraventricular tachycardia, and AV conduction, a central focus of interest revolved around ventricular arrhythmias, electrophysiologic testing, and drug evaluation for treatment. A glimpse of the logbook from that time indicates the variety of clinical conditions evaluated, including programmed extra-stimulation techniques (Figs. 13.2, 13.3, and 13.4). Interest in this specific field was central to Hartzler's eclectic skills and expertise. During EP studies in these patients, single, double, and triple extra-stimuli were delivered during sinus and paced rhythm to see if either sustained VT or VF could be initiated. Depending on the results of this, intravenous procainamide was used, and then repeat extra-stimuli were again delivered. The Mayo Clinic section of engineering designed the "rosewood box" which housed an advanced cardiac stimulator and was used for several years until smaller, more advanced devices became commercially available. The "EP service," as we were called then, spent countless hours both in the CCU and the EP lab drug testing patients with ventricular arrhythmias. Multiple conversations about double and triple extra-stimuli to induce a ventricular arrhythmia and the specificity and

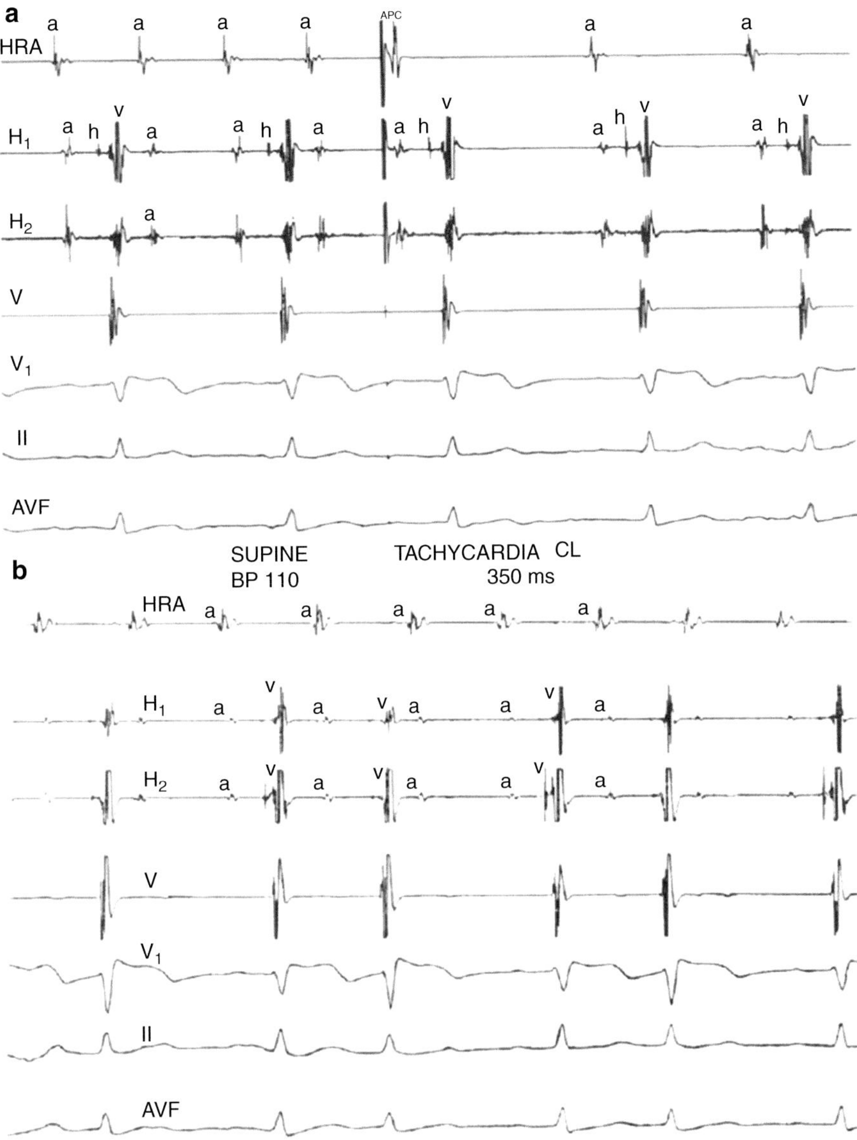

Fig. 13.12 (**a**) During EP study, in a patient with spontaneous SVT related to sinus node reentry, an APC terminates the arrhythmia. (**b**) In the patient in the supine position, tachycardia CL is 350 msec and BP is 110 mm systolic. (**c**) When the patient is upright, the CL decreases to 320 msec, and BP falls to 75 with resultant associated symptoms of near syncope. (From Hammill, S.C., et al. I Am Coll Cardiol 4 (1):65–71, 1984; used with permission)

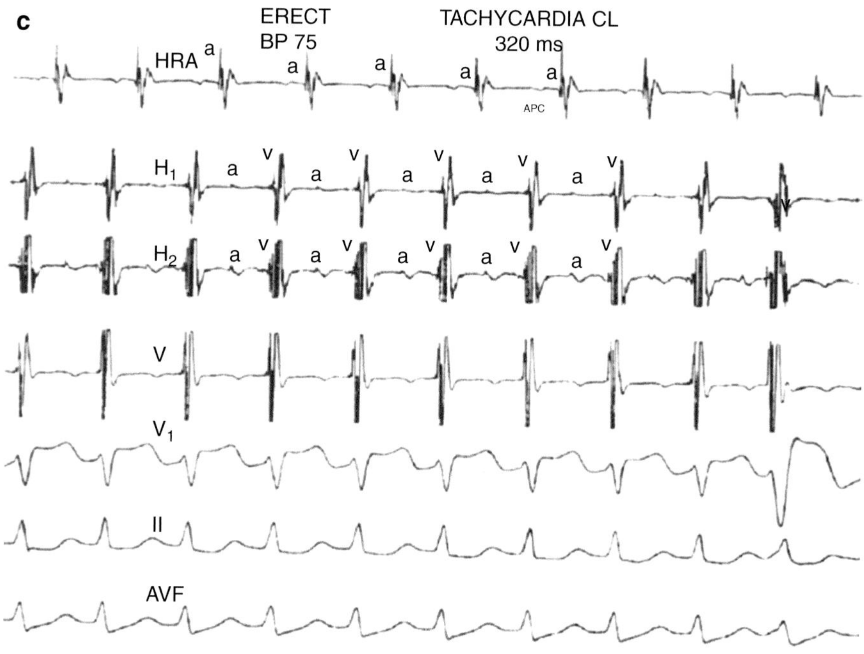

Fig. 13.12 (continued)

sensitivity of different techniques were explored as part of the strategy developed to treat these high-risk patients. Such discussions about sensitivity and specificity of inducible rhythms based on the use of multiple increasingly aggressive algorithms continue to the present time. After identifying the clinical arrhythmia, multiple drugs were administered in an attempt to find a medication that would preclude induction, in which case the patient would be treated with that approach.

Select patients with ischemic heart disease and persistent ventricular tachycardia despite serial drug testing underwent the procedure of endocardial resection and/or aneurysmectomy to eliminate the substrate that supported reentrant ventricular tachycardia. These surgical procedures were complex and included members from the EP team operating and interpreting the recordings derived from the epicardial and endocardial mapping systems being developed at the time and the cardiac surgical team headed by Dr. Hartzell Schaff.

In addition to drug testing, as mentioned, permanent pacemakers for termination of both supraventricular and ventricular tachycardia were tested. Throughout this time, there was active discussion about the potential for ablation of some of these ventricular rhythms. The brain child of Hartzler, details of patient characteristics, the concept, and inception were the focus of considerable thought, requiring the delivery of DC energy in the left ventricle using a quadripolar catheter after the ventricular arrhythmia had been mapped. The initial experience with ablation for ventricular tachycardia occurred under the direction of Hartzler and Holmes.

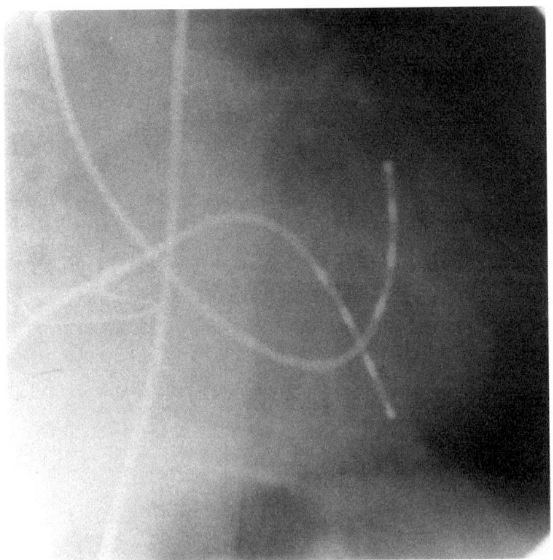

Figs. 13.13 and 13.14 Intracavitary VT ablation used DL energy. On Figure 13.14, during each shock the fluoroscopic image became blank

Subsequent to this, the procedure, while infrequent, laid the foundation for directed VT ablation and continued to be applied in very carefully selected patients. In 1985, a 60-year-old man was referred for drug-resistant sustained monomorphic ventricular tachycardia status post-single vessel LAD CABG with a patent graph but severe hypokinesis of the anterobasal, anterolateral, apical basal septal, and posterolateral segments. The EF was 40%. Medical therapy had included amiodarone, procainamide, Norpace, and beta-blocker. After extensive discussion by four EP physicians, Wood, Holmes, Hammill, and Osborn, the patient was taken to the catheterization laboratory. Quadripolar catheters were placed into both right and left ventricles (Figs. 13.13 and 13.14). Mapping was performed at eight separate locations during clinical VT, with the earliest point of activation in the anterolateral free wall of the left ventricle. Under general anesthesia, four 300-joule shocks were delivered through the distal electrode of the left ventricular catheter and exited through a back surface paddle. During each shock, as had been seen with earlier cases, the fluoroscopic image (Figs. 13.13 and 13.14) became blank as the image intensifiers were saturated for a brief time before returning to normal function. After the fourth shock, the patient had no spontaneous clinical tachycardia and that specific rhythm could not be induced. The patient did well in the hospital and 36 years later was still living as registered in Mayo Clinic records. These early procedures set the way for more targeted intervention which has now become standard of care.

This multi-stakeholder decade closed brightly with continued evolution of both diagnostic and therapeutic energy applied to improve the clinical outcome of a large number of patients using less invasive strategies of care and paving the way to more modern pacing and electrophysiologic techniques. A review of where we are and where we are going was published by Hammill, Sugrue, Gersh, Porter, Osborn, Wood, and Holmes (1986) [19].

References

1. Fye WB. Frederick A. Willius. Clin Cardiol. 2001;24:751–2.
2. Burchell HB. Observations on additional instances of a supernormal phase in the human heart. J Lab Clin Med. 1942;28:7–11.
3. Hanley PC, Vlietstra RE, Merideth J, et al. Two decades of cardiac pacing at the Mayo Clinic (1961 through 1981). Mayo Clin Proc. 1984;59:268–74.
4. Hayes DL, Furman S. Atrio-ventricular and ventriculo-atrial conduction times in patients undergoing pacemaker implant. Pacing Clin Electrophysiol. 1983;6:38–46.
5. Holmes DR Jr, Hayes DL, Gray JE, Merideth J. The effects of magnetic resonance imaging on implantable pulse generators. Pacing Clin Electrophysiol. 1986;9:360–70.
6. Hartzler GO, Holmes DR Jr, Osborn MJ. Patient-activated transvenous cardiac stimulation for the treatment of supraventricular and ventricular tachycardia. Am J Cardiol. 1981;47:903–9.
7. Hartzler GO. Treatment of recurrent ventricular tachycardia by patient-activated radiofrequency ventricular stimulation. Mayo Clin Proc. 1979;54:75–82.
8. Sugrue DD, McLaran C, Hammill SC, Gersh BJ, Mair DD, Holmes DR Jr. Refractory supraventricular tachycardia in the neonate: treatment with temporary antitachycardial pacing. Mayo Clin Proc. 1985;60:169–72.
9. Nishimura RA, Gersh BJ, Vlietstra RE, Osborn MJ, Ilstrup DM, Holmes DR Jr. Hemodynamic and symptomatic consequences of ventricular pacing. Pacing Clin Electrophysiol. 1982;5:903–10.
10. Nishimura RA, Gersh BJ, Holmes DR Jr, Vlietstra RE, Broadbent JC. Outcome of dual-chamber pacing for the pacemaker syndrome. Mayo Clin Proc. 1983;58:452–6.
11. Moe GK, Childers RW, Merideth J. An appraisal of "supernormal" A-V conduction. Circulation. 1968;38:5–28.
12. Holmes DR Jr, , Danielson GK, Gersh BJ et al. Surgical treatment of accessory atrioventricular pathways and symptomatic tachycardia in children and young adults. Am J Cardiol 1985;55:1509–1512.
13. Wood DL, Hammill SC, Danielson GK. Use of the cryoprobe to facilitate intraoperative electrophysiologic mapping by inhibiting sinus node function in automatic atrial tachycardia. Am J Cardiol. 1987;59:176.
14. Wood DL, Hammill SC, Holmes DR Jr, Osborn MJ, Gersh BJ. Catheter ablation of the atrioventricular conduction system in patients with supraventricular tachycardia. Mayo Clin Proc. 1983;58:791–6.
15. Kapoor WN, Hammill SC, Gersh BJ. Diagnosis and natural history of syncope and the role of invasive electrophysiologic testing. Am J Cardiol. 1989;63:730–4.
16. Hammill SC, Holmes DR Jr, Wood DL, et al. Electrophysiologic testing in the upright position: improved evaluation of patients with rhythm disturbances using a tilt table. J Am Coll Cardiol. 1984;4:65–71.
17. McLaran CJ, Gersh BJ, Sugrue DD, Hammill SC, Seward JB, Holmes DR Jr. Tachycardia induced myocardial dysfunction. A reversible phenomenon? Br Heart J. 1985;53:323–7.
18. Grogan M, Smith HC, Gersh BJ, Wood DL. Left ventricular dysfunction due to atrial fibrillation in patients initially believed to have idiopathic dilated cardiomyopathy. Am J Cardiol. 1992;69:1570–3.
19. Hammill SC, Sugrue DD, Gersh BJ, et al. Clinical intracardiac electrophysiologic testing: technique, diagnostic indications, and therapeutic uses. Mayo Clin Proc. 1986;61:478–503.

Chapter 14
1990s: EP and Pacing

Thomas M. Munger, Stephen C. Hammill, Douglas L. Packer, and Win-Kuang Shen

As the last decade of the twentieth century opened, two new heart rhythm leaders emerged at Mayo Clinic Rochester (MCR). These were Drs. Stephen Hammill and David Hayes, both to subsequently become presidents of the Heart Rhythm Society (formerly North American Society of Pacing and Electrophysiology [NASPE]).

This decade would see the emergence of new service lines of practice in the area of arrhythmology, including RF catheter ablation, nonthoracotomy ICD implantation, dedicated outpatient and inpatient arrhythmia services, a vigorous regional outreach clinical practice, the opening of heart rhythm services at the new sister clinics in Phoenix, Arizona, and Jacksonville, Florida, dedicated space for heart rhythm laboratory procedures on the St. Mary's Hospital, creation and expansion of basic and translational science labs, formal creation of CME programs and an EP Fellowship Program, and ultimately the formation of the core team for MCR heart rhythm as it exists today. This was also the time at which electrophysiology transitioned from a diagnostic specialty to a full-fledged medical and procedural therapeutic endeavor. This is that story.

T. M. Munger (✉) · S. C. Hammill · D. L. Packer
Department of Cardiovascular Diseases, Mayo Clinic, Rochester, MN, USA
e-mail: Munger.thomas@mayo.edu

W.-K. Shen
Department of Cardiovascular Diseases, Mayo Clinic, Phoenix, AZ, USA

© Mayo Foundation for Medical Education and Research, under exclusive license to Springer Nature Switzerland AG 2021
D. R. Holmes Jr., R. L. Frye (eds.), *The Mayo Clinic Cardiac Catheterization Laboratory*, https://doi.org/10.1007/978-3-030-79329-6_14

Mayo Clinic Rochester Leadership in Pacing and Electrophysiology

Dr. John Merideth had opened the Device Clinic at Mayo Clinic in 1971 and then became the first director of the pacemaker/EP group in 1974. As outlined in the prior chapter, he had spent time with Gordon Moe (a University of Minnesota graduate [1940]) in Utica, New York, during the 1960s, who would also later collaborate with Dr. Douglas Zipes and Dr. Jose Jalife. Downstate, at the time at the Staten Island Public Health Service Hospital, was Dr. Anthony Damato and a training/investigative program that would include multiple future leaders of clinical electrophysiology: Drs. Akhtar, Gallagher, Josephson, Mirowski, Prystowsky, Ruskin, and Scherlag, among others.

In 1972, Dr. James Maloney had performed the first His study at Mayo Clinic. Following this, the pacing and electrophysiology section was then led by Dr. Maloney in 1978, followed by Dr. David Holmes in 1980, and subsequently by Dr. Michael Osborn in 1984.

In 1988, Dr. Stephen Hammill became the EP lab director, and Dr. David Hayes became the device lab director. By now, Dr. Holmes had assumed directorship of the cardiac catheterization lab where he would devote the lion's share of his subsequent career.

Administrative minutes of the first 3 years of Steve's and David's tenure are archived in a booklet entitled "EP-PM Administrative Meeting Minutes, 1988–1990." In attendance at that first meeting, January 27, 1988, were Drs. Stephen Hammill, Doug Wood, Bernard Gersh, David Hayes, and Jan Christiansen, RN. Absent, but to be noted in future meetings, were Drs. David Holmes, Michael Osborn, Michael McGoon, Ronald Vlietstra, Co-Burn Porter (Peds), John Merideth, and Jane Trusty, RN.

Topics for that first meeting included setting meeting times; reviewing research protocols, CPI Ventak-P, CPI Endotak, and IV Amiodarone, and Pacesetter Sensalog (rate-responsive pacer); and centralization of appointment follow-up for ablation (which was still DC, since 1981) and ICD patients. Finally, budgeting for an OR mapping system and an electrophysiology (EP) computer database was initiated (Fig. 14.1).

The Administrative Playbook: 1988–1990

For the next 3 years, this "playbook" of group administrative activity would serve as the template for major initiatives of the next decade and beyond. Personnel, space, research topics, service lines, outreach, IT, and others are archived in the pages of this document:

- April 5, 1988: Dr. Marshall Stanton (training with Dr. Doug Zipes group in Indiana) was approved as a Mayo Clinic Scholar.
- April 5, 1988: Dr. Doug Packer was approved as clinician investigator.

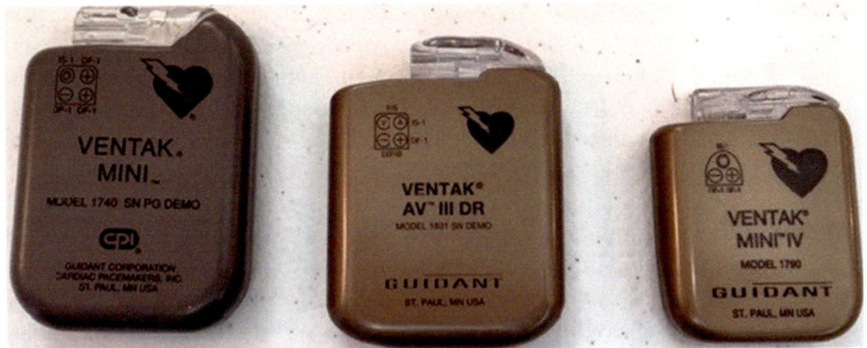

Fig. 14.1 During the 1990s, ICD implantation moved from the surgical suite to the electrophysiology laboratory. Here are three different versions of the CPI Ventak line, circa 1995–1999 with the device shown. The original MINI was smaller than the preceding Ventak-P (1988) and PRx (I, II, III, 1990–1994). The earlier versions weighed 180–235 g with displacements of 100–145 cc, whereas the MINI weighed only 125 g and had a volume of 68 cc. The MINI IV was only 78 g and had a volume of 39 cc

- April 5, 1988: EP-PM fellows were approved – 1 year clinical and 1–1.5-year research (Dr. Doug Wood had been the first fellow).
- June 1, 1988: Dr. Richard Rodeheffer (CHF) discussed a study to look at complex ectopy in DCM patients (placebo vs. amiodarone).
- July 6, 1988: Dr. Thomas Munger had expressed interest in a 2-year EP fellowship to Dr. Hammill.
- September 7, 1988: Initiation of the EP-PM Thursday Cath Conference.
- October 5, 1988: Dr. Munger – 1 year of NIH research which was to be undertaken with Dr. Packer who would soon be arriving from Duke.
- October 5, 1988: Clinical protocols for head up tilt and antiarrhythmic therapy for DCM patients were discussed.
- November 2, 1988: Bloom stimulators and recording systems were to be reviewed at AHA meeting.
- January 4, 1989: The ECG Lab database for Olmsted county was finalized.
- January 4, 1989: Dr. Packer begins at Mayo Clinic Rochester with translational lab space on Alfred-4 at St. Mary's Hospital.
- February 1, 1989: Dr. Vlietstra recommends a teaching video on pacemaker implant and EP studies be made for NASPE.
- February 1, 1989: Dr. Win Shen to begin his EP Clinical Fellowship in April 1989 a year after arriving back from Duke basic science training.
- February 1, 1989: The signal-averaged ECG was introduced into clinical practice at Mayo Clinic.
- March 1, 1989: Dr. Hayes comments on the need for an additional device implanter, and interest for this position had been expressed by Dr. Raul E. Espinosa, which was to be discussed with Dr. Hugh Smith, then chair of cardiology.
- March 1, 1989: Red Wing (joint U Minnesota-Mayo Clinic annual EP meeting) was discussed.

- March 1, 1989: Dr. Packer discussed preliminary thoughts about the "Buxton Protocol," a multicenter study of patients with nonsustained VT, low EF, and inducible VT randomized to treatment or nontreatment. This of course was to become the pivotal trial published a decade later, in December of 1999: Multicenter Unsustained Tachycardia Trial (MUSTT). MUSTT, along with the MADIT studies, would rapidly expand ICD indications in the early 2000s.
- May 10, 1989: Guidelines for the CV Division were proposed for the use of flecainide and encainide in anticipation of the August publication in NEJM of the Cardiac Arrhythmia Suppression Trial (CAST). The paradigm at the time was that if one suppressed ventricular ectopy in patients with DCM or post-MI, then one would reduce sudden death. Wray and Seltzer had hinted at the proarrhythmic effects of antiarrhythmic therapies by reporting on quinidine syncope in the early 1960s. Now, CAST had shown this for patients with coronary artery disease, and thus new local guidelines were required for the Mayo Clinic practice. And an FDA advisory followed which required legal input and alerts sent to our cardiologists and patients. This type of proactive review and action served as a template for device and lead recalls in the subsequent three decades.
- July 12, 1989: EP trainees expressed interest in a Classic EP Journal Club initiating.
- August 2, 1989: Isoproterenol was added to head up tilt testing for vasovagal syncope.
- October 4, 1989: Dr. Espinosa to begin on pacing service as a fellow in January–March 1990 and as a staff consultant in April–June 1990.
- October 4, 1989: Dr. Marshall Stanton became the first director of electrophysiology education. The Monday AM weekly AM/PM conference was to resume.
- October 4, 1989: Incremental 0.5 FTE MD was requested to begin a dedicated 1/2 day Heart Rhythm Clinic (HRC). The other 1/2 day would be dedicated to traditional cardiac clinic. The MD would do 15 arrhythmia consults per week (3 per day).
- October 4, 1989: The computerized EP report process was finalized. The worksheet would be completed during the case, given to Administrative Assistant Susan Wegman, and then she would enter the data, and the report would be placed in the paper record and a copy sent to the outside physician.
- November 1, 1989: Jeanette Ramaker, one of the original two EP techs moved to a data collection job with the Lavonne Hammes' cath lab group. Joyce Lewis, a surgical tech from CV surgery, was hired to replace Jeanette Ramaker.
- November 1, 1989: All weeks for the MD staff for 1990 were covered except those for AHA and ACC, a chronic problem for a group with multiple responsibilities at the national level and would be a recurring theme over the years.
- November 1, 1989: Comments were solicited about the formation of a dedicated Arrhythmia Hospital Service.
- December 13, 1989: The use of chemical ablation to treat VT and radiofrequency ablation to treat AVNRT and accessory pathways was discussed. Dr. Stanton was to travel to the University of Arizona to visit Dr. Frank Marcus, and Dr. Packer was to travel to the University of Oklahoma to visit Dr. Warren Jackman to discuss these energy sources and techniques.

- January 3, 1990: At the first administrative meeting of the decade were Drs. Hammill, Hayes, Osborn, McGoon, Stanton, Gersh, Packer, and Nurse Trusty. There were 12 weeks uncovered for HRC that year, the MUSTT protocol was to be reviewed by the CV research committee, and a schedule for the EP fellow to have 1 day off per week was instituted.
- February 21, 1990: It was noted that more patients were rapidly being referred in from the region, both Group Health in Minneapolis, Minnesota, and Sioux Falls, South Dakota. Access at Mayo Clinic was only 25% of other regional groups, and thus it was suggested access be increased dramatically (EP outreach) and provide excellent service (computerized reporting sent to referring MDs). Scott Finnesgard and Shu Hon Yu from the Mayo Clinic IT group were to facilitate the latter.
- March 14, 1990: Mayo Clinic began research protocol implantation of the Medtronic PCD which was an ATP/pacing/ICD combination device that eventually was approved in the 1992–1993 timeframe. The new Transvene lead that would follow in late 1990 would allow nonthoracotomy placement of ICDs. Additionally, CPI entered into their Phase III study of the Ventak-P investigational protocol and anticipated market release in late 1990 as well.
- March 14, 1990: A case of a patient's stroke in the EP lab was presented for quality assurance purposes. This process was to be replicated in the future with the development of the quality assurance section of pace/EP in subsequent decades.
- May 9, 1990: Lisa Fanning was appointed as "lead technician" position at the EP/PM lab at St. Mary's Hospital. This was a new position. Computer terminals were installed in the EP Reading Room on Alfred-6.
- May 9, 1990: Dr. Hammill had sent a request to Dr. Hugh Smith to add an FTE for creating an EP consult service (hospital) and increment the EP lab to three EP consultants, beginning in 1991.
- May 9, 1990: Dr. Packer reported that the RF ablation protocol had gone through CPC and was now at the Mayo Clinic IRB committee.
- September 5, 1990: Additional staff requests – EP-PM technician and EP studies coordinator. The EP computer system was to replace the EP logbook in 1991.
- December 5, 1990: The first nonthoracotomy PCD with intravascular leads was implanted in Room #70 (St. Mary's Hospital, Alfred-6). The patient was then taken to CV surgery to have the SQ patch placed, leads tunneled, DFT testing, and device implanted.
- December 5, 1990: The RF generator arrived in the late autumn with the first ablation performed by Drs. Packer/Hammill.

Pacing and Electrophysiology: Hammill and Hayes

Dr. Stephen Hammill had completed his EP Fellowship at Duke University in 1980, with Dr. John Gallagher. Steve looked at jobs at the University of Oklahoma and the University of Michigan (chief: Bertram Pitt) before arriving at Mayo Clinic Rochester. He interviewed with Drs. Holmes, Gersh, Osborn, and Hugh Smith.

The first cardiovascular surgeon he met after arriving in Rochester was at an OR mapping with Dr. Gordon Danielson (who had been doing surgical division of accessory pathways since 1972 at Mayo Clinic). (Dr. John Gallagher had always done these at Duke in the surgical theater with Drs. William Sealy and James Cox.) He remembers receiving the question, "Who are you?" during that initial case (Fig. 14.2); nonetheless Steve and Gordon would share hundreds of mapping cases over the next 20 years.

Another surgical colleague, Dr. Hartzell Schaff, was recruited the same month as Dr. Hammill and did much of the intraoperative ventricular tachycardia (VT) mapping and surgical ablation in the 1980s and 1990s. Dr. Schaff also did the first ICD implant at Mayo Clinic in 1985. To qualify for implant, a patient would have to survive two cardiac arrests, syncopal events, or sustained VT episodes, one without and one with amiodarone administration! The batteries on the first devices lasted a little over a year, were large displacement requiring thoracotomy and abdominal placement, and provided only unipolar waveform shocks. The first models weighed 250 g with a displacement of 145 cc, compared to contemporary devices weighing 80 g and volumes of 30 cc. Additionally, there was no bradycardia pacing, no antitachycardia pacing (ATP), and no diagnostic electrograms (EGMs). The zone rate cutoffs had to be customized and set at the factory and could not be changed.

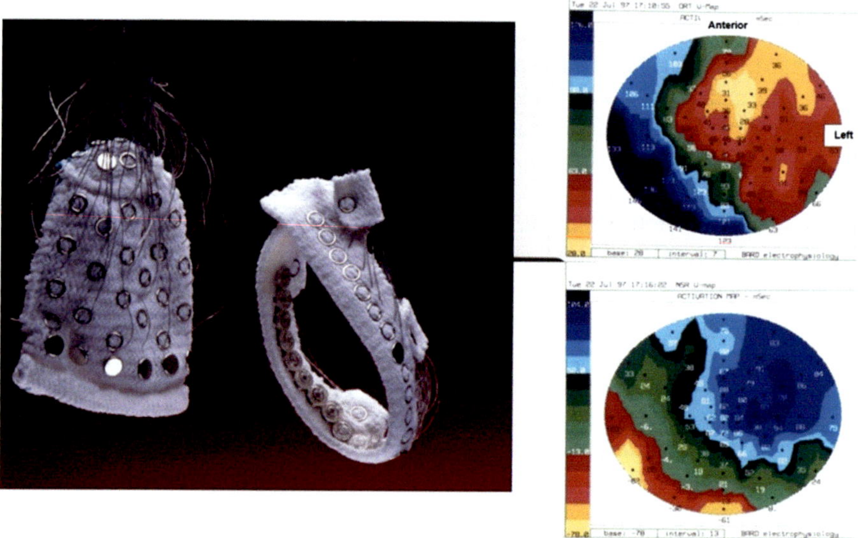

Fig. 14.2 By the 1990s, intraoperative mapping for WPW, which had been done since the late 1960s and early 1970s, had been automated by using these sock and AV ring multielectrode arrays with a computerized mapping system. This 1997 RV/LV epicardial map, in an Ebstein's patient undergoing tricuspid valve repair with Dr. Gordon Danielson, was created with the sock electrode array on the left. The top map shows earliest activation in *yellow* and *red* of the midventricular LV (left conduction system) with delay to the RV due to the patient's RBBB. The lower map, collected in orthodromic reciprocating tachycardia, demonstrates two retrogradely conducting accessory pathways on the right free wall and posterior septum of the RV

Steve recalls that there were a lot of extra connections to be made on the early ICD devices, a feature that prompted Hartzell to clear his throat and dryly observe that scientists worked on the device and everyone else had worked on the leads. Subsequently, programming of detection rate, energies, and duration of arrythmia until therapy were available by 1988. By 1990, biphasic waveforms were being developed with transvenous leads, and in 1993, the devices were miniaturized enough to move the packs from the abdomen to the pectoral area.

Delayed approval of the nonthoracotomy ICD devices in the early 1990s tweaked Steve's interest in what professional societies like NASPE (currently HRS) might bring to the table in regard to information for new technology approval and subsequent regulation and payment paradigms. He and David also saw this as an opportunity to work with colleagues in the industry to enhance research collaboration for better products. Thus, a Mayo Clinic scholarship program was developed for industry engineers to imbed those individuals within the Mayo Clinic practice to facilitate learning about deficiencies and enhancements that would be important from the clinicians' point of view.

The early 1990s was also a time to enhance the allied staff roles in the EP and pacing lab. To this day, advanced mapping on the Rochester campus is performed primarily by electrophysiology technicians, and programming and testing of implantable devices are done by device nurses. Industry staff function in supportive roles. Electrophysiology nurses in conjunction with fellows perform central venous access. The nurses were also responsible for stimulation during diagnostic and ablation studies, continuing to this day.

Dr. David Hayes completed his Internal Medicine and Cardiovascular Training at Mayo Clinic Rochester and worked with Dr. Jim Maloney as a participant in the Young Investigator competition at NASPE (established in 1979). To achieve expertise in device implantation and management, Dr. Hayes completed the last 6 months of fellowship before coming on the Mayo Clinic staff (via Dr. Bob Frye's direction and Dave Holmes' encouragement) in 1982 at the Montefiore Hospital in the Bronx, New York City. There he worked with Dr. Seymour Furman (who, with two colleagues, had placed the first endocardial pacemaker in 1958). He remembers his first encounter with Dr. Furman, who initially reminded David that he was tired of writing papers for his fellows. With that challenge, David hammered out a manuscript examining the AV and VA conduction times in patients undergoing pacer implant, further clarifying the mechanisms of pacemaker-mediated tachycardia (PMT) in the new age of dual-chamber pacing. He and Dr. Furman published this in January 1983. This collaboration would continue as Drs. Furman, Holmes, and Hayes would publish "A Practice of Clinical Pacing" in 1986 (now in its fifth edition) (Fig. 14.3).

In the Spring of 1983, after Dr. Hayes began his staff career at Mayo Clinic, under a NAPSE Fellowship, he traveled to the Clinic Val d'Or, Paris, France, to further his implantation skills; there, a surgeon did the implants, typically 10–12 implants per day using the cephalic technique. By the time he and Steve assumed directorships in the late 1980s, dual pacing was well established with multiple

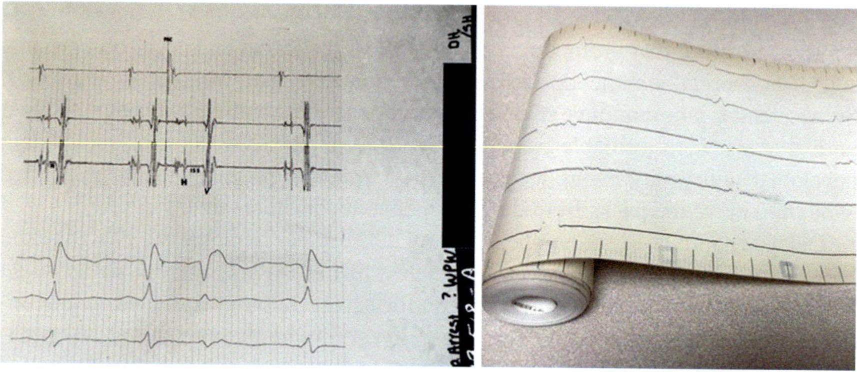

Fig. 14.3 The computer entered the EP lab in the early 1990s. This two-catheter (RA and HIS) study was performed by Drs. David Holmes and Steve Hammill in 1982 in a patient with out-of-hospital arrest. Note the prolonged HV interval of 155 msec. The rolling paper record was not always immediately available for review. Contemporary archiving uses cloud servers and discs with immediate retrieval and review and dozens to hundreds of channels of data available (as opposed to the 4–6 channels shown above)

candidate rate-responsive sensors under study, including accelerometers, dP/dT, QT, and the ventricular depolarization gradient (VDG).

As the 1990s opened, Dr. Ron Vlietstra was doing most of the extractions. With infections, lead failures like the 801 Telectronics Accufix J-lead fractures, and incremental endocardial hardware implantation, it became clear that new technology was required for extraction. Spectranetix (now part of Philips) introduced the laser sheath to facilitate extraction in the 1990s which immediately increased the success and tempered the risk of extraction (albeit not to zero). During this decade, devices became more miniaturized, and the initial primary prevention ICD trials were released (MADIT, 1996). During this decade a core of four implanters would finish the decade: Hayes, Osborn, McGoon, and Espinosa. This would change in the 2000s as indications further expanded for device therapies (Fig. 14.4).

One of the most cited papers of the group during this time was a study examining the interactions between implantable devices and the newly emerging cellular phone technologies. This was critically important to understand implantable device interactions with consumer wireless products in the complex electrical environments of the upcoming twenty-first century.

Dr. Hayes served as NASPE president from 1999 to 2000 and soon thereafter became division chair for cardiovascular medicine at Mayo Clinic Rochester. Important initiatives during that time (just after the 20th anniversary of NASPE) included moving the society to a larger platform by hiring a dedicated administive partner James Youngblood, and moving the headquarters from Massachusetts to Washington, DC. David and Steve also helped establish internal allied health education programs as well as similar programs with Pacesetter and then

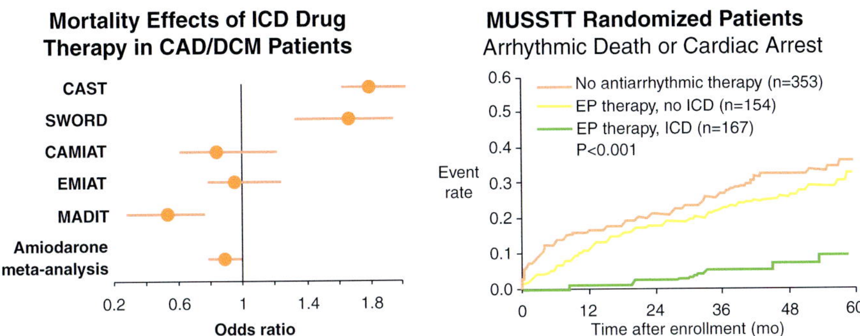

Fig. 14.4 During the 1990s, several trials of antiarrhythmic therapy (CAST/SWORD using flecainide, encainide, and D-sotalol) were shown to increase mortality in patients with ventricular arrhythmias, depressed EF, and coronary disease or dilated cardiomyopathy. Amiodarone appeared to offer mild benefit in meta-analysis, but the MADIT trial was one of the earliest to demonstrate the advantage of primary prevention ICD. MUSTT soon followed and confirmed this observation

Medtronic. Later colleagues, like Drs. Paul Friedman and Sam Asirvatham, would make similar contributions.

RF Catheter Ablation and the Multicenter Randomized Trial

As Dr. Doug Packer arrived at Mayo Clinic in 1989, there had been just two decades of surgical accessory pathway ablation and 8 years of DC catheter ablation for AV block creation and VT. RF ablation was just appearing in the literature as an alternative energy source for destruction of cardiac tissue to facilitate tachyarrhythmia treatment. Dr. Packer had always been interested as a child in tearing the wrecked cars of toy electric trains apart, and this led him to do electrical work on automobiles at his father's car dealership. He eventually went to Duke University for medicine, cardiology, and electrophysiology. There, Dr. Eugene Stead had been Department of Medicine chair for two decades and the founder of the Duke Cardiovascular Disease Research Database, the first of its kind and the resource for the Duke Clinical Research Institute (DCRI). Doug met Dr. Gallagher and Dr. Cox and met during faculty visits Drs. Zipes, Scheinman, Josephson, Prystowsky, and Klein. He was a contemporary of Dr. Gust Bardy (SCD-hEFT trial), worked in the research labs of Drs. Harold Strauss and Gus Grant, and trained just ahead of Drs. Ellenbogen, Curtis, Worley, and Chen. While on staff at Duke for 3.5 years following his EP fellowship, he worked with Dr. Rob Califf as CCU codirector. He bought Stephen Hammill's house in 1981 as Steve was leaving for Minnesota. He also networked with the fellows at Penn, Drs. Frank Marchlinski and John Miller.

After Dr. Packer arrived in 1989, he opened the translational laboratory at Alfred-4 at St. Mary's Hospital where his first two fellows were Drs. Jennifer Shannon and Thomas Munger. He redesigned the EP reporting system at Mayo Clinic. After acquisition of the initial radionics RF generator, the first RF WPW ablation was performed in 1990 (with guest Dr. Bill Miles from Indiana University), and all other arrhythmia targets followed in the next 5 years. During the 1990s, multiple tools came online to facilitate catheter ablation including 4-D mapping systems for which he received his first AHA Grant in 1993 with Dr. Rich Robb. Additionally, an intracardiac ultrasound (ICE) catheter was co-developed with Dr. James Seward in 1998 that immediately provided real-time information for transseptal puncture targeting, evaluation of hypotension and effusion, and lesion formation assessment. These tools were then used in tandem in the translational animal lab at St. Mary's Hospital to facilitate biophysics characterization of newer ablative energy sources like cryoablation as the decade closed.

The first AF catheter ablation at Mayo Clinic was in 1997 and was patterned after work Dr. James Cox had performed creating the MAZE III/IV. Dr. JJ Morris, as well as Drs. Schaff, Sundt, and Dearani, would use the COX surgical technique at Mayo Clinic in the early 1990s. Dr. John Swartz had done earlier work with nonsteerable catheters. As the group began linear ablation for AF before 4-D mapping was available, the archiving of ablations was left to the poor technicians sticking "paper dots" onto a transparency that was over the AP and lateral cameras of the X-ray screens! AF ablation also was the subject of an AHA grant. Soon thereafter, the Haissaguerre paper outlining the pulmonary vein isolation as a target (later termed wide-area-circling ablation (WACA) by Doug in 2003) complemented the linear paradigm, and the "catheter-MAZE" was born.

As mentioned above, the "Buxton Protocol" or what was to become the MUSTT trial came to Mayo Clinic with Dr. Packer and was published in NEJM in late 1999; it clearly documented that EP-guided drug therapy was inferior to ICD implantation for mortality in regard to ischemic patients with EF <40% and inducible VT that was drug refractory OR responsive. His experience with MUSTT and his prior work with the group at Duke would then serve the Mayo Clinic Group well in future participations within several trials: SCD-hEFT, HAT, and CABANA.

The 1990s as a Growth Engine

The decade would see the pacing and electrophysiology group begin the three-decade growth phase which continues to this day. In 1994, the lab space at the St. Mary's campus left Alfred-6 and moved to the new Mary Brigh add-on wings on the fourth floor (the current location). The new space housed up to 12 labs that was shared with the interventional cardiac catheterization lab, as well as a dedicated tilt lab. Initially, the HRS group occupied 3 labs, rooms 110, 111, and 112, while 105, 109, and 106 were added in more recent years. Several more faculty came on the staff during this decade, including Drs. Win Shen, Tom Munger, Robert Rea, Paul Friedman, Margaret Lloyd, and Arshad Jahangir. Robust basic science programs also grew this decade and will be covered in the next chapter. Additionally, EP outreach programs to North Dakota, Iowa, Wisconsin, and out-state Minnesota (Duluth) were created to facilitate referral, evaluation, and treatment in a clinical field that was exploding.

The Electrophysiology Fellowship grew from one fellow per year to two and at times had three. Dr. Shen facilitated developing an International Training Program and included MDs from abroad who would visit for 3–12 months for observation and targeted research projects while others would get formally trained (these countries included Australia, Ireland, Japan, Turkey, Israel, Hong Kong, Russia, India, Malaysia, Germany, and China, to name several). Dr. Michael Glikson from Sheba Medical Center trained with the group during this time and has provided a lifetime of international collaboration for multiple projects.

It was also during the 1990s that the pacing and electrophysiology section initiated their first CME meeting series. Dr. Stanton facilitated this with the first Mayo Clinic heart rhythm CME meeting in Napa Valley, California, in 1995. This has become the annual "Arrhythmias and the Heart" Hawaii meeting, attended regularly by over 300 participants and accompanied by no fewer than ten other CME offerings by Mayo Clinic faculty groups.

As the 1990s closed, a look back at the top Mayo Clinic Rochester HRS authors' papers in that decade documents the important concepts, issues, and studies from the HRS team (Appendix). The group had undergone rapid growth and was poised for the twenty-first century with active basic, translational, and clinical arrhythmology programs, and the educational backbone to complement those assets.

Mayo Clinic Rochester HRS Authors' 20 Top Cited Papers of the 1990s

1. Murphy JG, **Gersh BJ**, Mair DD, Fuster V, **McGoon MD**, Ilstrup DM, McGoon DC, Kirklin JW, Danielson GK. Long-term outcome in patients undergoing surgical repair of Tetralogy of Fallot. *NEJM* 1993; 329:593–9. **<u>CITATIONS: 791</u>**

   - *Includes section on late sudden cardiac death incidence in 161 TOF surgical patients followed for a mean of 21 years, many since the 1950s.*

2. Grogan M, Smith HC, **Gersh BJ, Wood DL**. Left ventricular dysfunction due to atrial fibrillation in patients initially believed to have idiopathic dilated cardiomyopathy. *Am J Cardiol* 1992; 69:1570–3. **<u>CITATIONS: 455</u>**

   - *The first reference in Martha's paper is Doug Packer's 1986 Duke study of tachycardia-induced cardiomyopathy (TICM) in eight patients: one with atrial tachycardia and seven with accessory pathways; another Mayo paper in 1985 with senior author DR Holmes had observed tachycardia myocardial dysfunction in four points with accessory pathways. Martha's 1992 paper included ten AF TICM patients and referenced that the last paper to site this phenomenon was from 1949 and commented that quinidine could provide relief from CHF in this cohort.*

3. **Munger TM, Packer DL, Hammill SC**, Feldman BJ, Bailey KR, Ballard DJ, **Holmes Jr., DR, Gersh BJ**. A population study of the natural history of Wolff-Parkinson-White Syndrome in Olmsted County, Minnesota, 1953–1989. Circulation 1993;87: 866–73. <u>**CITATIONS: 378**</u>

   - *An Olmsted County natural history study of 113 WPW patients followed over a mean of 12 years. Ages at detection ranged from birth to 77 years and a sudden death rate of 0.0015 per patient-year with none occurring in the half of patients who had no symptoms. Seven percent had structural heart disease. The incidence per year of newly diagnosed cases was 4 per 100,000.*

4. Ficker DM, So EL, **Shen WK**, Annegers JF, O'Brien PC, Cascino GD, Belau PG. Population-based study of the incidence of sudden unexplained death in epilepsy (SUDEP). *Neurology* 1998; 51:1270–4. <u>**CITATIONS: 365**</u>

   - *All patients with SUDEP 1934–1994 in Rochester, Minnesota, were compared to the expected rate of SCD in people ages 20–40 years. Nine cases were noted with a rate of 0.35 per 1,000 person-years, an incidence 24 times higher than the background rate of SCD.*

5. Nishimura RA, **Hayes DL, Holmes Jr., DR**, Tajik J. Mechanism of hemodynamic improvement by dual-chamber pacing. *JACC* 1995; 25:281–8. <u>**CITATIONS: 359**</u>

   - *Fifteen patients with DCM underwent variable AV interval settings with simultaneous Doppler echo, and catheterization generated hemodynamics which suggested diastolic MR should be avoided in these patients.*

6. Ommen SR, Odell JA, **Stanton MS**. Atrial arrhythmias after cardiothoracic surgery. *NEJM* 1997; 336:1429–34. <u>**CITATIONS: 359**</u>

   - *This concise paper reviewed contemporary medical and cardioversion management of POAF, a very frequent clinical arrhythmia, as well as the appropriate use of anticoagulation (warfarin). The paper also comments on recent FDA approval of ibutilide, an option for rapid AF/AFL.*

7. Wilkoff BL, Byrd CL, Love CJ, **Hayes DL**, Sellers TD, Schaerf R, Parsonnet V, Epstein LM, Sorrentino RA, Reiser C. Pacemaker lead extraction with the laser sheath: results of the pacing lead extraction with the excimer sheath (PLEXES) trial. *JACC* 1999; 33:1671–6. <u>**CITATIONS: 339**</u>

   - *Early extraction had relied on snare, traction, and telescoping rigid sheaths. This randomized trial of 301 patients with 465 chronic leads used the new laser sheath technology vs. conventional techniques. Success was 94% for laser vs. 64% for conventional. It should be noted there were potentially life-threatening complications in three laser patients and zero conventional patients.*

8. Low PA, Opfer-Gehrking TL, Textor SC, Benarroch EE, **Shen WK**, Schondorf R, Suarez GA, Rummans TA. Postural tachycardia syndrome (POTS). *Neurology* 1995; 45: S19–25. **CITATIONS: 326**

   • *This review described the Mayo Clinic system of grading the severity of the poorly understood disorder of orthostatic intolerance.*

9. Holmuhamedov EL, Jovanovic S, **Dzeja PP**, Jovanovic A, **Terzic A**. Mitochondrial ATP-sensitive K⁺ channels modulate cardiac mitochondrial function. *Am Physiol Soc* 1998; 275: H1567–76. **CITATIONS: 319**

   • *Direct evidence for mitochondrial K_{ATP} channel involvement in the regulation of mitochondrial metabolic functions was demonstrated. These channels are on the inner mitochondrial membrane. Elsewhere in the myocyte, they exist on the sarcolemma, where when opened, shortening of the action potential occurs, as well as a decrease in intracellular calcium, resulting in cardioprotection during ischemia.*

10. Nishimura RA, **Trusty JM**, **Hayes DL**, Ilstrup DM, Larson DR, Hayes SN, Allison TG, Tajik AJ. Dual-Chamber pacing for hypertrophic cardiomyopathy: A randomized, double-blind, crossover trial. *JACC* 1997; 29:435–41. **CITATIONS: 310**

    • *Nineteen patients with severe HCM underwent either DDD pacing for 3 months followed by AAI pacing for 3 months or the reversed order. Hemodynamic echo gradients were assessed as well as QOL scoring and exercise tolerance. Sixty-three percent in the dual arm had improvement but 41% also did in the AAI arm with 31% having no change in the DDD arm and 5% getting worse. It was also observed that there was symptomatic improvement in some patients without a gradient improvement, suggesting a placebo effect might also have been present.*

11. Paulmichl M, Li Y, Wickman K, **Ackerman M**, Peralta E, **Clapham D**. New mammalian chloride channel identified by expression cloning. *Nature* 1992; 356:238–41. **CITATIONS: 298**

    • *This new class of ion chloride channel was expressed in Xenopus oocytes. This was chloride-selective and an outward current. Its function was examined by site-directed mutagenesis which resulted in dependence on extracellular calcium concentration.*

12. **Terzic A, Jahangir A, Kurachi Y**. Cardiac ATP-sensitive K⁺ channels: regulation by intracellular nucleotides and K⁺ channel-opening drugs. *Am J Physiol* 1995; 269 (Cell Physiol. 38): C525–45. **CITATIONS: 268**

    • *The molecular structure of the K_{ATP} channel was now understood. The regulation of nucleotides by this channel was reviewed in several papers from outside and within the Mayo Clinic group.*

13. **Ackerman MJ**. The long QT-syndrome: Ion channel diseases of the heart. *Mayo Clin Proc* 1998; 73: 250–69. **CITATIONS: 251**

- *At that time, over 35 mutations in 4 ion channel genes – KVLQT1, HERG, SCN5A, and KCNE1 – had been identified (LQTS 1, 2, 3, and 5). Many more have been identified by Dr. Ackerman and others over the ensuing two decades.*

14. **Hayes DL**, Wang PJ, Reynolds DW, Estes III M, Griffith JL, Steffens RA, Carol GL, Findlay GK, Johnson CM. Interference with cardiac pacemakers by cellular telephones. *NEJM* 1997; 336:1473–9. **CITATIONS: 244**

    - *This was a multicenter prospective cross-over trial of 980 patients with PPMs and 5 different cellular phones (1 analog and 4 digital); the incidence of clinically important interference was 7%. This interference was not seen if the phone was placed over the ear. Since cellular phones were just coming to market at that time, the observations for device patients and the use of such consumer devices were significant.*

15. Driscoll DJ, Jacobsen SJ, **Porter CBJ,** Wollan, PC. Syncope in Children and Adolescents. *NEJM* 1997; 336:1473–9. **CITATIONS: 222**

    - *Using the Rochester Epidemiology Project, children seeking medical attention for syncope during 1950–1954 and 1987–1991 were examined. The incidence of syncopal patients seeking medical attention was 72 and 126 per 100,000 per year and was higher for females with an incidence in the 15–19-year age groups.*

16. **Ackerman MJ**, Tester DJ, **Porter CBJ**. Swimming, a gene-specific arrhythmogenic trigger for inherited Long QT Syndrome. *Mayo Clin Proc* 1999; 74:1088–94. **CITATIONS: 197**

    - *Thirty-five cases of autosomal LQTS with the DVLQT1 gene were confirmed with blood or molecular autopsy methods. Six of these patients had a personal or family history of drowning or near-drowning. One of these included a molecular autopsy of a 12-year-old girl who had died in 1976 from drowning.*

17. Bardy GH, Marchlinski FE, Sharma AD, Worley SJ, Luceri RM, Yee R, Halperin BD, Fellows CL, Ahern TS, Chilson DA, **Packer DL**, Wilber DJ, Mattioni TA, Reddy R, Kronmal RA, Lazzara R. Multicenter comparison of truncated biphasic shocks and standard damped sine wave monophasic shocks for transthoracic ventricular defibrillation. *Circulation* 1996; 94:2507–14. **CITATIONS: 186**

    - *In this prospective, randomized, blinded study, 294 patients eligible for analysis were studied at the time of ICD implantation testing. Equivalence was shown for a 200-joule monophasic damped sine wave pulse vs. a 130-joule truncated biphasic pulse. There was less ST segment shift seen 10 s after shock delivery in the biphasic group and was to have implications for upcoming AED cost, size, and weight.*

18. Oliva PB, **Hammill SC**, Edwards WD. Cardiac rupture, a clinically predictable complication of acute myocardial infarction: report of 70 cases with clinicopathologic correlation. *JACC* 1993; 22:720–26. **<u>CITATIONS: 170</u>**

   - *Patients who had rupture had a higher incidence of pericarditis, restlessness, repetitive emesis, and agitation than those without. Rupture was often associated with sudden transient hypotension and bradycardia and pseudonormalization of T wave inversions from their infarction.*

20. Spittell PC, *Hayes DL* . Venous complications after insertion of a transvenous pacemaker. Mayo Clin Proc 1992; 62:258–265. **<u>CITATIONS: 143</u>**

   - *This was an overall compendium of complications with transvenous pacer insertion over the prior 3 decades from 63 prior studies published in the timeframe of 1980-1990. Venous thromboembolism remained a signficant morbidity.*

29. **Shen WK**, Edwards WD, **Hammill SC**, Bailey KR, Ballard DJ, **Gersh BJ**. Sudden unexpected nontraumatic death in 54 young adults: a 30-year population-based study. *Am J Cardiol* 1995; 76:148–52. **<u>CITATIONS: 146</u>**

   - *In this well-surveyed study cohort in Olmsted County, Minnesota (aged 20–40), from 1960–1989 there were 54 patients. Men outnumbered women 2 to 1. A significant proportion in the 1980s had cocaine use. Seventeen percent had pathologic features of ARVC although six of the nine had other established causes of death.*

Excludes:	Guidelines, consensus statements, and letters
Includes:	Invited reviews at high IF (>7) journals and randomized clinical trials (if study PI is Mayo Clinic or <20 authors)
Citation Data:	Derived from SCOPUS, November–January 2020–2021; includes at least on Mayo Clinic HRS author at that time

Chapter 15
2000s: EP and Pacing

Thomas M. Munger, Stephen C. Hammill, Douglas L. Packer,
Win-Kuang Shen, Samuel J. Asirvatham, Paul A. Friedman,
and Hon-Chi Lee

Basic Science in Pacing and Electrophysiology at Mayo Clinic

Dr. Hon-Chi Lee arrived at Mayo Clinic Rochester in 2001. He had been recruited by Drs. Jamil Tajik (then CV division chair) and Veronique Roger (CV research) as well as Dr. Hayes (who was soon to become CV division chair). Part of his recruitment also included meeting with Dr. Andre Terzic for an hour at that year's AHA meeting. Dr. Lee had attended medical school at Harvard, did his residency at Stanford/MGH, and did a surgical clerkship at Brigham and Women's Hospital. When Lee finished his time at Stanford, during a job interview at Duke in 1988, he first met both Drs. Win Shen (who was working in Harold Strauss's lab) and Doug Packer (junior faculty). His interview panel also included Drs. Prystowsky and German. He also interviewed at Vanderbilt and Michigan, and eventually went to the University of Iowa, where he spent the first decade of his career. Dr. Lee studied the calcium channel, using patch clamp as the chief technique, and became an active device implanter upon his arrival. His original lab was located at Alfred-4 on the St. Mary's campus but moved to the Stabile Building downtown once that space was opened later in the decade.

Dr. Lee recalls attending the annual Society of General Physiologists meeting in the mid-1980s at the Marine Biological Laboratory at Woods Hole, where Drs. Arthur "Buzz" Brown and David Clapham were having a lively discussion about

T. M. Munger (✉) · S. C. Hammill · D. L. Packer · S. J. Asirvatham · P. A. Friedman
H.-C. Lee
Department of Cardiovascular Diseases, Mayo Clinic, Rochester, MN, USA
e-mail: Munger.thomas@mayo.edu

W.-K. Shen
Department of Cardiovascular Diseases, Mayo Clinic, Phoenix, AZ, USA

beta vs. gamma G-protein regulation of ion channels. This was his first exposure to Dr. Clapham, who had completed an undergraduate EE degree, done his residency at Brigham and Women's Hospital and worked there briefly before coming to Mayo Clinic Rochester, where he worked from 1987 to 1997.

Early in the 1980s, it was recognized that the cardiac catheterization and echocardiography laboratories had developed significant translational and basic science sister labs, with the likes of Drs. Paul VanHoutte, John Burnett, and others. While Dr. Osborn was still director in the mid-1980s, Steve Hammill worked with Drs. Hugh Smith (then CV division chair) and Ron Vlietstra (then research chair for CV) to begin building out similar sister labs for the Heart Rhythm group. To that end was Dr. Clapham's recruitment in the late-1980s. Soon thereafter also came Dr. Yoshi Kurachi from Osaka, Japan. Both of these ion channel laboratories served as incubators and immersion experiences for an entire group of fellows during the 1990s who would later join Mayo Clinic faculty and develop their own significant programs: Drs. Andre Terzic, Michael Ackerman, and Arshad Jahangir. After moving to Boston, Dr. Clapham eventually joined the National Academy of Sciences in 2006.

Dr. Ackerman graduated from Mayo Medical School in 1988 and received the PhD in 1993. His basic work in the Clapham lab occurred from 1994 to 1995. Pediatric training followed, including pediatric cardiovascular training, completed in 2000. The work with Clapham initially was with the newly cloned I_{K1} channel and then the chloride channel. By 1995, Dr. Mark Keating, then at the University of Utah, had discovered the *HERG* gene, responsible for LQT 2, and published two papers in NEJM about the findings; Dr. Ackerman discussed these findings with Dr. Clapham and the possibilities of understanding other diseases with genetic, protein, and functional analysis.

In November of 1996, on his first night on pediatric ICU call, a boy named Jonathan was admitted from a local Rochester sports complex following a drowning. His QT interval was 560 ms, clearly prolonged. Given the gravity of the event, his recent experiences in the Clapham lab, and the emerging science of LQT genetics, Mike decided that he would become a LQT ion channel specialist and have an associated laboratory to accompany the clinical program. The following year, Clapham moved to Harvard, and Dr. Steve Thibodeau, his postdoc, remained to work with Dr. Ackerman; Dave Tester, senior technician, also joined him in the lab. Their first genetic mutation associated with a channelopathy was discovered and published in 1998.

Dr. Dave Driscoll, then pediatric cardiology chair, and Dr. Jamil Tajik, adult cardiology chair, were brought into the discussion. While Dr. Keating would be discovering the next new gene, Dr. Ackerman's group would be examining the next new mutation associated with pathology. Dr. Tim Olson arrived in 1999 from Utah, where he had worked with Keating, and thus an early critical mass of "genetic arrhythmology/cardiology" was born at Mayo Clinic. Dr. Tajik liked the idea and wished to incorporate the new hypertrophic cardiomyopathy (HCM) service line into the program, and thus began a joint venture between the Department of Medicine and the Department of Pediatrics that continues to this day.

As the Human Genome Project completed in 2001, samples from around the country were sent to the Ackerman lab for analysis and eventually included patients with other channelopathies or structural diseases like CPVT, SQTS, ARVC, and DCM. Mayo Medical Ventures worked with Familion in 2004 to streamline the processes for analysis and allow access to the larger group of practitioners for these new genetic technologies via commercialization, and a newfound forte of the Mayo Clinic programs was realized. The Mayo Clinic strength of phenotype characterization was complemented with precise genetic information, providing another level of risk assessment, which then translated into more appropriate adjudication of risk for ICD implantation in channelopathy patients, athletic participation for such patients, and advanced medical and surgical therapies. Important collaborators off-site have included Dr. Craig January and colleagues at the University of Wisconsin, Drs. Art Moss, Peter Swartz, and Sylvia Priori on the International LQT registry, and a "genetic cardiologist" mentor, then at Texas Children's Hospital in Houston, Dr. Jeff Towbin. Currently, Dr. Ackerman is the director of the Windland Smith Rice Genetic Heart Rhythm Clinic and Laboratory and has served as the president of the Sudden Arrhythmia Death Syndromes (SADS) Foundation since 2006.

Dr. Andre Terzic met Dr. Mike Ackerman in the early 1990s on the Guggenheim seventh floor when Terzic was working with Dr. Yoshi Kurachi and Ackerman was working with Dr. Clapham. Dr. Terzic had joined Mayo Clinic following a fellowship in clinical pharmacology and received his PhD in Philadelphia at Thomas Jefferson and the University of Illinois in Chicago. While his early work was with ion channels, specifically the IK_{ATP} channel, his laboratory has subsequently focused on cardioprotection in heart failure, the genetics of stress tolerance, ion channel biology, and regenerative medicine and stem cell biology. He is the director of the Shannon Mayo Center for Regenerative Medicine and is director of the NIH Cardiovasology Program.

Dr. Jahangir completed his clinical fellowship in 1997 and worked with both Drs. Kurachi and Terzic. He joined Dr. Win Shen in Phoenix in 2011 and then Dr. Tajik at Aurora Health in Milwaukee, where he has been director of the Center for Integrative Research on Cardiovascular Aging and for AF Advanced Therapies.

Mayo Clinic HRS basic science has continued to grow and flourish in the past 35 years and is poised to augment further. According to Dr. Lee, between basic, translational, epidemiologic, and clinical research, the group in Rochester contributed nearly 200 peer-reviewed manuscripts to the medical literature just in the calendar year 2018.

Devices 2000s: CRT, Primary Prevention ICD, and Laser Extraction

As the 2000s opened, the device practice was about to explode. It was clear that device implantation, the tools developed for ablation and the cardiac cath lab in the 1990s, and anatomic observations from electrophysiology were all coming together.

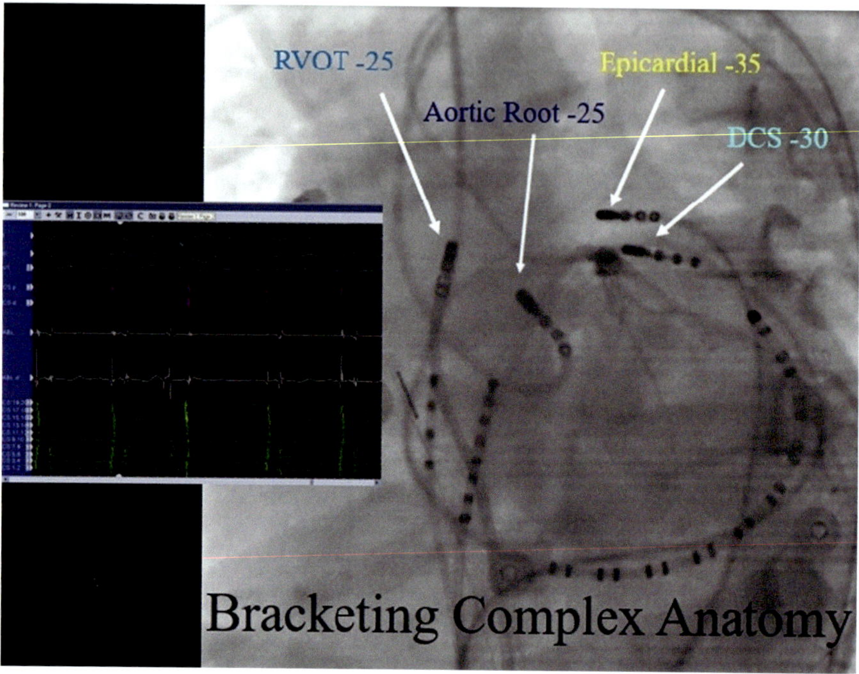

Fig. 15.1 Bracketing complex anatomy became routine in the 2000s, as PVC and VT targets moved from the RV outflow tract to the aortic root. X-ray imaging shows multiple intracardiac catheters in the aorta, coronary sinus, RV simultaneously in RA intracardiac ultrasound probe, 4D mapping-enabled ablation catheter, and left coronary artery injection. The PVC was epicardial and is shown on the inset

Cardiac resynchronization therapy (CRT) was being validated with multiple trials like MUSTIC, MIRACLE, PATH-CHF, CONTAK CD, COMPANION, and MADIT-CRT being completed (Fig. 15.1).

Dr. David Holmes recalls working with a newly arrived Dr. Sam Asirvatham in the late 1990s and Dr. Dave Hayes. The application of CRT was introduced by David Hayes. Given the requirement for the coronary sinus as the anatomic structure to facilitate delivery of LV leads and evaluation of left ventricular venous branches for placement were needed, the cardiac cath lab (Holmes) was involved in early procedures. These were carried out in room 106 with both the cath lab and pacing physicians working together, as the approaches used to access the lateral wall were those used in interventional cardiology procedures. Some of the procedures were lengthy. Dr. Holmes' first interaction with Asirvatham was in this setting during a long complicated procedure. They were both scrubbed, and Dr. Asirvatham introduced himself to Dr. Holmes in his soft voice. Holmes remembers struggling with the procedure, and then Asirvatham discussed the different structures around the space in which they were working, particularly the fact that they might have entered the vein of Marshall about which Dr. Holmes' knowledge was limited to say the least. After some time, they were able to satisfactorily finish the procedure. Dr. Holmes left the case with the glimpse into the incredible knowledge and prowess of this individual with his soft-spoken ways.

Dr. Asirvatham had practiced OB/GYN in India, where he would receive journals from the local medical school and where his interests were peaked by reading articles about cardiac electrophysiology and neurosurgery. He vividly recalls reading a paper from Drs. Ralph Lazzara and Warren "Sonny" Jackman in the late 1980s, which prompted more reading, particularly from this group at the University of Oklahoma. At that time, there was no electrosurgery for WPW in India, and Asirvatham wondered how to learn this field. He would go to the United States and retool to become an electrophysiologist; that was 1990. He went to Columbia in New York and then to the University of Wisconsin at Madison for the years 1992–1994. During his first CCU rotation, he remembers airlifting a patient with incessant WPW-related arrhythmias to Dr. Jackman's group. He then achieved his aspiration of cardiovascular training at Oklahoma in the years 1995–1998. Much of Dr. Asirvatham's education at Oklahoma, like his past, was via careful observation, which would generate ideas. This skill he would bring to Mayo Clinic in 1998 for a 2-year research fellowship.

Asirvatham became interested in Mayo Clinic from one of the Oklahoma fellows who subsequently did an interventional fellowship in Rochester; this fellow encouraged him to visit. He interviewed with Doug Packer and Marshall Stanton at an ACC meeting to seal the deal. He never interviewed with Steve Hammill, Rick Nishimura (who was program director), or Jamil Tajik. During his first 5 years on the Mayo Clinic staff (2000–2005), Asirvatham performed over 1000 cardiac dissections with the cardiac pathologist Dr. William Edwards, who facilitated access to the specimens; each specimen required 5 hours of processing for dissection and photography. Dr. Paul Friedman also assisted with photography during this time. This was well over a 2-year intensive project and amplified Asirvatham's deep knowledge of cardiac anatomy and his subsequent work in his own translational research program. He has maintained his contact with his former teachers at Oklahoma for meetings and research interests. Dr. Benjamin Scherlag has visited Asirvatham's Rochester lab to offer suggestions about fat pad autonomic physiology, among other topics. Dr. Asirvatham's acumen as an educator is legendary and was recently recognized by the ACC.

In addition to the CRT trials, the primary prevention trials supporting the use of ICD (SCD-HeFT and MUSTT) and several high-profile lead and device malfunctions (Telectronics Accufix 801 Atrial J-lead: 1995) requiring extractions, the clinical demands for the practice ballooned. While Drs. Rea, Lloyd, Asirvatham, and Cha had been added in the late 1990s and early 2000s, there remained unmet needs, and thus Drs. Shen, Munger, and Friedman joined for implantation of devices in the early 2000s.

Dr. Margaret Lloyd had attended medical school at the University of Nebraska, in her home state. She remarks the "light system" for the outpatient clinics at Mayo Clinic was also present in Lincoln, and this tweaked her interest in Mayo.

She did 2 years of translational research with Dr. Burnett in the heart failure group, additionally working with Drs. Redfield, Clavell, and Grogan. She then helped open the Mankato, MN, Mayo Clinic Health System practice in 1995–1997 (where Dr. Wood was CEO at the time), did an EP fellowship, and then joined the device group in 1998 with emphasis on heart failure. Dr. Lloyd did 6 months of additional pacing during her fellowship, and just after Dr. Hayes began the CRT program at Mayo Clinic, she went to Europe (as he had) for 2 months in Paris learning CRT. She also worked at "French Outreach" in Lyon and Marseilles. Training in Paris was with Drs. Daniel Gras and Phillipe Ritter (the latter, a leader of the European Cardiostim meeting, now with the Bordeaux group).

One of the more memorable of the lead recalls was the Telectronics Accufix 801 atrial J-lead. It had a retention wire within the J to holds its shape. Unfortunately, because of a spontaneous break in the retention wire (4–6% annually), there was an annual risk of protrusion of 1.5% and a smaller risk of death. The leads required surveillance, which involved Drs. Hayes, Holmes, and Lloyd. This continued several years. Now, the device group has managed multiple recalls, warnings, and alerts concerning hardware, software, and firmware, which require internal assessment and action plan implementation.

DFT testing became less routine as the decade closed. Extractions increased as device infection guideline recommendations expanded their use and laser techniques further improved. CRT also became easier to perform and eventually would be included in half of all ICD systems implanted. Besides the technical challenges with CRT implantation, programming for optimization of settings was also important. Dr. Raul Espinosa, who had joined the core group in 1990 after Dr. Ron Vlietstra left, assumed this task. He noted that during the first 5 years of his career, it was pure pacing, 2–3 cases a day with a downtown PPM clinic in the afternoon and hospital consults either in the morning or late evening; consultants took a week at a time on the rotation. Espinosa also recalls doing DFT testing with monophasic waveforms, requiring over 20 VF inductions until a successful vector was found. Dr. Espinosa created the CRT registry with Paul Friedman and got IRB approval and initiated this rich database for the group. By the early 2000s, the practice had gotten so busy a second operator was added each day.

Ablation 2000s: AF Ablation and Epicardial VT Ablation Come of Age

Meanwhile, Doug Packer had gained additional experience working with DCRI on the MUSTT, HAT, and SCD-HeFT trials. The concept of a randomized clinical trial examining AF ablation came quite early after the procedure was being undertaken clinically in the later 1990s. Packer wrote the protocol and grant in the early 2000s and, as the procedure matured a bit more, submitted to the NIH. He worked closely with Drs. Kerry Lee, Dan Mark, and Jeanne Poole (with whom he had collaborated on Bardy's SCD-HeFT trial). He realized he had not yet created a name for his study as he was running down a hallway at the annual HRS sessions in New Orleans to present the concepts for the trial. On the way there, he considered the acronym CANADA vs. CABANA. The latter stuck. The protocol would commence in 2009 with nurse Kristie Monahan at Mayo Clinic Rochester responsible for administrating the trial. During the decade of the 2000s, cryoablation, especially for pediatric patients, came of age after the publication of the multicenter "FROSTY" trial that the group participated in for SVT.

In 2004, Drs. Friedman and Munger visited for a week at the labs of Drs. Eduardo Sosa and Mauricio Scanavacca in Sao Paulo, Brazil, to learn the technique Dr. Sosa had pioneered to percutaneously enter an intact normal pericardial space; this was becoming a critical skill for epicardial VT ablation, particularly in patients with ARVC and DCM (in addition to Chagas patients, not readily seen in Minnesota!). Epicardial approaches would also be used in the following decade to close the left atrial appendage and for placement of device systems. At the close of the decade, Mayo Clinic and other groups were just beginning to use robotics systems for ablation: the Hansen robot and the Stereotaxis magnetic system. Dr. Munger would eventually perform over 200 AF ablations with the Hansen robotic system.

Dr. Asirvatham's work examining muscle sleeves within the two great cardiac arteries complemented findings in the clinical lab; Drs. Shen, Asirvatham, and Munger would place a circle-mapping array at the base of the aorta in a patient with PVCs and would further characterize the single potentials Dr. Kuck in Germany had published (Figs. 15.2 and 15.3).

In the year 2004–2005, Steve Hammill served as HRS (formerly NASPE) president following, Drs. Jim Maloney in 1991–1992 and Dave Hayes in 1998–1999. During this time, Hammill remembers his time as president as a time of transition

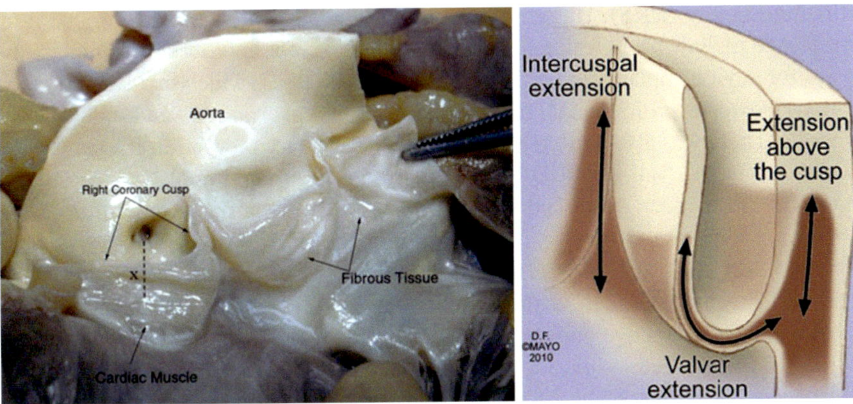

Fig. 15.2 Muscular extensions into the great vessels as demonstrated in the aorta several millimeters into the vessel. These muscle extensions can be the source for multiple arrhythmia syndromes (and thus ablation targets), including PVCs, ventricular tachycardia, atrial fibrillation, atrial tachycardia, and WPW. (Courtesy: SJ Asirvatham, MD)

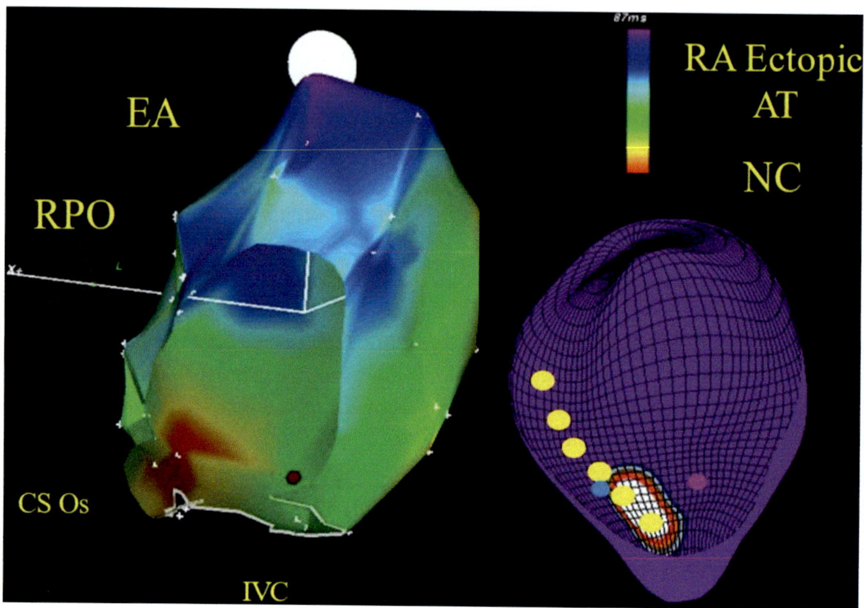

Fig. 15.3 Circa 2000, simultaneous 4D electroanatomic (EA) and noncontact (NC) activation mapping of a right atrial (RA) peri-coronary sinus os atrial tachycardia (AT). Right posterior oblique (RPO) projection. Earliest breakout in *red* on *left* map and *white* on *right* map

within the society, from its origins at Massachusetts General Hospital in 1979, to moving in 1984 to Wellesley, MA, in 1989 to Newton, MA, and that year to Washington, DC. At that same time, the new official journal *Heart Rhythm* was launched. This occurred just a year after the renaming of NASPE to the Heart Rhythm Society (HRS). Hammill presided over the restructuring of the board of trustees to include past presidents, creating guidelines for appropriate training pathways for device implantation by non-electrophysiologists (which involved collaboration between professional societies, industry, government, and educational boards). There was also work with CMS to cover primary prevention ICD implants, which led to the National ICD Registry working group and public advocacy and education for sudden death and atrial fibrillation. In Rochester, Hammill used the time to rename the electrophysiology and pacing service lines to simply "Heart Rhythm Services," aka, Mayo HRS. Additionally, by the end of the decade, HRS had two hospital services: a primary arrhythmia service and a consult service. During the decade active outreach practices in North Dakota, Minnesota, Iowa, and Wisconsin flourished, while independent HRS practices in Florida, Arizona, and Wisconsin further grew. In 2006, after 18 years as section chief, Steve Hammill turned the reigns of the section over to Dr. Packer.

Allied Health Staff in Pacing and Electrophysiology at Mayo Clinic

Lisa Fanning was the third EP technician hired into the group and has had the longest career, serving to this day, now over 40 years. Lisa graduated from high school in 1976 and took a 1-year surgical technician training through Mayo Clinic Rochester the year after. In November of 1977, she applied for a surgical position, and there were none to be found at Mayo Clinic. At that time, the entire Mary Brigh wing of St. Mary's Hospital was being built.

Fanning applied for a clinic job at the ECG lab instead. And then the supervisor there indicated that the Cardiac Cath Lab was hiring a third pacing and electrophysiology technician to join Ms. Colleen Byrne (Spring Valley, MN) and Ms. Jeannette Raymaker. Both individuals would leave for other pursuits, Colleen for nurse's training and Jeannette for the cardiovascular research unit. Lisa would remain and be the tech supervisor for over 20 years until Ms. Jes Evjen Harris assumed the role in 2016.

From those very early days in the late 1970s, she recalls working with Dr. Don Hagler (interventional pediatric CV and still with the group), as well as the CV fellows, Dr. Michael McGoon and Dr. Mark Callahan. McGoon eventually joined the group in device implantation for nearly 30 years and served as president of the Pulmonary Hypertension Association. He was the son of Dr. Dwight McGoon, the Mayo Clinic cardiac surgeon. Dr. Mark Callahan eventually joined as an echocardiographer in Rochester and passed prematurely in 2011. He was the son of Dr. John A Callahan, another Mayo Clinic cardiologist and echocardiographer. Dr. Munger recalls working with senior Dr. Callahan in the ECG laboratory in the Plummer Building in 1987, during his early fellowship, and recalls arrhythmia/interventional papers Callahan had published on digitalis visual toxicity effects, the use of echo for facilitating pericardiocentesis, and early ICU monitoring for arrhythmias. These included publications with Drs. EH Wood, JC Broadbent, DC McGoon, JW Kirklin, HJ Swan, AJ Tajik, and JW Seward.

Let's return to allied health staff in the EP/PPM labs. Dr. Maloney had just left when Lisa Fanning joined the group. While the Alfred-6 wing became the base of operations for EP/PPM (rooms 70 and 71), she was initially assigned to scrub into cases for single-chamber PPM implants with Drs. Osborn, Broadbent, Vlietstra, and Holmes. Dr. John Merideth, who directed the creation of the outpatient device clinic, also taught Ms. Jane Trusty, RN, how to do thresholds on devices in OR implants with surgeons. Thus was born the paradigm of the Mayo Clinic nursing staff performing lead testing in the cases (rather than relying on industry reps).

In the outpatient clinic was Ms. Sharon Neubauer, RN. Ms. Darlene Miller was the administrative assistant. This then transitioned to Ms. Ann Dreblow, who also put in orders for pacemaker devices and reps if needed (Intermedics, CPI,

Medtronic)—a current function of our supply chain group and Fanning. In 1985, Ms. Trusty was the individual who ordered the first ICD for implantation. Induction of ventricular fibrillation (VF) for defibrillation threshold testing (DFT) was facilitated by an AC fibrillatory device that Mayo Clinic bioengineering had created. Fanning also recalls that during VT inductions in the EP lab (doing serial drug testing), the tech would try to terminate the rhythm with overdrive pacing under the direction of the MD, and, if unable to do so, would summon anesthesia to the room to facilitate urgent cardioversion.

Ms. Kelly Griffin would be added and later went to the Mayo Clinic Florida campus as it opened, only to return to Rochester in the 2000s. Ms. Kathy Hynes initially worked part-time in the summer before being hired full time. The technicians operated the stimulators during EP studies until this was changed to the RNs in the 2000s. Ms. Jean Thomas replaced Griffin after her transfer to Florida, and later came others like Rita Eggenberger, Joyce Lewis, Lori Finley, Dave Vandeberg, and Craig Swiggum.

In 1994, when operations moved from Alfred-6 to Mary Brigh-4 (current location), there were just 6 EP/PM technicians, while now there are nearly 30. Ms. Jane Trusty was the nursing supervisor, and besides Sharon Neubauer, the nursing group included Mary Jane Rasmussen, Susan Grice, Jan Christiansen, and then Doug Beinborn, who had been working on the new interventional unit and eventually would be operations manager for over 20 years. Over the years the secretarial support transitioned through many individuals, including Susan Wegman, Mary Foster, Chris Bork, Linda Otis, Mary Ellen Hasenfus, and currently Chris Nelson. Fanning recalls working with the first EP fellow, Dr. Doug Wood, who has had several roles at Mayo Clinic, including CEO of the Mankato practice, vice-chair of the Department of Medicine, and AMA president for the State of Minnesota. Other early EP fellows in the 1980s included Drs. R. Wayne Kreeger, John Haas, Declan Sugrue, Bob Lemery, and Pierce Vatterott. Drs. Win Shen and Jenny Shannon were the last fellows trained before RF ablation began, while Drs. James Kappler and Thomas Munger were the first fellows trained during/after RF ablation began. The fellows would assist the attending clinicians reading the "roll records" created by the E for M recording machines (in conjunction with real-time oscilloscopes); one had to be particularly careful when changing a roll of paper not to burn fingers on the heat element in the recorder. Later, Z-stacks of paper were used for recording studies (Drs. Shen and Munger recall terming studies done with Doug Packer as "Packer-Stackers"). The lab transitioned from paper EGM, archiving to its first computer system called "EP LAB," to the Prucka GE computer system in the early 1990s (that is used to this day).

In the early days, the technicians and nurses took it upon themselves to self-teach EP and pacing, since there were no formal training programs. In the late 2000s, the RCES or RCIS certifications were created and expected for all technicians working in the Mayo Clinic labs. Additionally, it may take up to a year to fully train an EP or device nurse now, and many have taken the HRS exam for allied health members; currently, there are nearly 40 EP and device nurses between outpatient heart rhythm, genetics, device clinics, and inpatient laboratories. Dr. Asirvatham has enhanced

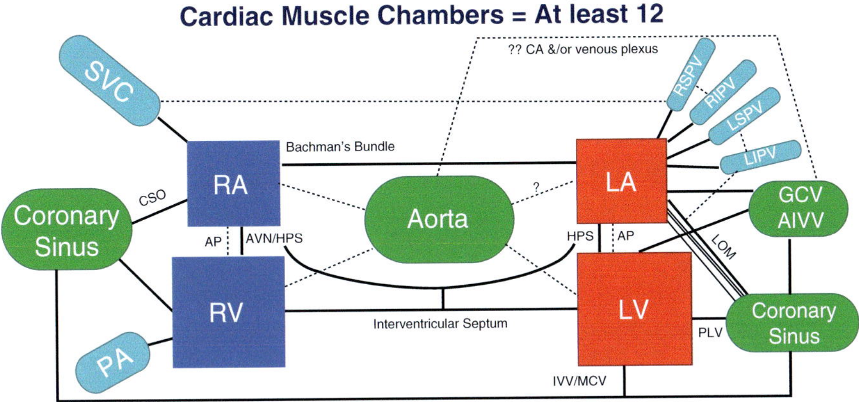

Fig. 15.4 The traditional heart to the electrophysiologist of the 1990s had four muscle chambers. By the end of the 2000s, it was clear the heart had at least 12 distinct "muscular chambers" that could act as triggers or reentrant structures, and many interconnected electrically: superior vena cava (SVC), coronary sinus os (CSO), pulmonary artery (PA), right atrium (RA), right ventricle (RV), left atrium (LA), left ventricle (LV), accessory pathway (AP), right superior pulmonary vein (RSPV), left superior pulmonary vein (LSPV), right inferior pulmonary vein (RIPV), left inferior pulmonary vein (LIPV), greater cardiac vein (GCV), anterior interventricular vein (AIVV), ligament of Marshall (LOM), posterior lateral vein (PLV), middle cardiac vein (MCV), atrioventricular node (AVN), His-Purkinje system (HPS), coronary arteries (CA). This figure does not include the autonomic nerve plexuses that also serve many of these structures

education for the technical staff. Fanning recalls a benchmarking Cleveland Clinic site visit in 2007 with Dr. Munger, nurse Grice, and Doug Beinborn. To this day, she comments that the real strengths of the Mayo Heart Rhythm program has been the integrated team, mission dedication, clinician thoroughness, and a specialized allied health staff, who are maximally educated and trained to the highest levels of their licensures (Figs. 15.4 and 15.5).

Mayo Clinic Rochester HRS Authors' 20 Top Cited Papers of the 2000s

1. Bardy GH, Lee KL, Mark DB, Poole JE, **Packer DL**, Boineau R, Domanski M, Troutman C, Anderson J, Johnson G, McNulty SE, Clapp-Channing N, Davidson-Ray LD, Fraulo ES, Fishbein DP, Luceri RM, Ip JH. Amiodarone or an implantable cardioverter-defibrillator for congestive heart failure. *NEJM* 2005; 352:225–37. **CITATIONS: 4752**

   - *The SCD-HeFT trial followed the MUSTT and MADIT studies supporting the use for primary prevention ICD implants in NYHA II-III CHF patients with EF of 35% or less, regardless of ischemic or nonischemic etiology. Amiodarone offered no benefit over placebo. The subsequent DANISH study*

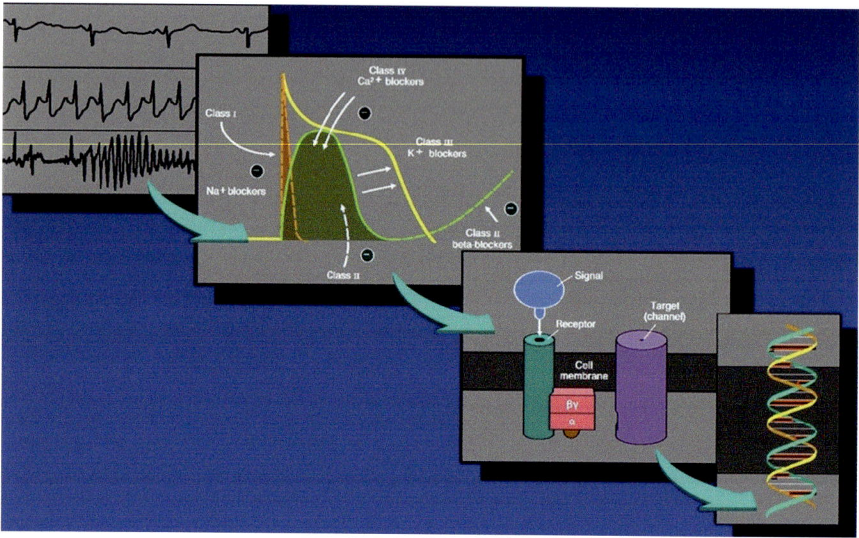

Fig. 15.5 The unification of arrhythmogenic syndromes, often causing catastrophic sudden death with basic electrophysiology and ion channels. Ultimately, the human genome accelerates in this decade after publication of the human genome project with its attendant technical advances. (Courtesy: MJ Ackerman, MD)

> *would be more equivocal in older patients due to a higher use of ACE/ARB and CRT in the next 15 years.*

2. Abraham WT, Fisher WG, Smith AL, Delurgio DB, Leon AR, Loh E, Zocovic DZ, Packer M, Clavell AL, **Hayes DL**, Ellestad M, Messenger J. Cardiac resynchronization in chronic heart failure. *NEJM* 2002; 346:1845–53. <u>**CITATIONS: 3913**</u>

   - *The MIRACLE trial was one of several randomized studies done at the turn of the millennium examining the use of CRT in heart failure patients. In this study, 453 patients with NYHA II-III CHF and EF 35% or less with QRSD of greater than or equal to 130 msec were randomized to CRT or control for 6 months. The CRT group experienced improvement in 6-min walk distance, functional class, QOL, and fewer hospitalizations. Success of implant was 92%.*

3. Cappato R, Calkins H, Chen S-A, Davies W, Iesaka Y, Kalman J, Kim Y-H, Klein G, **Packer D,** Skanes A. Worldwide survey on the methods, efficacy, and safety of catheter ablation for human atrial fibrillation. *Circulation* 2005;111: 1100–05. <u>**CITATIONS: 1175**</u>

   - *This summarizes results of 777 surveyed global centers with 181 that responded and 100 that had ongoing programs in the time period 1995–2002. The survey demonstrated technique evolution from RA compartmentalization and focal trigger ablation in the 1990s to electrical PV disconnection in the early 2000s. Major complications were present in 6%.*

4. Poole JE, Johnson GW, Hellkamp AS, Anderson J, Callans DJ, Raitt MH, Reddy RK, Marchlinski FE, Yee R, Guarnieri T, Talajic M, Wilber DJ, Fishbein DP, **Packer DL**, Mark DB, Lee KL, Bardy GH. Prognostic importance of defibrillator shocks in patients with heart failure. *NEJM* 2008; 359:1009–17. **CITATIONS: 989**

   - *In the SCD-HeFT ICD cohort (N = 811), a follow-up of nearly 4 years showed 33% with at least one shock: 128 appropriate, 87 inappropriate, and 54 a mixture. The hazard ratios for risk of death were 5.7 for appropriate shock patients and 2.0 for inappropriate shock patients compared to no shock. Progressive CHF was the most common reason for death.*

5. Maron BJ, **Shen WK**, Link MS, Epstein AE, Almquist AK, Daubert JP, Bardy GH, Favale S, **Rea RF**, Boriani G, Estes III M, Spirito P. Efficacy of implantable cardioverter-defibrillators for the prevention of sudden death in patients with hypertrophic cardiomyopathy. *NEJM* 2000; 342:365–73. **CITATIONS: 785**

   - *A multicenter collection of 128 HCM patients judged to be at high SCD risk was followed an average of 3 years (ages: 8–82 years). Incidence of appropriate shocks at 5 years was 15% and 40% in the primary and secondary prevention groups.*

6. Maron BJ, Thompson PD, **Ackerman MJ**, Balady G, Berger S, Cohen D, Dimeff R, Douglas PS, Glover DW, Hutter Jr., AM, Krauss MD, Maron MS, Mitten MJ, Roberts WO, Puffer JC. Recommendations and considerations related to preparticipation screening for cardiovascular abnormalities in competitive athletes. *Circulation* 2007; 115:1643–55. **CITATIONS: 752**

   - *This review of the available research concerning athletic participation in patients with underlying structural or inherited arrhythmia syndromes further identified customized recommendations. Epidemiologic studies following this paper additionally have enhanced patient tailored recommendations.*

7. Gami AS, Pressman G, Caples SM, Kanagala R, Gard JJ, Davison DE, Malouf JF, Ammash NM, **Friedman PA**, Somers VK. Association of atrial fibrillation and obstructive sleep apnea. *Circulation* 2004; 110:364–7. **CITATIONS: 744**

   - *The percentage of OSA patients who had AF was higher than the general population (49% vs. 32%) and had implications for the epidemic of obesity (OSA) and AF in the population.*

8. Kanagala R, Murali NS, Friedman PA, Ammash NM, Gersh MJ, Ballman KV, Shamsuzzaman ASM, Somers VK. Obstructive sleep apnea and the recurrence of atrial fibrillation. *Circulation* 2003; 117:2589–94. **CITATIONS: 700**

- *Following cardioversion, the recurrence rate at 1-year follow-up in untreated OSA patients was 82%, compared to 42% in treated patients, and 53% in a control group of patients who had not been sleep tested.*

9. Sohail MR, Uslan DZ, Khan AH, Friedman PA, Hayes DL, Wilson WR, Steckelberg JM, Stoner S, Baddour LM. Management and outcome of permanent pacemaker and implantable cardioverter-defibrillator infections. *JACC* 2007; 49:1851–9. **CITATIONS: 480**

   - *This retrospective Mayo Clinic review of all device infections admitted to hospital from 1991 to 2003 was done: 189 patients (138 PPM and 51 ICD). Coagulase-negative staph was present in 42% and S. aureus in 23%, with 69% having pocket infection and 23% endocarditis. Complete extraction was performed in 98%, with a cure rate of 96% achieved with device removal and antibiotics. This prompted guideline recommendations for CIED removal when feasible with infection.*

10. Cappato R, Calkins H, Chen S-A, Davies W, Iesaka Y, Kalman J, Kim Y-H, Klein G, Natale A, **Packer D**, Skanes A. Prevalence and causes of fatal outcome in catheter ablation of atrial fibrillation. *JACC* 2009; 53:1798–803. **CITATIONS: 411**

   - *Fatal outcomes from 162 of 546 worldwide centers were identified for the years 1995–2006. Thirty-two deaths (0.98 per 1000 patients) were noted in 45,115 procedures in 32,569 patients. These included tamponade (8), stroke (5), atrio-esophageal fistula (5), and pneumonia (2), with multiple other causes for the other 12 deaths. These figures would be important benchmarks when evaluating quality and safety programs for AF catheter ablation and research studies.*

11. Vatta M, **Ackerman MJ**, Ye B, Makielski JC, Ughanze EE, Taylor EW, Tester DJ, Balijepalli RC, Foell JD, Li Z, Kamp TJ, Towbin JA. Mutant Caveolin-3 induces persistent late sodium current and is associated with long-QT syndrome. *Circulation* 2006; 114:2104–2112. **CITATIONS: 388**

   - *Using PCR, HPLC, and direct DNA sequencing, 905 unrelated patients referred for LQTS genetic testing were examined for mutations on the CAV3 locus. In mutants, a gain of function for the late sodium current was observed, similar to that seen in LQT3 and the SCN5A mutations.*

12. **Ackerman MJ**, Siu BL, Sturner WQ, Tester DJ, Valdivia CR, Makielski JC, Towbin JA. Postmortem molecular analysis of SCN5A defects in sudden infant death syndrome. *JAMA* 2001; 286:2264–9. **CITATIONS: 384**

   - *Postmortem molecular review of 93 SIDS cases were carried out for years 1997–1999 from the Arkansas State Crime Lab. DNA was extracted from frozen myocardium. Two of the 92 (2%) had a mutation in SCN5A that could have contributed to SIDS.*

13. **Olson TM,** Alekseev AE, Liu XK, Park S, Zingman LV, Bienengraiber M, Sattiraju S, Ballew JD, **Jahangir A, Terzic A**. Kv1.5 channelopathy due to KCNA5 loss-of-function mutation causes human atrial fibrillation. *Hum Mol Genetics* 2006; 152,185–91. **CITATIONS: 353**

   - *Loss of function in the KCNA5 mutation was found to be a risk factor for atrial repolarization diminution and AF. This mutation was present in a family with AF and absent in 540 unrelated controls.*

14. Calkins H, Epstein A, **Packer D,** Arria A, Hummel J, Gilligan DM, Trusso J, Carlson, Luceri R, Kopelman H, Wilber D, Wharton JM, Stevenson W. Catheter ablation of ventricular tachycardia in patients with structural heart disease using cooled radiofrequency energy. *JACC* 2000; 35: 1905–14. **CITATIONS: 320**

   - *Cooling of the RF ablation tip had been shown to produce larger myocardial lesions. In 146 patients with VT, this was tested. Forty-one percent of patients had no VT inducible at the end of the case with acceptable safety (although complications were twofold higher than for SVT studies).*

15. Bunch TJ, White RD, **Gersh, JB,** Meverden RA, Hodge DO, Ballman KV, **Hammill SC, Shen WK, Packer DL**. Long-term outcomes of out-of-hospital cardiac arrest after successful early defibrillation. *NEJM* 2003; 348:2626–33. **CITATIONS: 291**

   - *This Olmsted County study of 200 patients who presented with SCD between 1990–2001 and received early defibrillation demonstrated that survival rate was similar to age-, sex-, and disease-matched controls who had not had a cardiac arrest. Most had near-normal QOL, with the exception of reduced vitality.*

16. **Jahangir A**, Lee V, **Friedman PA, Trusty JM**, Hodge DO, Kopecky SL, **Packer DL, Hammill SC, Shen WK, Gersh BJ**. Long-term progression and outcomes with aging in patient with lone atrial fibrillation. *Circulation* 2007; 115:3050–6. **CITATIONS: 289**

   - *A previously characterized Olmsted County cohort with AF documented from 1950 to 1980 was further followed. Overall survival of the lone paroxysmal cohort was similar to age-matched Minnesota controls. Age and coincident HTN increased the risk of thromboembolic complications late.*

17. Tester DJ, **Ackerman MJ**. Postmortem long QT syndrome genetic testing for sudden unexplained death in the young. *JACC* 2007; 49:240–6. **CITATIONS: 287**

   - *For the years 1998–2004, 49 cases of SUD, of which 30 were male and average age of 14 years, were examined using PCR, HPLC, and direct DNA sequencing. Ten patients had LQTS mutations. Women were more common than men, and half had death during sleep. One-third of relatives had similar mutations.*

18. **Kapa S,** Tester DJ, Salisbury BA, Harris-Kerr C, Pungliya MS, Alders M, Wile AAM, **Ackerman MJ**. Genetic testing for long-QT syndrome: distinguishing pathogenic mutations from benign variants. *Circulation* 2009; 120:1752–60. <u>**CITATIONS: 258**</u>

   • *Mutations for KCNQ1 (LQT1), KCNH2 (LQT2), and SCN5A (LQT3) were compared between 388 cases (LQT diagnostic score > 3 and/or QTc greater than or equal to 480 msec) and more than 1300 controls. Missense mutations were the most common in 78, 67, and 89% and >95% in controls. Mutations in the transmembrane, linker, and pore-encoding portions of the genome for KCNQ1 and KCNH2 were high probability of association with disease.*

19. Ozcan C, **Jahangir A, Friedman PA**, Patel PJ, **Munger TM, Rea RF, Lloyd MA, Packer DL**, Hodge DO, **Hayes DL, Gersh BJ, Hammill SC**. Long-term survival after ablation of the atrioventricular node and implantation of a permanent pacemaker in patients with atrial fibrillation. *NEJM* 2001; 344:1043–51. <u>**CITATIONS: 251**</u>

   • *In this retrospective study, 350 patients were followed for 3 years after AVNA and pacing in the years 1990–1998 and were matched for survival against a group that was age- and sex-matched in the Minnesota population for 1970–1990. Survival was lower than this group, and predictors included MI, CHF, and cardiac meds after ablation. Without these risks, survival was similar.*

20. **Packer DL**, Keelan P, **Munger TM**, Breen JF, **Asirvatham S**, Peterson LA, **Monahan KH**, Hauser MF, Chandrasekaran K, Sinak LJ, **Holmes Jr., DR**. Clinical presentation, investigation, and management of pulmonary vein stenosis complicating ablation for atrial fibrillation. *Circulation* 2005; 111:546–54. <u>**CITATIONS: 215**</u>

   • *Twenty-three patients with 34 stenoses pulmonary veins from atrial fibrillation ablation comprised this review. Clinical presentation of dyspnea, cough, and chest pain was noted. Technical repair with PTVA and BMS stents was reviewed.*

Excludes:	Guidelines, consensus statements, and letters
Includes:	Invited reviews at high IF (>7) journals and randomized clinical trials (if study PI is Mayo or <20 authors).
Citation Data:	Derived from end note (SCOPUS), October 21, 2020; includes at least one Mayo HRS author at that time.

Chapter 16
2010s: EP and Pacing

Thomas M. Munger, Douglas L. Packer, Win-Kuang Shen,
Samuel J. Asirvatham, Paul A. Friedman, Peter A. Noseworthy,
Yong-Mei Cha, and Suraj Kapa

The Fourth HRS President, CABANA, and Proton Ablation

For 2010–2011, Dr. Doug Packer served as president of the Heart Rhythm Society, joining Jim Maloney, Dave Hayes, and Stephen Hammill. He had assumed directorship of the Rochester Labs in 2006 and had launched CABANA. Dr. Eric Prystowsky, an old mentor and friend from Duke, had encouraged Doug to pursue this. During his tenure, the offerings at HRS diversified with initiation of venues such as AF Summit, VT Summit, Poster Town, Court Room Debate formats, and invited Live Cases.

During the preceding decade, there had been dramatic growth in the professional organization, such that it was no longer seen as an appendage of the American College of Cardiology to entities such as FDA, CMS, and AMA RUC (RVS [resource-based relative value scale] Update Committee) but as a separate professional society with unique concerns to its members. Thus, HRS obtained its own voice at CMS and RUC. This was critical as government regulatory overview came into full activity that year with the US Senate Finance Committee reviewing professional societies and hospitals alike and the passage of Physician Payments Sunshine Act (PPSA), section 6002 of the Affordable Care Act (ACA). Over 400 hospitals underwent audit for primary prevention ICD implantation appropriateness in the

T. M. Munger (✉) · D. L. Packer · S. J. Asirvatham · P. A. Friedman · P. A. Noseworthy
Y.-M. Cha · S. Kapa
Department of Cardiovascular Diseases, Mayo Clinic, Rochester, MN, USA
e-mail: Munger.thomas@mayo.edu

W.-K. Shen
Department of Cardiovascular Diseases, Mayo Clinic, Phoenix, AZ, USA

D. R. Holmes Jr., R. L. Frye (eds.), *The Mayo Clinic Cardiac Catheterization Laboratory*, https://doi.org/10.1007/978-3-030-79329-6_16

setting of elevated troponins. Dr. Rob Rea, then device director (following Dave Hayes), audited over 450 Mayo patients and only found two that fell outside parameters. Auditing and quality reporting evolved into the CMS ICD NCDR program. Beginning with Doug, and continuing during Dr. Tom Munger's tenure, a Mayo HRS quality program that captures the entire HRS practice, has been instituted, and adjudicates and reports a myriad of patient quality factors, including complications, clinical outcomes, supply costs, length of stay, patient satisfaction, shared decision-making, and ultimately value. In addition to domestic items, Doug fostered international relationships between HRS and its equivalent societies abroad (ECAS, EHRA, APHRS, LAHRS, and ESC) (Fig. 16.1).

During the rest of the decade, the CABANA trial, with its patient recruitment, randomization, and 5-year follow-up, was directed from Rochester in collaboration with Kerry Lee and Dan Mark at Duke. CABANA eventually had over 2200 AF patients randomized between catheter ablation and anti-arrhythmic drugs. While the trial did not show a survival benefit, it clearly demonstrated ablation superiority for AF burden and hospitalization. From CABANA, we have CABANA-CHF to study the subgroup analysis that did suggest particular efficacy for patients with AF and CHF together (Figs. 16.2 and 16.3).

In parallel, Doug has collaborated with the group at CERN in Europe concerning the use of ionizing radiation to ablate cardiac tissue for arrhythmia management, without the use of catheters. This work has been extensive at the translational level and bringing together several disciplines including clinical electrophysiology, radiation oncology, multimodality cardiac 4D imaging, and tissue characterization and pathology and histology. These collaborations have been critical to understand this new electrophysiology research frontier as to provide foundational work in particle

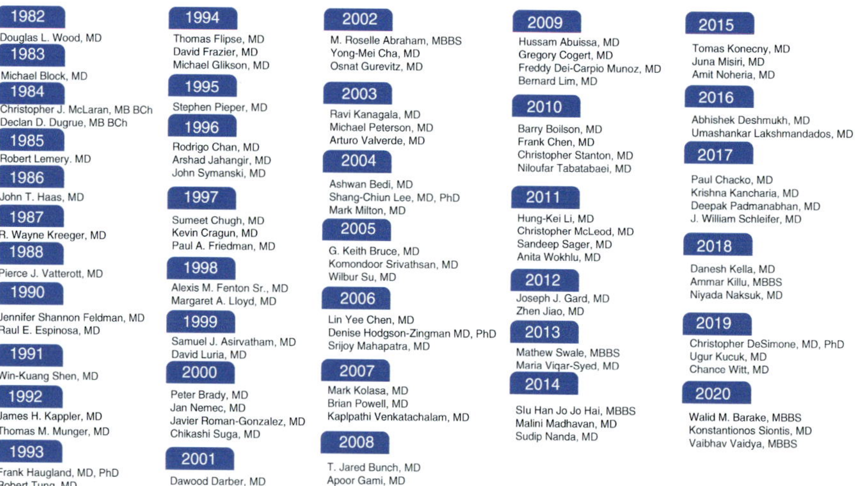

Fig. 16.1 Fellows trained after Mayo Rochester HRS Fellowship program established: 1982–2020. (Courtesy: MA Lloyd, MD)

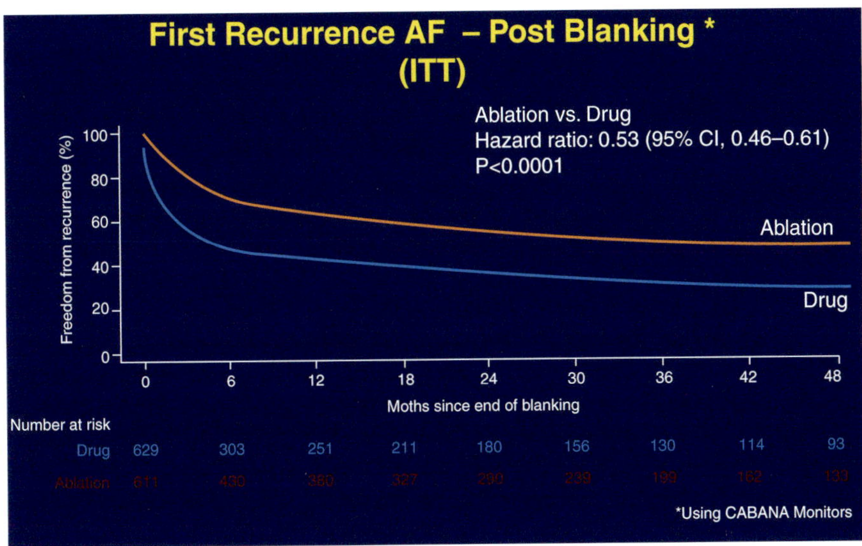

Fig. 16.2 Using intention to treat analysis, the recurrence of AF was reduced significantly compared to patients randomized to antiarrhythmic drug therapies ($p < 0.0001$). (Courtesy: DL Packer, MD)

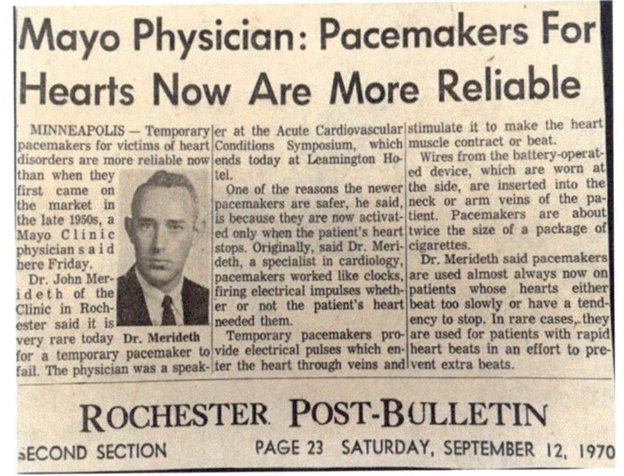

Mayo Physician: Pacemakers For Hearts Now Are More Reliable

MINNEAPOLIS — Temporary pacemakers for victims of heart disorders are more reliable now than when they first came on the market in the late 1950s, a Mayo Clinic physician said here Friday.

Dr. John Merideth of the Clinic in Rochester said it is very rare today for a temporary pacemaker to fail. The physician was a speaker at the Acute Cardiovascular Conditions Symposium, which ends today at Leamington Hotel.

One of the reasons the newer pacemakers are safer, he said, is because they are now activated only when the patient's heart stops. Originally, said Dr. Merideth, a specialist in cardiology, pacemakers worked like clocks, firing electrical impulses whether or not the patient's heart needed them.

Temporary pacemakers provide electrical pulses which enter the heart through veins and stimulate it to make the heart muscle contract or beat.

Wires from the battery-operated device, which are worn at the side, are inserted into the neck or arm veins of the patient. Pacemakers are about twice the size of a package of cigarettes.

Dr. Merideth said pacemakers are used almost always now on patients whose hearts either beat too slowly or have a tendency to stop. In rare cases, they are used for patients with rapid heart beats in an effort to prevent extra beats.

Dr. Merideth

ROCHESTER POST-BULLETIN

SECOND SECTION   PAGE 23 SATURDAY, SEPTEMBER 12, 1970

Fig. 16.3 Dr. John Merideth, a half-century ago, quoted in the Rochester Post Bulletin, discussing how pacemakers, which had just been out a bit more than a decade, were getting more and more reliable. That was the case in 1970 and is the case now in 2020. As the past decade had proceeded, the use of leadless pacemakers, subcutaneous ICDs, and multipolar CRT was adopted

physics, particle ablation biophysics, imaging and gating targeting technologies, and lesion assessment to maximize efficacy and safety. Dr. Robert Foote, in radiation oncology at Rochester, has been critical in assembling the teams required for this evolving endeavor. From the successful "noninvasive" AVN ablation in pigs in 2015 (performed in Heidelberg, Germany) to the first patients being treated at Mayo Clinic in Rochester in 2020, this frontier of therapeutics looks promising, extending beyond photonics, to protons, and carbon particles. He received the ACC Distinguished Translational Scientist Award in 2019 (of note, Dr. Asirvatham also received the Distinguished Teacher of the Year Award that same year at the same ACC meeting).

Administrative Realignments During the 2010s

Dr. Richard Gorlin, the son of a mechanical engineer, famed for developing the Gorlin formula for understanding valvular stenosis, had left Harvard in 1974 and became chief of medicine at Mt. Sanai in New York City. Five years later, Dr. Win Shen enrolled at New York Medical College, familiarized himself with their famed medicine chair (who also was formative in understanding hibernating myocardium), and became interested in cardiology and subsequently electrophysiology. In addition to Dr. Gorlin, another giant, Dr. David Scherf, in the field of electrocardiography and dual AVN physiology, had been at New York Medical College. Scherf had left the Vienna Department of Medicine (Chaired by Wenckebach) in 1938 and spent the rest of his life through 1977 at New York Medical College. From this medical school in the northeast, Win sought training in 1983 at Mayo Clinic in Rochester. As an intern, he approached Dr. Steve Hammill for a research project which was on trans-telephonic monitoring, and he collaborated with RN Sharon Neubauer and Dr. David Holmes, publishing the results in 1987. Dr. Shen also met with Dr. Dwight McGoon, who had stopped cardiac surgical operating but still maintained an office in the Plummer Building, about another project on sudden death in patients with double outlet right ventricle (DORV).

With Dr. Shen's interest in electrophysiology set, he inquired about a basic science experience, and Steve suggested going to his alma mater (Duke) for that; as in an earlier chapter, the basic science electrophysiology at Mayo Clinic was just in its infancy with the arrival of Dr. Clapham, and hence Win travelled to Raleigh-Durham, where he worked 2 years as an NIH scholar under Dr. Harold Strauss. That was 1986. Drs. Packer and Marcus Wharton (subsequent EP chief at Duke) and Jodie Hurwitz (Penn-Texas) were just finishing their fellowships. Dr. Joe Hill was a Duke medical student (MD-PhD) who Win met, and is now Willerson CV chair at UTSW and editor-in-chief of *Circulation*.

Many visitors passed through Duke in those years: Drs. Hon Chi Lee and Eduardo Marban visited for job interviews. Drs. Larry German and Eric Prystowsky were there briefly as interim EP directors. And as the Duke clinical EP program was in flux, Dr. Shen returned to Rochester in 1988 to complete cardiology and EP training and join the group in 1991, at the dawn of RF ablation. Given his patch clamp experience at Duke, he worked briefly with Dr. Yoshi Kurachi. He met Drs. Terzic, Jahangir, Tung, and Munger during those early years and, after deciding to devote his work to clinical science, transferred his two patch clamp stations over to

Andre Terzic. Dr. Shen then turned his attention to the epidemiology and mechanisms of vasovagal syncope and sudden death. He studied adenosine in the head-up tilt protocol, as well as incremental dosing of isoproterenol during that maneuver. Drs. Bob Frye and Hugh Smith served as controls in the adenosine tilt paper. Later in the 1990s he would team up with Drs. Rob Rea and Barry Maron (then in Minneapolis) to examine the natural history of HCM patients with ICDs (both from a primary prevention and secondary prevention standpoint). Dr. Shen again highlighted the importance that thorough phenotyping had been a strength in the Rochester practice, and now this could be leveraged when studying a new aspect of an old disease, hypertrophic cardiomyopathy (HCM), which had only been characterized in 1958. Win recalls the concept of "publication resilience" working with Dr. Maron during submission to NEJM. The manuscript was initially rejected, and the quote was, "This is not acceptable," from Barry. This required a call to the chief editor, a review of the paper, and then a complete rewrite, with it being eventually accepted. He had a similar experience when publishing his work on the 20-year natural history of AV nodal catheter ablation and pacing in the early 2000s, also to NEJM. Using adjunctive Olmsted County databases, from one of our fellows, Dr. Phil Patel proved key to the paper's final acceptance.

Dr. Shen also fostered the visiting clinician program for electrophysiologists, beginning in the 1990s to this day. As the invasive field progressed from a diagnostic procedure in the late 1980s to fully therapeutic by the late 1990s, international interest ballooned. This prompted many Mayo Clinic HRS members to create international exchange academic programs to Asia (China, Russia, India, Japan, Israel, Malaysia, Hong Kong, and Turkey), Central/South America (Mexico, Brazil, Argentina, Chile), Australia, and South Africa during the subsequent decades. Some of these exchanges continue to this day. International clinicians would visit Rochester for 3–12 months to observe procedures, attend educational offerings, and publish research. These also included physicians from Europe and within the United States and Canada.

In the early 2010s, Dr. Shen moved to Mayo Clinic in Phoenix and assumed chair of the cardiovascular department for the next 8 years (turning over the helm to Dr. Luis Scott recently), while remaining busy with his research, educational, and clinical duties. During his tenure, the Mayo Clinic in Arizona practice grew dramatically, particularly in HRS, circulatory failure, transplantation, and regional outreach; the new medical school opened, and incremental research positions within the department were added. Several new educational meetings (partnering with Dr. Komandoor Srivathsan) that see attendance increase every year were created. Dr. Shen continues to visit Rochester annually for practice and research activities.

Dr. Thomas Munger arrived at the Mayo Clinic campus in September of 1983, as a visiting medical student from the University of Vermont for a clinical rotation in rheumatology (a medical student from Tulane was also on the rotation and would later be a colleague in circulatory failure, Dr. Margaret Redfield). As a medical student in Vermont, he had spent a 1-month elective studying cardiac pathology with Dr. Nick Hardin and reading ECGs with Dr. Frans J. Th. Wackers (whose career in nuclear medicine was mostly at Yale except for 1981–1984 when he was faculty at Vermont). Dr. Wackers graduated from the University of Amsterdam and trained in cardiology from 1974 to 1977 with Drs. Dick Durrer and Hein Wellens, both fathers of clinical EP in Europe. His enthusiasm for the ECG was infectious, and stimulated Dr. Munger, to pursue cardiology and subsequently electrophysiology as a career.

Dr. Munger met Dr. Shen in 1988 during their echo rotation and found they had common interests. Win had just returned from Duke. Tom visited with Steve Hammill in 1989 to discuss his interest in EP, and Steve teamed him up with soon to arrive Doug Packer to do basic research with Purkinje fibers. The work eventually elucidated potential CAST (Cardiac Arrhythmia Suppression Trial) proarrhythmic mechanisms for antiarrhythmic drugs in the setting of ischemia. This was a 2-year NIH-sponsored fellowship followed by a clinical EP year. In the summer of 1992, Dr. Munger joined the HRS group. Dr. Munger recalls visiting with Dr. John Boineau on a job interview to St. Louis in 1991 about John's own research experience with intraoperative mapping with Dr. Sealy at Duke and Dr. Cox at Barnes.

Tom published an Olmsted County WPW paper of the long-term natural history of the disease from the 1950s to the 1980s, just at the dawn of RF catheter ablation. Dr. Munger expanded the regional outreach practice for HRS and expanded the educational curriculums for IM and CV over the next 10 years, eventually adding multiple administrative roles in the 2000s including vice-chair for education under Dave Hayes and clinical operations for HRS under Steve Hammill and Doug Packer.

Steve Hammill directed Tom to both professional society and federal committee work on coding, reimbursement systems, supply management and contracting, and medical ethics, as well as internal Mayo Clinic projects involving capital equipment and space. With no formal MBA, but the background for one, Dr. Munger assumed chair of the HRS Division in 2016 following Doug Packer.

During the latter half of the 2010s, additional faculty have been added (currently the division has 22 members). Additionally, there has been increased research and education time for faculty members, the initiation of a quarterly quality and safety report, creation of an annual visiting professorship (Dr. Frank Marchlinski and Dr. Ken Ellenbogen the first two), transitioning of the group through incremental lab projects, conversion and convergence of all Mayo Clinic sites to the EPIC medical record, and guidance through the COVID-19 pandemic. All the while, with enhanced fiduciary results, multiple programs have been further cultivated, to the point now that HRS is one-third of the entire Department of Cardiovascular Medicine and has an expanding regional, national, and international reach.

Dr. Paul Friedman became chair of the Mayo Clinic Department of Cardiovascular Medicine in Rochester in 2018. Paul had an electrical engineering background and a keen eye for gadgetry and innovation. He was educated at Stanford. And while at the University of Washington for an anesthesiology internship, he caught the cardiology bug and returned to California for his medicine residency. Wanting to move closer to family in Chicago, he decided to explore Mayo Clinic. Dr. Friedman met Drs. Marshall Stanton and Rick Nishimura during an initial visit to Rochester. He arrived in 1993 for a year research on ICD shock waveform science with Marshall on Alfred-9, and then completed the CV/EP fellowship in 1997 at which time he joined the HRS group.

Over the years, Dave Hayes has teamed up with several coauthors for device textbooks including David Holmes, Peg Lloyd, Sam Asirvatham, and Paul. Tom and Paul's week-long visit to Brazil in 2004 led to a rich experience with epicardial mapping and ablation that was subsequently archived in various manuscripts by Dr. Ammar Killu. Paul also recalls asking an old Mayo Clinic/Duke alumnus, Dr. Seth Worley, to visit Rochester to teach the Mayo Clinic group about venoplasty in the coronary sinus for facilitation of LV lead placement in the late 2000s. He then made a site visit to Lancaster, PA, with pacing nurse Tracy Webster and Dr. Yong-Mei Cha to observe Dr. Worley perform the procedures in order to bring the up-to-date techniques back to Mayo Clinic; this included balloon venoplasty, venous stenting, wire snaring techniques, and cutting balloons. Dr. Friedman and Dr. Michael Glikson have had an extensive collaboration between Mayo Clinic and Sheba Medical Center in Tel Aviv, culminating in more than 70 papers. Dr. Friedman is no stranger to early adoption of new technology, including the SQ ICD, the leadless pacer, and recently dozens of Nanostim leadless pacer extractions. He has teamed up frequently with Dr. Asirvatham to innovate new devices for the invasive labs.

Paul has served on the Board of Trustees at HRS and served as Device Lab director after Dr. Rob Rea and before the current director, Dr. Yong-Mei Cha. As Paul peers forward for the department, he sees cutting-edge innovation in the digital space. As Mayo Clinic aims to create its own platform by 2030, Dr. Friedman perceives technology as a tool to enhance early detection of disease through wearable diagnostics, AI neural networks (he has hired AI engineers to imbed within CV and HRS), home health sensors, and digital patient education widgets, allowing enhanced individualized awareness and compliance.

Quality and Safety in the Electrophysiology Laboratory

Dr. Rob Rea became device director after Dave Hayes stepped down (and Mike McGoon had been interim). He had trained in EP at the Medical College of Virginia, did a fellowship in sympathetic microneurography in Europe, and went to the University of Iowa and then Mayo Clinic in Arizona for a year, before coming to Rochester in 1995. During the 2010 DOJ investigations of device implantation appropriateness, Rob championed the audit process for the practice and with Dr. Dave Bradley, has provided standardization of reporting and adjudication of quality metrics for the contemporary Mayo Clinic practice. Dave joined the HRS Division in 2005 after training at the Universities of Minnesota and Michigan as well as the Howard Hughes Institute at the NIH. He became interested in EP listening to Dr. Fred Morady's fellows in the early 1990s and pursued cardiology and EP at Johns Hopkins, training under Dr. Hugh Calkins. He received the MSc in public health at Hopkins and has performed meta-analysis of RCTs in regard to CRT. One of his memories at Hopkins was seeing the list of the first ten patients who underwent implantation of Dr. Mirowski's ICD invention in the early 1980s.

Pediatric and Adult Congenital Electrophysiology

Congenital heart surgery at Mayo Clinic dates back to the days of Dr. C. Walton Lillehei at the University of Minnesota, where he performed the first open-heart operation in 1952, the first with cross-circulation in 1954, and the first battery-powered pacemaker in 1958 (created by Earl Bakken, Medtronic's founder). Dr. John Kirklin began the Mayo Clinic program in 1955, followed soon thereafter by Dr. Dwight McGoon and then subsequently Drs. Gordon Danielson, Francisco Puga, Joseph Dearani, and Richard Daly.

With congenital heart surgery and improved survival came late arrhythmias, and as EP evolved the specialist to treat pediatric patients and adults with congenital heart disease became critical. In 1984, Dr. Co-Burn Porter joined as the first pediatric electrophysiologist. He had trained at Texas Children's Hospital where Drs. Denton Cooley, Art Garson, and Paul Gillette practiced.

At Co-Burn's retirement in 2010, another pediatric electrophysiologist came to Mayo Clinic from Texas. Dr. Bryan Cannon was a fifth-generation Texan and thought he never would move from his home state. He had also trained at Texas Children's and actually took over Dr. Art Garson's office when he departed. He had been on staff there for 7 years when the call to Rochester came. The pediatric EP community is quite small with 300 in the country and only 5 in Minnesota; on his visit, he was impressed with the commitment to patients and education, and that was enough. Bryan has served as president of PACES (Pediatric and Congenital Electrophysiology Society) where he lobbied for pediatric EP to be represented in all guidelines that were published by HRS or ACC. With Dr. Phil Wackel (Duke trained), he treats the pediatric population and a fair number of adult patients. They both find easier access to cutting technology at a Heart Rhythm center that treats both adults and children. Dr. Cannon comments that now, many more adults with arrhythmias in the setting of repaired congenital heart lesions exist than children.

While a number of adult specialists have treated the adult with congenital heart disease arrhythmias over the years at Mayo Clinic, in the last 10 years, dedicated adult electrophysiologists now serve that population, first Dr. Chris McLeod (who is now at Mayo Clinic in Florida with Dr. Fred Kusumoto [current HRS President] and colleagues) and Dr. Malini Madhavan. Dr. Madhavan completed medical school in India in 2004 and came to Mayo Clinic the following year to do a visiting student rotation for a month on gastroenterology. She then met Dr. Jahangir who mentored her interest in cardiology. Dr. Madhavan then did her training in Rochester. She was even thinking about interventional cardiology before attending a Dr. Asirvatham conference, and then it was electrophysiology without a doubt! She has worked closely with Drs. Carole Warnes and Heidi Connolly to be truly an expert in congenital lesions with the nuances required to ablate and place devices in such patients. Dr. Madhavan has several active protocols in the area.

Implantable Device Practice in Its Sixth Decade

In 2014, Dr. Yong-Mei Cha became pace director after Dr. Friedman transitioned to vice-chair of the Department of Cardiovascular Medicine. She trained in San Diego, California, with Drs. Greg Feldt (UCLA) and Peng-Sheng Chen (Duke, current editor-in-chief of the *Heart Rhythm Journal*) as research fellow in 1991, coming from Beijing. Dr. Chen went to Cedars-Sinai in Los Angeles a couple years later, but Dr. Cha continued another 2 years with Dr. Feldt for a total of 4 years. From there, residency was at St. Louis University. Dr. Cha got assurances from Drs. Nishimura and DeMaria at UCSD that she would be accepted for training and was left with a decision between lots of snow in Minnesota or the West Coast once again. She chose Mayo Clinic.

She trained from 1998 to 2002 and worked with Drs. Shen, Redfield, and Terzic on arrhythmogenesis and heart failure. This, plus her earlier work with Dr. Chen, subsequently fostered her work with sympathetic modulation and arrhythmias and her current NIH grant on the use of CRT in patients with EF 35–50% and the associated metabolomics. During her tenure as device director, she has standardized pacing and ICD practice protocols, overseen multiple device recalls, brought new technologies into practice like peri-Hisian pacing, leadless pacing, and substernal pacing ICD, and participated in several HRS consensus guideline groups (Fig. 16.3).

At the conclusion of 2020, Dr. Michael Osborn retired from the HRS division after 43 years at Mayo Clinic. His father was a Mayo Clinic anesthesiologist and father-in-law an orthopedist who remembers when Dr. Michael DeBakey visited to learn vascular surgical techniques. In the years after WWII, the surgeons at Mayo Clinic operated 6 days a week. Mike trained at the University of Minnesota and UTSW at Parkland. After a stint in the USAF and Minneapolis for 3 years, he began CV training in 1977. Dr. Geoff Hartzler (who after being on the Mayo Clinic staff would move his practice to Kansas City to join other former Mayo Clinic staff members there) told him to consider electrophysiology, and he did. Three weeks before joining the staff, pacer implants moved from surgery to cardiology, and his training lasted for 2 weeks, joining Drs. Maloney, Holmes, and Broadbent. Dr. Osborn was proactive with bringing lead problems forward to Medtronic and other vendors which he would do his entire career; he and Rob Rea would become the consummate lead extractors. Dr. Bernard Gersh would join the staff in the 6 months before Mike and participated in the EP practice until the early 1990s. At that time Mike would transition to just implants for the rest of his career. He participated in the training of Drs. Hayes, McGoon, and Espinosa who formed the core group of implanters from 1990 to the early 2000s. He also was the PI for the use of amiodarone when it first was introduced and followed 504 patients until FDA approval. The site visit has always been important, and Mike recalls doing a site visit to U Penn in

1982 to see Drs. Leonard Horowitz and Mark Josephson to understand VT mapping and begin this at Mayo Clinic with newly arrived staff member Dr. Hartzell Schaff. Mike would serve as EP/pace director from 1984 to 1988 and served on multiple Mayo Clinic committees, including surgical committee for years, and was always the voice of reason for strategic planning.

Big Data, Artificial Intelligence, and Augmented Reality in HRS

Dr. Peter Noseworthy trained at Toronto General and then spent 9 years in Boston doing genetic GWAS research into QT repolarization, and receiving his IM/CV/EP training at MGH. EP training was under Dr. Jeremy Ruskin, also an alumnus of Anthony D'Amato's USPHS program at Staten Island, New York. From interest in genetic data evolved his subsequent interest in larger datasets, the type that Optum could deliver. Upon arrival to Mayo Clinic in 2013, he networked with Dr. Veronique Roger and the newly created Center for the Science of Health Care Delivery to understand the use of clinical treatments like ablation and DOACs in large populations. His understanding of big data was then used to auger Doug Packer's CABANA project. Peter ran a parallel study to CABANA with much larger datasets that were matched for the patients randomized in CABANA. When the datasets at the DCRI were unlocked, it was uncanny for them to see that the results in the big data study mirrored that of the much smaller randomized clinical trial (RCT). This was clearly a win for a properly designed big data study that might be used as a surrogate for a more time consuming and costly RCT. In 2016, Dr. Noseworthy transitioned into directorship of the ECG and monitoring lab of HRS. Nearly ten million ECGs in the Mayo Clinic database served as data to feed a neural network and an artificial intelligence algorithm. The neural network can predict age, gender, and ejection fraction from just analysis of the 3 s 12-lead ECG! This work of discovery, published in 2019, has already been cited over 100 times. Prospective trials of the algorithms are being run in primary care settings and will serve as templates for further utility of AI in the Heart Rhythm domain.

Dr. Suraj Kapa also joined the Heart Rhythm Division, in 2013. Like many in the group, Suraj had had a keen interest in mathematics and physics from an early age. His brother-in-law, who was training in EP at the University of Michigan, asked him how he used a Fourier transform. Dr. Kapa's interest was tweaked about such a specialty that would have such arcane questions. Thus, after completing medical school in New Jersey, he came to Mayo Clinic for residency in 2006 with the idea that he wanted to innovate after doing a student rotation at Mayo Clinic in gastroenterology.

Following medicine, Suraj went to Philadelphia, U Penn, for cardiology and EP training. There he trained with Dr. Frank Marchlinski's group. He met Doug Packer in 2009 before going to Penn but on the return trip to Mayo Clinic talked with Dave Hayes, Sam Asirvatham, and then CV chair, Dr. Chet Rihal. Dr. Kapa has created a sarcoid-arrhythmia multidisciplinary clinic service line. He has been an integral part of AI projects, translational research with new catheter technologies like Boston Scientific's "Direct Sense" RF catheter which is based on local impedance measurements, novel energy sources like particles, and electroporation. Additionally, he has set up the augmented reality/virtual reality (AR/VR) program for HRS that has the potential to revolutionize medical education, at a distance consultation, procedural planning, imaging interpretation, and robotics. Dr. Kapa surmises that AR/VR will integrate datasets that heretofore have been hard-siloed, yielding discovery.

The Future of Mayo Clinic in Rochester HRS Labs

Other colleagues have joined the HRS practice in the last 5 years including Drs. Siva Mulpuru, Abhishek Deshmukh, Ammar Killu, Christopher DeSimone, and Konstantinos Siontis. In addition, our regional colleagues are becoming more and more integrated with the Rochester practice, research, and education missions and include Dr. Freddy Del-Carpio Munoz of LaCrosse, WI, and Dr. Vaibhav Vaidya of Eau Claire, WI.

There are currently 37 active Heart Rhythm faculty at the 6 campuses in Arizona, Florida, Wisconsin, and Minnesota. Active electrophysiology graduate training programs are present in Rochester, Phoenix, and Jacksonville, and these have graduated over 100 fellows these past 4 decades (Fig. 16.1). Today, the Rochester HRS group sees nearly 10,000 outpatients per year and performs >350,000 ECGs and Holter exams annually, as well as 3500 invasive EP procedures. As of 2019, 27 clinical research protocols were active, and nearly 200 peer-reviewed papers were attributable to Mayo Clinic HRS faculty.

Steve Hammill believes strongly that the success of Mayo Clinic HRS has been tied to the culture of the Mayo Clinic itself. If you invest in people, equipment, education, collegiality, and discovery, in a setting where physicians are salaried, only good things happen. Doug Packer suggests that technology is critical and will always evolve, but we should never trade in our knowledge of electrophysiology first principles, and those should be a given. The electrophysiologist should learn how to learn (and unlearn) over time!

Dr. William Mayo said, "The best interest of the patient is the only interest to be considered, and in order that the sick may have the benefit of advancing knowledge, union of forces is necessary." HRS arrhythmology teams at Mayo Clinic are those "union of forces," as they serve patients and integrate and push the boundaries of discovery ever into a bright future.

Mayo Rochester HRS Author's 20 Top Cited Papers of the 2010s

1. Cappato R, Calkins H, Chen S-A, Davies W, Iesaka Y, Kalman J, Kim Y-H, Klein G, Natal A, **Packer DL**, Skanes A, Ambrogi F, Biganzoli E. Updated worldwide survey on the methods, efficacy, and safety of catheter ablation for

human atrial fibrillation. *Circ Arrhythm Electrophysiol* 2010; 3:32–8. **CITATIONS: 1364**

This update on the data collected in the prior decade demonstrated that patients treated with AF catheter ablation in the 2003–2006 timeframe at 18-month median follow-up achieved asymptomatic status without anti-arrhythmic drugs 70% (16,309 patients) of the time. Major complications had dropped to 4.5%.

2. **Packer DL**, Kowal RC, Wheelan KR, Irwin JM, Champagne J, Guerra PG, Dubuc M, Reddy V, Nelson L, Holcomb RG, Lehmann JW, Ruskin JN. Cryoballoon ablation of pulmonary veins for paroxysmal atrial fibrillation. *JACC* 2013; 61:1713–23. **CITATIONS: 500**

The STOP-AF trial was the pivotal study of efficacy and safety for the cryoballoon device used today for pulmonary vein isolation. At 1 year, treatment success with the device was 69.9% compared with 7.3% for drug therapy. Seventy-nine percent of the drug arm crossed over. Phrenic nerve palsies occurred in 11.2% of patients with 25/29 having resolved at a year.

3. Natale A, Reddy VY, Monir G, Wilber DJ, Lindsay BD, McElderry HT, Kantipudi C, Mansour MC, Melby DP, **Packer DL**, Nakagawa H, Zhang B Stagg RB, Boo LM, Marchlinski FE. Paroxysmal AF catheter ablation with a contact force sensing catheter. *JACC* 2014;111: 1100–05. **CITATIONS: 259**

The SMART-AF multicenter trial examined the efficacy and safety of this contact force sensing catheter for PAF ablation. Tamponade occurred in four patients. The more the investigator stayed within the designated contact force parameters, the better the freedom from recurrence. Average force was 18 ± 9 g.

4. Yao X, Abraham NS, Sangaralingham LR, Bellolio F, McBane RD, Shah ND, **Noseworthy PA**. Effectiveness and safety of dabigatran, rivaroxaban, and apixaban versus warfarin in nonvalvular atrial fibrillation. *J Am Heart Assoc* 2016; 359;5: e003725 doi: 10.1161. **CITATIONS: 231**

This study used a large US insurance database with both Medicare Advantage and privately insured patients to compare real-world efficacy and safety of DOACs vs. each other and against warfarin in nonvalvular AF. Apixaban was associated with lower risks of both stroke and major bleeding.

5. Reddy VY, Exner DV, Cantillon DJ, Doshi R, Bunch TJ, Tomassoni GF, **Friedman PA**, Estes III, M, Ip J, Niazi I, Plunkitt K, Bander R, Porterfield J, Ip JE, Dukkipati SR. Efficacy of implantable cardioverter-defibrillators for the prevention of sudden death in patients with hypertrophic cardiomyopathy. *NEJM* 2015; 373:1125–35. **CITATIONS: 225**

A multicenter trial of the St. Jude Nanostim leadless pacemaker which was successfully implanted in 504/526 patients (96%). Lead dislodgement was present in 1.7% and perforation in 1.3%. Leadless technology has become much more prevalent in the 6 years since this report and has been shown to be advantageous for reducing in particular infections related to pacing.

6. Blume GG, **McLeod CJ**, Barnes ME, Seward JB, Pellikka PA, Bastiansen PM, Tsang TSM. Left atrial function: physiology, assessment, and clinical implications. *Eur J Echocardiogr* 2011; 12:421–30. **CITATIONS: 214**

   Multiple echocardiographic measurements and biomarkers important for characterizing LA function are suggested for enhanced prognostication in AF.

7. Harmon KG, Asif IM, Maleszewski JJ, Owens DS, Prutkin JM, Salerno JC, Zigman ML, Ellenbogen R, Rao AL, **Ackerman MJ**, Drezner JA. Association of atrial fibrillation and obstructive sleep apnea. *Circulation* 2015; 132:10–19. **CITATIONS: 211**

   From the NCAA database (2003–2013), the incidence and characterization of sudden deaths were reported. A total of 4,242,519 athlete-years with 514 SCDs were noted. Accidents in occurred in 257; medical causes were present in 147. There were 79 SCDs. Black athletes and males had a threefold increased SCD rate over white athletes and females. At autopsy, the most common causes were unexplained (25%) and HCM (8%). Men's basketball, soccer, and football had the highest rates of SCD; for women's sports, the most likely were X-country, volleyball, and swimming. Insurance claims only identified 11% of the SCDs.

8. Yao, X, Abraham NS, Alexander C, Crown W, Montori VM, Sangaralingham LR, Gersh MJ, Shah ND, **Noseworthy PA**. Effect of adherence to oral anticoagulants on risk of stroke and major bleeding among patients with atrial fibrillation. *J Am Heart Assoc* 2016; 5: e003074 doi: https://doi.org/10.1161/JAHA.115003074. **CITATIONS: 208**

   Using a retrospective cohort analysis of a US commercial insurance database, 66,661 AF patients had been initiated on warfarin, dabigatran, rivaroxaban, or apixaban between 2010 and 2014; 1.1 median years of follow-up was available. Anticoagulation compliance was poor and only moderately improved with DOACs.

9. Kapplinger JD, Landstrom AP, Salisbury BA, Callis TE, Pollevick GD Tester DJ, Cox MGPJ, Bhuiyan Z, Bikker H, Wiesfeld ACP, Wauer RNW, van Tintelen JP, Jongbloed JDH, Calkins H, Judge DP, Wilde AAM, **Ackerman MJ**. Distinguishing arrhythmogenic right ventricular cardiomyopathy/dysplasia-associated mutations from background noise. *JACC* 2011; 57:2317–27. **CITATIONS: 205**

This study examined genetic variation in health controls for the ARVC susceptibility genes. Rare missense mutations should be interpreted in the context of location, sequence conservation, and ethnicity as they rarely are associated with the phenotype. Mutations were present in 58% of patients and 16% of controls, while "radical" mutations were present in 43% of ARVC cases while only 0.5% of controls.

10. Domingo-Medeiros A, Tan BH, Crotti L, Tester DJ, Eckhardt L, Cuoretti A, Kroboth SL, Song C, Zhou Q, Kopp D, Schwartz PJ, Makielski JC, **Ackerman MJ**. Gain-of-function mutation S422L in the KCNJ8-encoded cardiac KATP channel Kir6.1 as a pathogenic substrate for J-wave syndromes. *Heart Rhythm* 2010; 7:1466–71. **CITATIONS: 202**

One BrS and one ERS case had this mutation. Both cases were negative for mutations otherwise producing Brugada and early repolarization syndromes.

11. **Packer DL**, Mark DB, Robb RA, **Monahan KH**, Bahnson TD, Poole JE, **Noseworthy PA**, Rosenberg YD, Neal J, Mitchell B, Flaker GC, Pokushalov E, Romanov A, Bunch J, Noelker G, Ardashev A, Revishvili A, Wilber DJ, Cappato R, Kuck KH, Hindricks G, Davies W, Kowey PR, Naccarelli GV, Reiffel JA, Piccini JP, Silverstein AP, AL-Khalidi HR, Lee KL. Effect of catheter ablation vs antiarrhythmic drug therapy on mortality, stroke, bleeding, and cardiac arrest among patients with atrial fibrillation: The CABANA randomized clinical trial. *JAMA* 2019; 321:1261–74. **CITATIONS: 197**

This prospective trial included over 2200 patients randomized to either ablation or drugs, followed out to 5 years. No difference in the primary endpoint was noted. Crossover from drugs to ablation occurred in 28%. A significant reduction in hospitalization, recurrent AF, and QOL was noted for ablation. A trend favoring ablation for the primary end point was seen in CHF patients.

12. **Hayes DL,** Boehmer JP, Day JD, Gilliam III FR, Heidenreich PA, Seth M, Jones PW, Saxon LA. Cardiac resynchronization therapy and the relationship of percent biventricular pacing to symptoms and survival. *Heart Rhythm* 2011; 8:1469–75. **CITATIONS: 193**

A group of 36,935 patients were followed via remote monitoring to examine the mortality relationship. The greatest reduction in mortality occurred with >98% biventricular pacing. AF and ventricular ectopy were typically responsible.

13. Al-Khatib SM, Hellkamp A, Curtis J, Mark D, Peterson E, Sanders GD, Heidenreich PA, Hernandez AF, Curtis LH, **Hammill S**. Non-evidence-based ICD implantations in the United States. *JAMA* 2011; 305:43–9. **CITATIONS: 189**

This retrospective cohort study of cases submitted to the NCDR-ICD registry between 2006 and 2009 was examined which included 111,707 patients. Patients who received ICD off-label were assessed to be 23%. The number varied dramatically by site and whether the physician was an EP MD (lower).

14. Yao X, Shah ND, Sangaralingham LR, Gersh BJ, **Noseworthy PA**. Non-Vitamin K antagonist oral anticoagulant dosing in patients with atrial fibrillation and renal dysfunction. *JACC* 2017; 69: 2779–90. **CITATIONS: 186**

This study contained 14,865 AF patients from a large US administrative database who received a DOAC between 2010 and 2015 with normal dosing and adjusted for renal dysfunction. There were 1473 with renal indication for reduc-

tion of dose (43% were partially overdosed). In those with preserved renal function, 13% were underdosed. This group did have a higher risk of stroke.

15. Seet RCS, **Friedman PA,** Rabinstein AA. Prolonged rhythm monitoring for the detection of occult paroxysmal atrial fibrillation in ischemic stroke of unknown cause. *Circulation* 2011; 124:477–86. **CITATIONS: 180**

This review suggested that cardiac monitoring may be an important surveillance strategy for detection of PAF for early treatment and prevention of TIAs and stroke due to thromboembolic events.

16. Wokhlu A, **Monahan KH,** Hodge DO, **Asirvatham SJ, Friedman PA, Munger TM, Bradley DJ,** Bluhm CM, Haroldson JM, **Packer DL**. Long-term quality of life after ablation of atrial fibrillation. *JACC* 2010; 55:2308–16. **CITATIONS: 149**

In this Mayo Clinic study, 502 symptomatic AF patients were examined after ablation for QOL. QOL improved in all groups at 2-year follow-up, including those who were drug/AF-free (72% of the cohort) and those with recurrence, on/off drugs.

17. **Del Carpio Munoz F**, Syed FF, Noheria A, **Cha YM, Friedman PA, Hammill SC, Munger TM, Venkatachalam KL, Shen WK, Packer DL, Asirvatham SJ**. Characteristics of premature ventricular complexes as correlates of reduced left ventricular systolic function: study of burden, duration, coupling interval, morphology, and site of origin of PVCs. *J Cardiovasc Electrophysiol* 2011; 22:79198. **CITATIONS: 132**

Seventy Mayo Clinic patients with no other cause of cardiomyopathy underwent PVC ablation. Seventeen had reduced EF, and this group was compared to those with preserved EF. Those with reduced EF had higher PVC burden (29 vs. 17%), wider PVC (154 vs. 146 msec), and higher prevalence of multiform PVCs (88 vs. 58%). VT$_{ns}$, sinus rhythm QRSD, and coupling PVC interval were not predictive.

18. Wokhlu A, Hodge DO, **Monahan KH, Asirvatham SJ, Friedman PA, Munger TM, Cha YM, Shen WK, Brady PA,** Bluhm CM, Haroldson JM, **Hammill SC, Packer DL**. Long-term quality of life after ablation of atrial fibrillation. *J Cardiovasc Electrophysiol* 2010; 21:1071–8. **CITATIONS: 125**

In this Mayo Clinic study, 774 AF ablation patients were examined over 3-year follow-up. At 2 years, AF elimination was 71% in PAF patients and 61% in persistent AF patients. Independent predictors of recurrence were diabetes, persistent AF pattern, and LA size >45 mm, with a trend including HTN, DCM, and HCM.

19. Attia ZI, **Kapa S,** Lopez-Jimenez F, McKie PM, Ladewig, DJ, Satam G, Pellikka PA, Enriquez-Sarano M, **Noseworthy PA, Munger TM, Asirvatham SJ,** Scott CG, Carter RE, **Friedman PA**. Screening for cardiac contractile dys-

function using an artificial intelligence-enabled electrocardiogram. *Nature Med* 2019; 25:70–4. **CITATIONS: 101**

This initial artificial intelligence (AI) paper from the group used the Mayo Clinic ECG and Echo databases. A convolutional neural network was ECG-trained and tested on 52,870 patients. The ECG algorithm predicted EF ≤35% with a sensitivity ROC curve of 0.93. Simple diagnostic tests like the ECG potentially can be used to screen for LV dysfunction in a population and is being tested.

20. Sriram CS, Syed FF, Ferguson ME, Johnson JN, Enriquez-Sarano M, Cetta F, **Cannon BC, Asirvatham SJ, Ackerman MJ**. Malignant bileaflet mitral valve prolapse syndrome in patients with otherwise idiopathic out-of-hospital cardiac arrest. *JACC* 2013; 62:222–30. **CITATIONS: 100**

Of 1200 patients (2000–2009) evaluated at the Mayo Clinic LQTS genetic clinic, 24 had experienced SCD (16 women). MVP was found in 42% and related to female gender, MVP, high burden, particularly multifocal (outflow papillary muscle).

Excludes:	Guidelines, consensus statements, and letters
Includes:	Invited reviews at high IF (>7) journals and randomized clinical trials (if study PI is Mayo Clinic or <20 authors).
Citation Data:	Derived from End Note (SCOPUS), October 21, 2020; includes at least one Mayo Clinic HRS author at that time.

Chapter 17
Cardiac Surgery and the Cardiac Cath Lab

Hartzell V. Schaff

Introduction

The establishment and growth of cardiac surgery at Mayo Clinic paralleled the development of the cardiac cath lab. Prior to 1955, cardiovascular surgical procedures were primarily extracardiac and included pericardiectomy, systemic-to-pulmonary artery shunts for cyanotic congenital heart disease, repair of coarctation of the aorta, closure of patent ductus arteriosus, and correction of vascular anomalies [1–6]. Intracardiac repair was limited to closed mitral valve commissurotomy and repair of atrial septal defects using the atrial well technique [7–9]. In March 1955, John Kirklin, M.D. and associates closed a ventricular septal defect in a 5-year-old girl with the aid of the Mayo Gibbon heart-lung apparatus, expanding the possibility of intracardiac repair to a wide spectrum of conditions. Availability of surgical treatment of heart disease was an important stimulus for cardiologists and physiologists to accurately identify cardiac diseases and understand pathophysiologic mechanisms.

It is impossible to reflect on the cardiac cath lab and the early development of cardiac surgery without some amusement as regards the recent rediscovery of "heart teams" [10–12]. Mayo Clinic is a multispecialty institution where teamwork has always been a hallmark of clinical practice. This is especially true in cardiovascular disease and is capsulized in a 1951 article in *Minnesota Medicine* where Dr. Kirklin wrote, "Before mention is made of the indications for and the results of operation, it should be emphasized that the surgical treatment of mitral stenosis, as of other cardiovascular lesions, is an enterprise which in our institution requires the utmost in co-operation between the various individuals involved. We are completely dependent upon our cardiologists for the preoperative evaluation of the condition of these

H. V. Schaff (✉)
Department of Cardiovascular Surgery, Mayo Clinic, Rochester, MN, USA
e-mail: schaff@mayo.edu

D. R. Holmes Jr., R. L. Frye (eds.), *The Mayo Clinic Cardiac Catheterization Laboratory*, https://doi.org/10.1007/978-3-030-79329-6_17

patients. Their great care in arriving at the diagnosis and their constant and complete co-operation in preoperative and postoperative management have been indispensable to us at the Mayo Clinic. Dr. Earl Wood has supervised the cardiac catheterization in all the patients we have operated upon, and his analysis and interpretation of these data are of tremendous assistance to us" [5]. Collaboration between cardiovascular surgery, cardiology, and the cath lab is further illustrated in the first report of open-heart operations at our clinic, which included coauthors from surgery, cardiology, anesthesiology, engineering, and physiology [13]. There has always been a "heart team" at our clinic.

Cardiac Surgery and the Cardiac Cath Lab: Early Years

Close cooperation between the cardiac cath lab and surgery predated the advent of open-heart surgery. As discussed in detail in other chapters of this book, clinical investigations of cardiovascular disease evolved from the physiologic studies of Dr. Earl Wood who, in the investigation of G forces during World War II, pioneered fundamental diagnostic techniques and applied these to human studies of cardiac disease [14–16]. An early collaboration with Dr. O. T. Clagett led to investigations of the hemodynamics of patients undergoing repair of coarctation of the aorta [17, 18]. Physiologic evaluation of surgical patients in the cath lab was expanded to incorporate normal controls as well as patients who had undergone coarctation repair [19, 20]. These detailed studies included dye curve sampling to measure circulation time and estimate blood volume and cardiac output as well as simultaneous intra-arterial pressure measurements from the radial and femoral arteries. The investigators found that the circulation time to the femoral artery in patients with coarctation was similar to that of normal patients, but the velocity of circulation above the coarctation was increased above normal. Further, surgical repair of the coarctation tended to restore normal circulation times.

In another study of surgical patients undergoing closure of patent ductus arteriosus, Wood and Clagett determined that blood flow through the ductus was approximately 40% of cardiac output. In seven patients with patent ductus, moderate degrees of exercise led to greater pulse pressure compared to normal controls. As expected, closure of a patent ductus arteriosus caused an immediate increase in systolic and diastolic systemic arterial pressures [21].

These physiologic studies of surgical patients provided important information and concepts that are used today. A classic study by Connolly, Kirklin, and Wood established the close relationship between pulmonary artery wedge pressure and left atrial pressure. They investigated 17 patients with an atrial septal defect in the cath lab and 12 patients intraoperatively who were undergoing mitral valve commissurotomy for rheumatic mitral stenosis [22]. Their paper concluded, "…the pulmonary artery wedge pressure pulse is a reasonably accurate reflection both in magnitude and in the contour of the left atrial pressure pulse in man during normal respiration and also during assisted respiration at operation."

With the advent of open-heart surgery, the physiologic studies [23] became more focused on cardiac diagnosis in preparation for surgical correction. Indeed for the first 25 years of cardiac surgical practice, surgeons were dependent upon colleagues in the cath lab for hemodynamics assessment and for imaging of the heart and great vessels through contrast ventriculography, contrast aortography, and pulmonary angiography. These specialized radiographic studies required input from colleagues in radiology with a special interest in cardiac disease, most notably Owings W. Kincaid, M.D. [24] and George D. Davis, M.D.

Importance of the Cardiac Cath Lab to Care of Cardiac Surgical Patients

Most cardiac surgeons understand the close early relationship between our specialty and the cardiac cath lab, but few are aware of the fundamental contributions to intra-operative and postoperative care that derived from investigations by Dr. Wood and his associates; these might be considered the unexpected benefits of research. Indeed, many of the techniques for hemodynamic monitoring used today were developed or refined from the physiologic studies of G forces in the human centrifuge and subsequently during catheterization for cardiac diagnosis [15, 16, 25].

Studies of blood pressure in men subjected to G forces in the human centrifuge required remote monitoring and recording, and to solve this problem, Lambert and Wood adapted the Statham strain gauge manometer for direct recording of arterial pressure [26, 27]. Radial and femoral artery cannulations for continuous pressure measurement are routine procedures used in virtually every cardiac surgical patient today, during and after an operation. In current practice, devices for analysis of arterial waveforms estimate stroke volume and provide "continuous" information on cardiac output and peripheral resistance. Arterial waveform analysis and its relation to cardiac output were an early interest of Mayo Clinic investigators in the cath lab who described a method for beat-to-beat estimation of changes in stroke volume from central and peripheral arterial pressure recording calibrated against a single determination of cardiac output by the Fick method or dye dilution curves [28].

Noninvasive measurement of blood oxygen saturation is ubiquitous in hospitalized patients, and its use is considered the standard of care for cardiac surgical patients in the operating room and in the intensive care unit. Photoelectric plethysmography too was refined by Wood and associates, who modified the device described by Millikan [29] to create an ear oximeter initially for use in the study of physiologic responses to G force [30].

Indicator dilution dye curves were employed extensively for the measurement of cardiac output in physiologic studies and in clinical cardiac catheterization for detection and quantification of intracardiac shunts [31, 32]. These same methods were used intraoperatively to confirm closure of septal defects and to quantify valvular regurgitation before and after repair [33, 34]. Indeed, monitoring completeness of intracardiac repair with double-sampling dye curves was standard in our operating rooms until the advent of intraoperative transesophageal echocardiography [35, 36].

There is also a connection between the Mayo Clinic Cath Lab and the flow-directed pulmonary artery catheter used in most open cardiac procedures in our clinic and elsewhere [37, 38]. Dr. H. Jeremy Swan was a research fellow working with Earl Wood's group, who subsequently joined the Mayo Clinic staff. He established the clinical cath lab at St. Mary's Hospital and was director of that unit until 1965, when he was recruited to the position of chief of cardiology at Cedars-Sinai Hospital in Los Angeles. During his time at Mayo Clinic, Dr. Swan had an interest in pulmonary circulation [39–44] and performed many right heart catheterizations, a foundation for his later development, with Willy Ganz, of the eponymous balloon-tipped catheter flow-directed pulmonary artery catheter [45–47].

Cardiac Surgery and the Cardiac Cath Lab in Contemporary Practice

For 30 years the close collaboration between cardiac surgeons and the cardiac cath lab benefited both specialties and provided a unique working relationship. So what has changed? Well, everything. One fundamental aspect of collaboration is a dependency of workers on one another, and with the rapid evolution of percutaneous techniques, cardiologists are no longer reliant on cardiac surgeons to manage a wide range of structural cardiovascular diseases. Indeed, the focus of most cardiologists in the cath lab is on interventions, and the current generation of trainees interested in cardiac catheterization aspires to careers as interventional cardiologists.

At the same time, advances in noninvasive imaging with echocardiography, computed tomography (CT), and cardiac magnetic resonance imaging have greatly reduced the need for diagnostic studies in the cath lab in preparation for cardiac surgery. At one time, a patient with mitral valve regurgitation might undergo cardiac catheterization with contrast ventriculography to assess the degree of valve leakage and have coronary arteriography to screen for associated coronary artery disease. In current practice, such patients are assessed with Doppler echocardiography, and patients without symptoms of ischemic heart disease may have CT angiography to evaluate for coronary artery disease. In the current era, the assessment of mitral valve regurgitation in the cath lab is reserved for patients who have conflicting data from Doppler echocardiography or unusual clinical presentations [48].

The evolution of the relationship between cardiac surgery and the cardiac cath lab is evident from considering two common conditions: obstructive coronary artery disease (CAD) and valvular aortic stenosis. There are other examples, but these illustrate the changing practice landscape. Coronary artery bypass surgery was widely used in the late 1970s and through the next decade, and cardiologists in the cath lab at Mayo Clinic were experts in angiographic techniques. With the rapid development of balloon coronary angioplasty [49] and subsequently intracoronary stents, coronary artery disease in most patients can be managed percutaneously. The relative value of percutaneous coronary intervention (PCI) versus coronary artery bypass grafting (CABG) for different patient subsets has been studied exhaustively and debated widely. But today most patients with CAD who require revascularization receive PCI, especially those with single or double vessel involvement. Surgical revascularization is generally reserved for those patients with more extensive coronary atherosclerosis [50, 51] and for patients who have received PCI but have restenosis. The shift in revascularization strategy to PCI whenever possible has impacted the attitudes of cardiologists and changed the relationship of surgeons with the cardiac cath lab. Professional pride may lead some interventional cardiologists to view surgical referral for CABG as a defeat. And for surgeons, not only are there fewer patients selected for surgical revascularization, but those who are referred are often more difficult to manage because of older age, more advanced coronary atherosclerosis, comorbidities, and prior PCI [52–54].

A similar change in the relationship between surgery and the cardiac cath lab has occurred in the management of patients with valvular aortic stenosis. While catheterization for hemodynamic assessment of the severity of valve narrowing is rarely necessary, for an increasing proportion of patients requiring valve intervention, transcatheter aortic valve replacement (TAVR) has supplanted open surgery. Anticipating the potential practice disruption of the new technology, manufacturers and regulators were careful to involve both cardiac surgeons and interventional cardiologists in the initial rollout and trials of this novel procedure.

Currently, in the United States, payors follow CMS guidelines for reimbursement for TAVR, which mandate the involvement of both a cardiac surgeon and an interventional cardiologist experienced in the evaluation and treatment of patients with aortic stenosis. Operators from both specialties are expected to evaluate patients independently prior to a procedure and to jointly participate in the technical aspects of TAVR. The cardiac surgeon and the interventional cardiologist are the core of the structural heart team, and there is general consensus that patients benefit from multidisciplinary review and counseling before TAVR. But the presence of both specialists during every procedure can create inefficiencies, and it seems inevitable that TAVR will be done by one operator in the future [55]. In Germany, TAVR has been performed in hospitals without onsite cardiac surgery backup [56]. Thus, as happened with PCI for coronary artery disease, TAVR for treatment of aortic valve stenosis will reduce the need for open surgery. These advances in technology in the cath lab have clearly benefited patients, but as is the case with most complex diseases, there are many situations where potential advantages of one procedure over another are not clear, and shared decision-making with the patient regarding TAVR should include input from surgeons and cardiologists.

These technological advances in cardiovascular diseases have had an unwanted impact on resident education that is not widely appreciated outside our specialty. As mentioned previously, many percutaneous solutions for structural heart disease have reduced the need for relatively simple cardiac surgical procedures (secundum atrial septal defect closure, single and double CABG, isolated aortic valve replacement), and these operations are the most useful for technical training of cardiothoracic surgical residents. Coupled with work-hour restrictions, the fewer number of relatively straightforward cardiac surgical cases has reduced the operative experience of current residents; the impact of this on future practice is unknown but is unlikely to improve the technical proficiency of trainees. Practice changes may also alter the education of fellows in cardiovascular disease. Focus on interventional techniques in the cath lab can reduce the breadth of exposure and understanding of detailed hemodynamic assessment that is necessary for the evaluation of complex patient conditions [57–60].

Technology and subspecialization have affected didactic educational activities as well. For example, the cardiac catheterization conference was once a clinical conference broadly attended by cardiologists and by all cardiac surgeons and available residents. Discussion of challenging cases included input from senior cardiologists whose shared experience and wisdom were not available in other venues. But with rapid advancement in technology, conference topics have focused more on procedural aspects of care and have become less valuable to those not involved in the interventional practice.

The relationship of cardiac surgery and the cath lab at Mayo Clinic has evolved with advances in technology and disease management, and initial close collaboration now may appear, in many areas, to be cooperative competition. But real progress is always associated with some discomfiture, and patients are the ultimate benefactors of the changing landscape.

References

1. Harrington SW, Barnes AR. Diagnosis and surgical treatment of chronic constrictive pericarditis. South Surg. 1940;IX:459–84.
2. Harrington SW. Chronic constrictive pericarditis: partial pericardiectomy and epicardiolysis in twenty-four cases. Ann Surg. 1944;120:468–85.
3. Clagett OT. Surgical considerations in tetralogy of Fallot. Proc Staff Meet Mayo Clin. 1947;22:180–2.
4. Kirklin JW, Clagett OT. Vascular "rings" producing respiratory obstruction in infants. Proc Staff Meet Mayo Clin. 1950;25:360–7.
5. Kirklin JW. Surgical treatment of diseases of the heart and great vessels. Minn Med. 1951;34:865–70.
6. Clagett OT, Kirklin JW, Ellis FH Jr, Cooley JC. Surgical treatment of patent ductus arteriosus. Surg Clin North Am. 1955;Mayo Clinic No:965–73.
7. Kirklin JW. Surgical treatment of mitral stenosis. Proc Staff Meet Mayo Clin. 1952;27:357–60.

8. Kirklin JW. A useful instrument for mitral commissurotomy. Proc Staff Meet Mayo Clin. 1951;26:176–7.
9. Barrattboyes BG, Ellis FH Jr, Kirklin JW. Technique for repair of atrial septal defect using the atrial well. Surg Gynecol Obstet. 1956;103:646–9.
10. Sintek M, Zajarias A. Patient evaluation and selection for transcatheter aortic valve replacement: the heart team approach. Prog Cardiovasc Dis. 2014;56:572–82.
11. Halaby R, Nathan A, Han JJ. Establishing an interdisciplinary research model among trainees: preparing for a heart team future. J Am Coll Cardiol. 2020;76:2565–8.
12. Head SJ, Kaul S, Mack MJ, Serruys PW, Taggart DP, Holmes DR Jr, et al. The rationale for heart team decision-making for patients with stable, complex coronary artery disease. Eur Heart J. 2013;34:2510–8.
13. Kirklin JW, Dushane JW, Patrick RT, Donald DE, Hetzel PS, Harshbarger HG, et al. Intracardiac surgery with the aid of a mechanical pump-oxygenator system (gibbon type): report of eight cases. Proc Staff Meet Mayo Clin. 1955;30:201–6.
14. Wood EH, Geraci JE. General and special technics in cardiac catheterization. Proc Staff Meet Mayo Clin. 1948;23:494–500.
15. Wood EH. Special instrumentation problems encountered in physiological research concerning the heart and circulation in man. Science. 1950;112:707–15.
16. Wood EH. Evolution of instrumentation and techniques for the study of cardiovascular dynamics from the thirties to 1980, Alza lecture, April 10, 1978. Ann Biomed Eng. 1978;6:250–309.
17. Hallenbeck GA, Wood EH, Clagett OT. Apparatus for recording physiologic variables during operations on man, with observations on changes of blood pressure during resection for coarctation of the aorta. Surg Clin North Am. 1948;28:851–9.
18. Hallenbeck GA, Wood EH, Clagett OT. Changes in radial arterial blood pressure during surgical resection of coarctation of the aorta. Fed Proc. 1948;7:49.
19. Hallenbeck GA, Wood EH, Burchell HB, Clagett OT. Coarctation of the aorta; the relationship of clinical results to cardiovascular dynamics studied before, during, and after surgical treatment. Surg Gynecol Obstet. 1951;92:75–80.
20. Beard EF, Wood EH, Clagett OT. Study of hemodynamics in coarctation of the aorta using dye dilution and direct intraarterial pressure recording methods. J Lab Clin Med. 1951;38:858–72.
21. Taylor BE, Pollack AA, Burchell HB, Clagett OT, Wood EH. Studies of the pulmonary and systemic arterial pressure in cases of patent ductus arteriosus with special reference to effects of surgical closure. J Clin Invest. 1950;29:745–53.
22. Connolly DC, Kirklin JW, Wood EH. The relationship between pulmonary artery wedge pressure and left atrial pressure in man. Circ Res. 1954;2:434–40.
23. Burchell HB, Wood EH. Physiologic measurements in cardiac malformations. Mod Concepts Cardiovasc Dis. 1948;17:25.
24. Earnest F. Owings Wilson Kincaid. Am J Roentgenol. 2010;195:532.
25. Wood EH. Prevention of the pathophysiologic effects of acceleration in humans: fundamentals and historic perspectives. IEEE Eng Med Biol Mag. 1991;10:26–36.
26. Lambert EH, Wood EH. Direct determination of man's blood pressure on the human centrifuge during positive acceleration. Fed Proc. 1946;5:59.
27. Lambert EH, Wood EH. The use of a resistance wire, strain gauge manometer to measure intraarterial pressure. Proc Soc Exp Biol Med. 1947;64:186–90.
28. Warner HR, Swan HJC, Connolly DC, Tompkins RG, Wood EH. Quantitation of beat-to-beat changes in stroke volume from the aortic pulse contour in man. J Appl Physiol. 1953;5:495–507.
29. Millikan GA. Speed of response of arterial oxygen saturation to rapid change in equivalent altitude. Fed Proc. 1946;5:74.
30. Wood EH, Geraci JE, Groom DL. Photoelectric determination of blood oxygen saturation in man. Fed Proc. 1948;7:137.
31. Wood EH, Swan HJ, Marshall HW. Technic and diagnostic applications of dilution curves recorded simultaneously from the right side of the heart and from the arterial circulation. Proc Staff Meet Mayo Clin. 1958;33:536–53.

32. Swan HJC, Wood EH. Localization of cardiac defects by dye-dilution curves recorded after injection of T-1824 at multiple sites in the heart and great vessels during cardiac catheterization. Proc Staff Meet Mayo Clin. 1952;28:95–100.

33. Toscano-Barboza E, Kirklin JW, Swan HJ, Wood EH. Applications of indicator-dilution technics in clinical surgery. Proc Staff Meet Mayo Clin. 1957;32:509–17.

34. Orszulak TA, Schaff HV, Danielson GK, Piehler JM, Pluth JR, Frye RL, et al. Mitral regurgitation due to ruptured chordae tendineae. Early and late results of valve repair. J Thorac Cardiovasc Surg. 1985;89:491–8.

35. Hagler DJ, Tajik AJ, Seward JB, Schaff HV, Danielson GK, Puga FJ. Intraoperative two-dimensional Doppler echocardiography. A preliminary study for congenital heart disease. J Thorac Cardiovasc Surg. 1988;95:516–22.

36. Click RL, Abel MD, Schaff HV. Intraoperative transesophageal echocardiography: 5-year prospective review of impact on surgical management. Mayo Clin Proc. 2000;75:241–7.

37. Lee M, Curley GF, Mustard M, Mazer CD. The Swan-Ganz catheter remains a critically important component of monitoring in cardiovascular critical care. Can J Cardiol. 2017;33:142–7.

38. Judge O, Ji F, Fleming N, Liu H. Current use of the pulmonary artery catheter in cardiac surgery: a survey study. J Cardiothorac Vasc Anesth. 2015;29:69–75.

39. Beck W, Swan HJ, Burchell HB, Kirklin JW. Pulmonary vascular resistance after repair of atrial septal defects in patients with pulmonary hypertension. Circulation. 1960;22:938–46.

40. Swan HJ, Burchell HB, Wood EH. Effect of oxygen on pulmonary vascular resistance in patients with pulmonary hypertension associated with atrial septal defect. Circulation. 1959;20:66–73.

41. Burchell HB, Edwards JE, Shepherd JT, Swan HJ, Wood EH. Clinical, physiological, and pathological considerations in patients with idiopathic pulmonary hypertension. Br Heart J. 1957;19:70–82.

42. Swan HJ, Marshall HW, Wood EH. The effect of exercise in the supine position on pulmonary vascular dynamics in patients with left-to-right shunts. J Clin Invest. 1958;37:202–13.

43. Heath D, Swan HJ, Dushane JW, Edwards JE. The relation of medial thickness of small muscular pulmonary arteries to immediate postnatal survival in patients with ventricular septal defect or patent ductus arteriosus. Thorax. 1958;13:267–71.

44. Swan HJ, Zapata-Diaz J, Burchell HB, Wood EH. Pulmonary hypertension in congenital heart disease. Am J Med. 1954;16:12–22.

45. Swan HJ, Ganz W, Forrester J, Marcus H, Diamond G, Chonette D. Catheterization of the heart in man with use of a flow-directed balloon-tipped catheter. N Engl J Med. 1970;283:447–51.

46. Ganz W, Donoso R, Marcus HS, Forrester JS, Swan HJ. A new technique for measurement of cardiac output by thermodilution in man. Am J Cardiol. 1971;27:392–6.

47. Swan HJ. Cardiac surgery and hemodynamic monitoring. Can Anaesth Soc J. 1982;29:336–40.

48. Breen TJ, Jain CC, Tan NY, Miranda WR, Nishimura RA. Paroxysmal severe mitral regurgitation. Mayo Clin Proc. 2021;96:86–91.

49. Vlietstra RE, Holmes DR Jr, Smith HC, Hartzler GO, Orszulak TA. Percutaneous transluminal coronary angioplasty: initial Mayo Clinic experience. Mayo Clin Proc. 1981;56:287–93.

50. Deb S, Wijeysundera HC, Ko DT, Tsubota H, Hill S, Fremes SE. Coronary artery bypass graft surgery vs percutaneous interventions in coronary revascularization: a systematic review. JAMA. 2013;310:2086–95.

51. Head SJ, Davierwala PM, Serruys PW, Redwood SR, Colombo A, Mack MJ, et al. Coronary artery bypass grafting vs. percutaneous coronary intervention for patients with three-vessel disease: final five-year follow-up of the SYNTAX trial. Eur Heart J. 2014;35:2821–30.

52. Altarabsheh SE, Deo SV, Hang D, Haddad OK, Cho YH, Markowitz AH, et al. Coronary artery bypass grafting after percutaneous intervention has higher early mortality: a meta-analysis. Ann Thorac Surg. 2015;99:2046–52.

53. Chocron S, Baillot R, Rouleau JL, Warnica WJ, Block P, Johnstone D, et al. Impact of previous percutaneous transluminal coronary angioplasty and/or stenting revascularization on outcomes after surgical revascularization: insights from the imagine study. Eur Heart J. 2008;29:673–9.

54. Barakate MS, Hemli JM, Hughes CF, Bannon PG, Horton MD. Coronary artery bypass grafting (CABG) after initially successful percutaneous transluminal coronary angioplasty (PTCA): a review of 17 years experience. Eur J Cardiothorac Surg. 2003;23:179–86.
55. Giri JS, Szerlip M, Devireddy C, Cox DA, Kavinsky C, Genereux P, et al. SCAI 2018 think tank proceedings: "what should the role of the surgeon be in TAVR, both as a co-operator and in-patient evaluation for TAVR?". Catheter Cardiovasc Interv. 2019;93:178–9.
56. Eggebrecht H, Bestehorn M, Haude M, Schmermund A, Bestehorn K, Voigtländer T, et al. Outcomes of transfemoral transcatheter aortic valve implantation at hospitals with and without on-site cardiac surgery department: insights from the prospective German aortic valve replacement quality assurance registry (AQUA) in 17 919 patients. Eur Heart J. 2016;37:2240–8.
57. Talreja DR, Nishimura RA, Oh JK, Holmes DR. Constrictive pericarditis in the modern era: novel criteria for diagnosis in the cardiac catheterization laboratory. J Am Coll Cardiol. 2008;51:315–9.
58. Lloyd JW, Nishimura RA, Borlaug BA, Eleid MF. Hemodynamic response to nitroprusside in patients with low-gradient severe aortic stenosis and preserved ejection fraction. J Am Coll Cardiol. 2017;70:1339–48.
59. Reddy YNV, Murgo JP, Nishimura RA. Complexity of defining severe "stenosis" from mitral annular calcification. Circulation. 2019;140:523–5.
60. Miranda WR, El Sabbagh A, Nishimura RA, Rihal CS. Mitral stenosis assessment using left atrial pressure via radial approach: an alternative to Transseptal puncture. JACC Cardiovasc Interv. 2019;12:2430–1.

Chapter 18
2020 and Beyond: The Future Catheterization Laboratory

Mohamad Alkhouli

The glory of medicine is that it is constantly moving forward, that there is always more to learn

    William J. Mayo

In the prior chapters, we enjoyed reading about the incredible history of the catheterization laboratory at Mayo Clinic. We learned about its evolution from a small lab that offers basic diagnostics to a sophisticated 14-room suite that routinely performs surgical-like interventions. We also learned about the gifted individuals whose innovation, hard work, and discipline enabled the lab to overcome many challenges and become one of the leading reference labs in the world. In this section, we provide a futuristic vision of the major component of the catheterization laboratory encompassing the three shields of clinical practice, research, and education.

Imaging in the cath Lab

The interplay between cardiac catheterization and noninvasive imaging has been both fascinating and dynamic. Historically, cardiac catheterization was the first means to provide diagnostic data in patients with suspected valvular or congenital heart diseases. Echocardiography then emerged to supply the same information noninvasively, leading to an initial decline in catheterization procedures until PCI

M. Alkhouli (✉)

Department of Cardiovascular Diseases, Mayo Clinic, Rochester, MN, USA

e-mail: Alkhouli.mohamad@mayo.edu

D. R. Holmes Jr., R. L. Frye (eds.), *The Mayo Clinic Cardiac Catheterization Laboratory*, https://doi.org/10.1007/978-3-030-79329-6_18

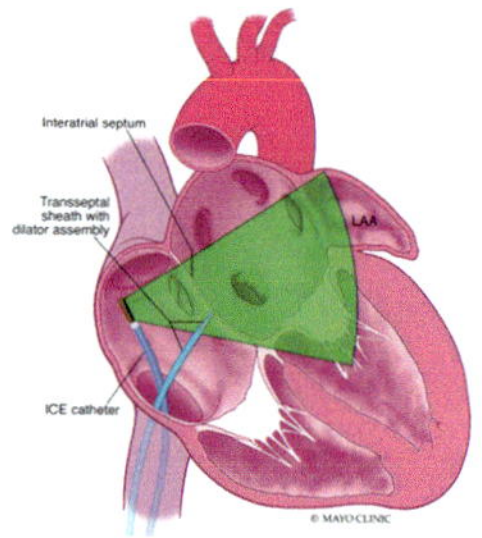

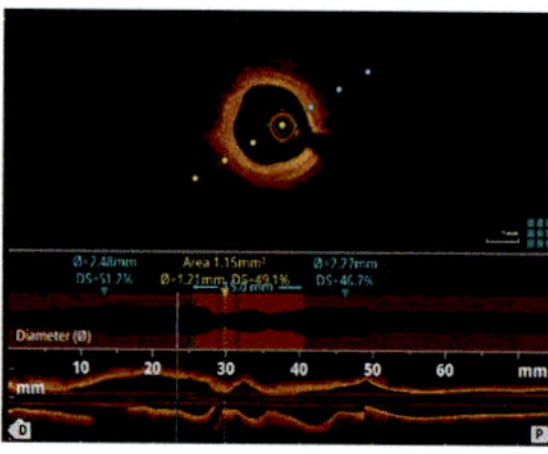

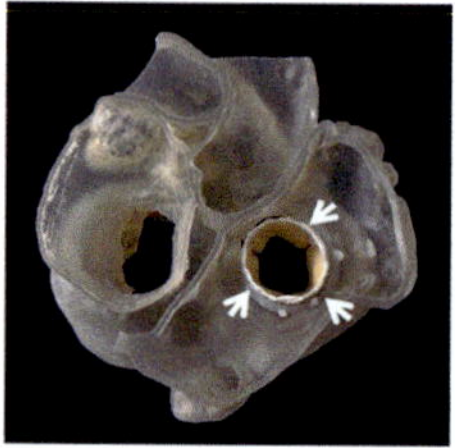

Fig. 18.1 Modern imaging modalities in the cath lab

materialized and flourished in the late 1970s. Since then, imaging in the cath lab has taken a quantum leap forward (Fig. 18.1).

A. *Intravascular Imaging:* Intravascular ultrasound (IVUS) and optical coherence tomography (OCT) have revolutionized our ability to appreciate detailed vascular anatomy and plaque characteristics both in the coronaries and in the peripheral vasculature. Although data supporting the improved outcomes with intravascular imaging-guided PCI are overwhelming, the utilization of IVUS and OCT remains uncommon in the United States [1–4]. This is likely multifactorial due to the time constraints, the modest reimbursement, and the lack of smooth integration of intravascular and cine imaging systems. In addition, residual technical challenges remain as important barriers to the adoption of routine intravascular imaging. For example, while IVUS has an excellent depth penetration and quantitative performance, its ability to characterize vulnerable plaque and thrombus is quite limited. OCT, on the other hand, still requires a blood-free medium and subsequently a high contrast load, a fair amount of manual processing, and a non-negligible learning curve [4]. Affordable hybrid IVUS/OCT imaging catheters with coregistration, automated processing, and imaging through blood capabilities are expected to lead to a growing use of intravascular imaging in the near future.

B. *Imaging for SHD Interventions:* Contemporary 2D and 3D transthoracic and transesophageal echocardiography provides outstanding guidance for transcatheter structural heart disease (SHD) interventions. Indeed, routine and complex SHD interventions have become entirely dependent on adequate echocardiographic images. Future procedural imaging for SHD interventions will likely mark two major advances. First, multimodality imaging will continue to be the backbone for planning of SHD interventions. However, those will be increasingly integrated and displayed in modern intuitive ways (3D-printed models, virtual and augmented reality software, etc), which would improve case planning and allow the creation of custom-made devices to address complex anatomies (e.g., unusual serpiginous paravalvular leak or large multilobulated left atrial appendage [LAA]). Second, imaging modalities that allow a minimalistic approach to SHD interventions will be progressively refined and adopted. For example, the value of intracardiac echocardiography (ICE) in facilitating LAA and intra-atrial septal defect closure under moderate sedation has led to an increasing use of ICE in the cath lab despite the lack of any meaningful technological advancement in ICE in the last 20 years [5, 6]. Recognizing this unmet need and the potential to further expand ICE guidance to other transcatheter valvular therapeutics has recently fueled major recent investments in enhancing the capabilities of ICE catheters [7]. Newer catheters with biplane and 3D/4D imaging abilities are currently being introduced to the market and will likely lead to major changes in intraprocedural guidance of SHD interventions.

High-Risk PCI

Following decades of disruptive innovation, routine PCIs have now reached a relative steady state [8]. However, the management of the complex coronary artery disease (CAD) continues to evolve. Indeed, technological advancements afforded interventional cardiologists (IC) the ability to tackle coronary lesions that were previously deemed exclusively surgical or even inoperable. This included PCI of left main, multivessel, or severely calcified lesions and chronic total occlusions (CTOs), as well as complex PCI in patients with valvular disease, ventricular dysfunction, or cardiogenic shock (Fig. 18.2) [9–11]. A special term for this type of interventions was recently coined (clinically indicated high-risk PCI; CHIP), which was accompanied with a rapid proliferation in training programs, conferences, and seminars dedicated to the teaching and promotion of CHIP. A parallel notable growth occurred in the utilization of mechanical circulatory support (MCS) pumps, atherectomy, reentry devices, and other tools dedicated to support CHIP. There are still challenges which remain to be addressed. First, while the safety of CHIP is now well documented, the clinical utility of those interventions has not yet been established, an issue that has given rise to controversies and ongoing debates. Second, certain lesion subsets remain difficult to tackle despite the remarkable progress in technology. For example, tools and techniques to treat calcific CAD and in-stent restenosis remained largely undeveloped for many years [12]. The advent of lithotripsy balloons, however, has revived the interest in calcium modification. Given the excellent early reported performance of lithotripsy balloons, this technique might be the focus of many investigations and refinement in the near future [13]. Third, considering the substantial cost, time, and radiation exposure associated with CHIP interventions,

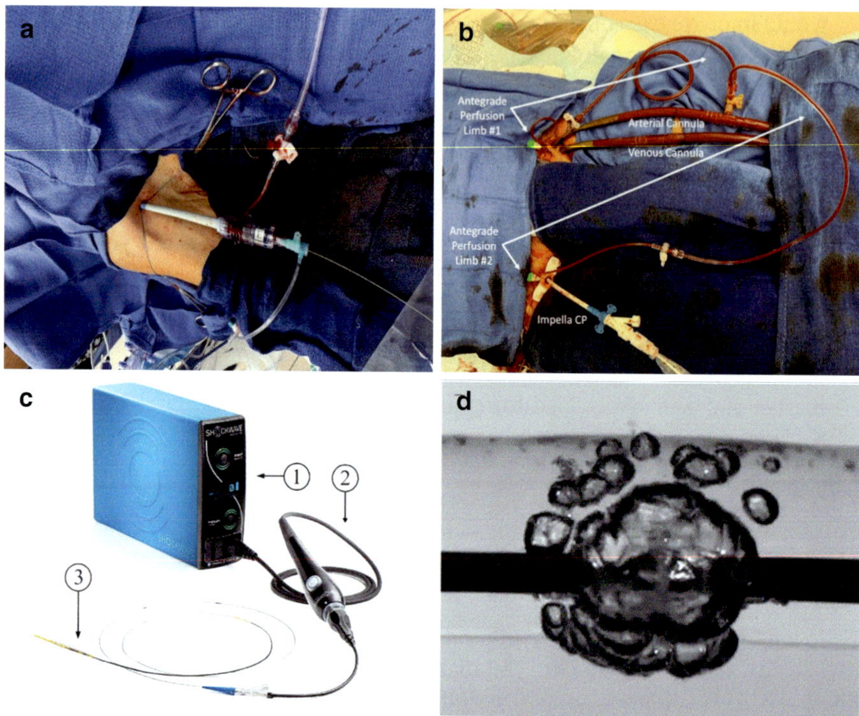

Fig. 18.2 High-risk PCI in contemporary labs. (**a**) Percutaneous axillary access for combined unprotected left main PCI and transcatheter aortic valve replacement. (**b**) Percutaneous extracorporeal membrane oxygenation and left ventricular venting. (**c**) Lithotripsy facilitated revascularization in heavily calcified lesions. (**d**) In vitro illustration of lithotripsy. (Reprinted with permission [Kereiakes et al. Am Heart J. 2020;225:10–18])

logistical issues related to job market, cath lab flow, and reimbursement need to be resolved for the sustainability and growth of CHIP programs. Whether the field of CHIP will continue to thrive or atrophy depends on our success in addressing those remaining challenges.

Disease-Based Care Teams

The heart team concept was pioneered in the early PCI era to allow a balanced and evidence-based approach to CAD [14]. This approach has gained strong support by professional societies and is now embedded as a Class I recommendation in most guidelines. Despite the limited scientifically controlled data supporting a clinical benefit to the "heart team," in actual practice it has improved and solidified interdisciplinary relationships and resulted in improved ability to evaluate risk-benefit issues even in complex CAD. These successes have resulted in expanding the scope to extend the heart team concept to other patient populations and disease entities. Initiatives were called on to establish care teams for valvular disorders (heart valve team), vascular disease, cardiogenic shock (CS), and pulmonary embolism [11] with variable success. While the journey of the "heart valve" team was extraordinarily successful, multidisciplinary team decisions in other venues (e.g., vascular disease management) remained rare despite its proven impact on clinical outcomes [15]. Collaborative teams for cardiogenic shock and pulmonary embolism resulted in modest success amid issues related to the limited clinical data, personal availability, and sustainability. Unfortunately, the future will only bring additional challenges such as the diminishing reimbursement and the increasing territorial focus of each specialty, which may erode even the most established and successful teams. Furthermore, as disruptive transcatheter technologies (e.g., TAVR) become more of a commodity, debates are arising on the clinical need for multiple operators in such cases. Professional societies and other stakeholders will need to invest in redefining multidisciplinary collaboration to salvage and advance what has been proven to be one of the most key determinants of patient outcomes: disease-based care teams.

Artificial Intelligence (AI)

The interest in AI applications in cardiovascular medicine has grown considerably recently, and Mayo Clinic cardiologists have been on the forefront of AI research. AI-enabled ECG algorithms developed at Mayo Clinic have achieved excellent performance in identifying hypertrophic cardiomyopathy, left ventricular dysfunction, aortic stenosis, and atrial fibrillation during sinus rhythm [16, 17]. Similar progress has been made in cardiovascular imaging, with AI algorithms now capable of providing accurate automated reads, detecting subtle findings, and providing prognostic information [16]. Although the utilization of AI in most cath labs has been limited to date, its potential future applications are numerous. Table 18.1 lists the possible useful AI tools in the cath lab for the foreseeable future.

Personalized Care

The complexity of both patients referred to the cath lab and cardiac therapeutics offered in the lab often leads to uncertainties in appropriate patient and procedure selection, as well as periprocedural management. Hence, future interventional practices will feature an increasing emphasis on personalized risk assessment, cardiac prostheses, and adjunctive medical therapy.

Risk Assessment Risk prediction models have become increasingly popular [22, 23]. Numerous scores are now available to predict the risk of adverse events in the setting of acute illness (GRACE ACS score, etc) or with cardiac interventions (TAVR in-hospital mortality risk calculator, Mayo Clinic PCI risk score, etc). However, most of these risk scores predict a single outcome (i.e., mortality), encompass a limited number of conditions and procedures, and are not provided in an intuitive interface for patient use. Efforts need to focus on constructing simple, credible, and readily available risk assessment tools that can be used by both the physician and the patient alike. Mandeep Singh et al. have shown that several post-PCI adverse events (not only mortality) can be predicted from patient baseline multi-morbidity. This approach, if externally validated, might provide a simple approach for risk prediction using traditional risk factors. Another futuristic approach would utilize AI-enhanced algorithms to predict short- and long-term outcomes using routinely collected data. For example, an ECG-AI model was able to predict future cardiomyopathy in patients with normal ventricular function and to predict long-term mortality after cardiac surgery [17]. Eventually, an AI-based automated risk assessment tool that incorporates all data elements available in electronic health records (risk factors, vital sings, results of cardiac testing, etc) will likely prevail and become an essential component of every patient's assessment.

Cardiac Prostheses 3D printing has improved our ability to understand and treat complex structural and congenital heart defects. To date, 3D-printed models have allowed in vitro testing of a procedural feasibility (e.g., paravalvular leak closure) and the prediction of peridevice leak after TAVR or LAA occlusion. However, it is

Table 18.1 Future Application of Artificial Intelligence in the cath Lab

1. Rapid point-of-care tools for diagnosis of acute cardiovascular events or monitoring of chronic disease
2. Risk stratification of AMI (e.g., ECG identification of occluded culprit vessel, impending shock)
3. Determining patient's candidacy for pragmatic clinical trials
4. Automated iterative gantry positioning to optimize imaging
5. Assessing patient's frailty and rehab potential using wearable trackers and health monitors
6. Analyzing coronary lesion characteristics using angiographic data only [18, 19]
7. Early recognition of catheter dampening using CNN automated waveform analysis [20]
8. Wire-free algorithms to detect functionally significant stenoses [21]
9. Online segmentation, quantification, and coregistration of intracoronary imaging (IVUS, OCT)
10. AI, virtual and augmented reality for planning and guidance of structural heart interventions
11. Robotic transcatheter interventions

likely that the wealth of patient-specific anatomical details afforded by multimodality imaging will be further improved and integrated to allow the development, refinement, printing, and implantation of personalized tissue or polymer-based valves and other intracardiac devices [24].

Periprocedural Management The majority of procedures in the cath lab require adjunctive periprocedural antiplatelet and/or anticoagulation therapy. The optimal drug combination before, during, and after the procedure remains controversial, and national and international practices vary considerably. In addition, the increasing complexity of patients referred for catheter-based therapy (older, need for concomitant procedure, polypharmacy, bleeding risk, etc) has led to an ongoing management conundrum. The integration of genotype-guided therapy, time-varying risk assessment models, and patient decision aid tools will likely become a hallmark of future cath lab daily practice [22, 25].

Sensor Technology

Ambulatory monitoring for clinical events and their precursors is rapidly growing. In the HF field, for instance, interest in remote assessment of volume status to reduce HF hospitalizations has led to the pioneering of purpose-specific implantable monitors. CardioMEMS (Abbott, Abbott Park, IL), an implantable wireless pulmonary artery pressure monitoring device, demonstrated lower rates of HF and all-cause hospitalization vs. standard of care across a broad range of patients with symptomatic HF [26, 27]. In patients presenting with acute myocardial infarction, the AngelMed Guardian System (Anel Medical Systems, Eatontown, NJ) resulted in a markedly reduced prehospital delay to care (1.6 vs. 12.7 h, $p < 0.089$) compared with patients who did not have remote monitoring (Fig. 18.3) [28]. It is anticipated that the sensor technology will further expand in scope, quality, and quantity. We can speculate on a few target applications: (a) Pressure sensors will develop further to allow continuous monitoring of valvular regurgitation, intracardiac pressure, and vascular impedance. Those will become standalone low-profile implantable or optional add-on pieces to transcatheter valves, clips, occluders, and pacing wires. (b) Rhythm monitors that can now be incorporated into wearables (e.g., Apple Watch) will undergo several refinements to become capable of detecting subtle but clinically meaningful rate and rhythm disturbances. This will have a substantial impact on managing patients at risk for major arrhythmias such as those at risk for complete heart block after transcatheter aortic valve replacement (TAVR). (c) Smart sensors that allow iterative modification of procedural strategies will emerge. For example, a rhythm sensor incorporated in the frame of a transcatheter valve can sense the rising tension on the conduction system during valve deployment and allow for a modification of valve technique to mitigate the need for permanent

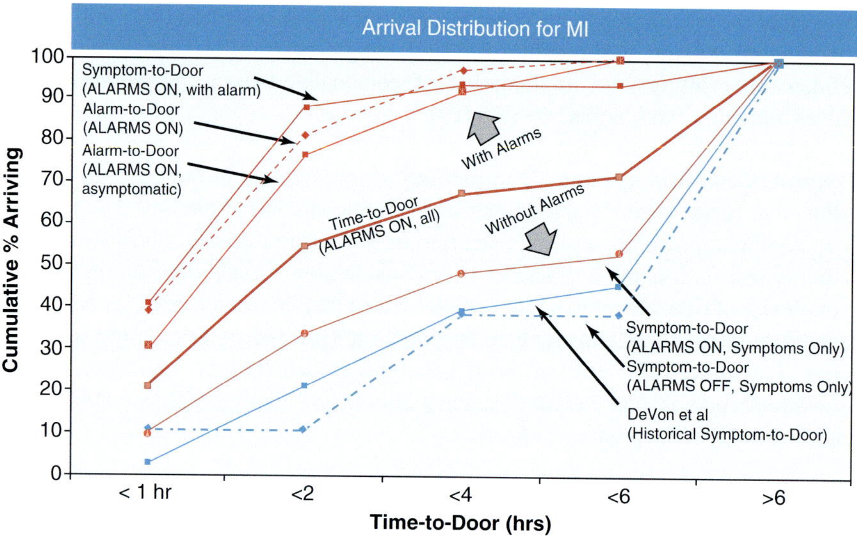

Fig. 18.3 Future of sensor technology. Distribution of arrival time in patients with myocardial infarction with versus without remote monitoring using the AngelMed Guardian System. (Reprinted with permission [Holmes et al. J Am Coll Cardiol. 2019:22;74(16):2047–2055])

pacemakers (balloon auto-deflation in balloon-expandable systems and repositioning in self-expandable systems). (d) Sensors to detect cerebral embolic debris in high-risk patients might become a reality and may allow tailored medical or interventional therapy to reduce stroke risk [29].

Valvular Heart Interventions

Transcatheter valvular therapeutics have sustained an unprecedented evolution in their number, scope, and complexity. To date, over half a million patients have undergone TAVR, and >100,000 patients received the MitraClip device worldwide. Furthermore, a large number of inventions to treat mitral and tricuspid valve regurgitation (MR, TR) are currently being evaluated in preclinical and clinical studies. Yet, the SHD interventional field is still considered in its infancy. Certain issues with TAVR such as pacemaker rates, stroke, coronary access, and durability still need to be resolved. Similarly, mitigating the anatomical challenges with transcatheter mitral and tricuspid valve repair and replacement therapies remains an area of ongoing research.

The next wave of innovations in transcatheter valve interventions will likely be characterized by:

(a) Emphasis on pathophysiology. The swift proliferation of transcatheter repair and replacement devices overshadowed our incomplete understanding of the valvular disease. This is especially true with functional regurgitant lesions, namely, MR and TR [20]. However, with randomized clinical trials revealing contradictory results, and with the high reported residual morbidity and mortality after complex transcatheter treatment of MR and TR, there is a growing recognition of the need to further our understanding of the pathophysiology of valve disease. Fortunately, this is already underway; a considerable body of literature started to surface documenting the utility of novel imaging techniques (e.g., 4D MRI), flow dynamics, and valve stress testing in improving our comprehension of the etiology, dynamicity, and clinical impact of MR and TR (Fig. 18.4). Similar studies have also shown the extent and impact of the altered aortic root geometry after TAVR and its possible association with leaflet thrombosis, valve durability, and coronary flow impediment. Research in this area may lead to the development of more physiological and patient-specific transcatheter solutions which may be associated with superior clinical outcomes. Benefactor awards at the Mayo Clinic Cath Lab have been granted to incorporate multimodality imaging and invasive hemodynamics to better understand functional MR and TR. In addition, a growing collaboration between Mayo Clinic Cath Labs and flow dynamic engineers across the country has been initiated, aiming to pioneer novel devices/interventions that may restore normal physiology and flow dynamics.

(b) Expansion of transcatheter microsurgery. Until recently, all transcatheter interventions have been limited to the implantation of artificial devices (valve, plug, etc) to treat a specific pathology. Tissue modification, akin to what is possible with cardiac surgery, remains in uncharted territory. In the last few years, nonetheless, transcatheter electrosurgery techniques (e.g., BASILICA, LAMPOON, etc) were invented to address certain anatomical challenges with TAVR and TMVR (Fig. 18.4) [30]. The purview of such techniques has been limited due to their intricacy and technical challenges. However, we speculate that transcatheter leaflet modification techniques will continue to improve by incorporating new energy sources (e.g., laser, cryoablation, etc) and novel imaging modalities such as scanning fiber endoscopy, terahertz imaging, and OCT. The anticipated success of these interventions will open the door to experiment additional surgical-like procedures (e.g., transcatheter complex leaflet repair, tumor removal, etc) which may further transform the field of SHD interventions.

(c) New paradigms for device development and outcomes research. The relative explosion of SHD technologies in recent years uncovered major impediments to bringing a new device to clinical use such as the excessive costs and significant delays in regulatory processes. The early feasibility study (EFS) initia-

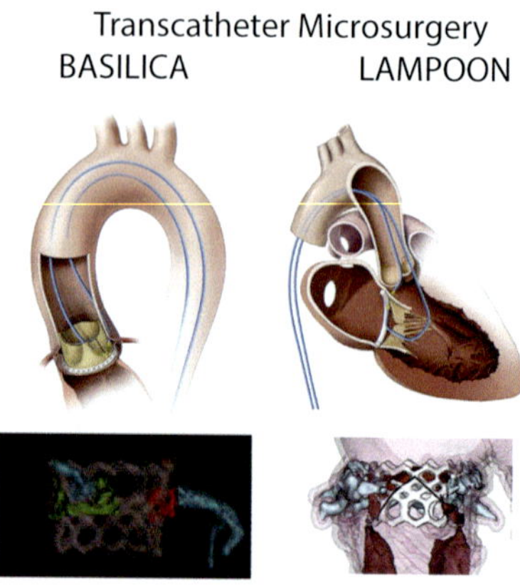

Fig. 18.4 Advanced transcatheter valve intervention concepts. Left, Cardiac magnetic resonance-derived path line visualization of cardiac blood flow. Future transcatheter valve therapies aiming to restore normal physiology will heavily incorporate flow dynamics imaging. Right, Illustration of current transcatheter electrocautery procedures. BASILICA; bioprosthetic or native aortic scallop intentional laceration to prevent iatrogenic coronary artery obstruction. LAMPOON; intentional laceration of the anterior mitral valve leaflet to prevent LVOT obstruction. (Reprinted with permission [Sengupta et al. JACC Cardiovasc Imaging. 2012;5(3):305–16, and Khan et al. Am Coll Cardiol. 2020:31;75(12):1455–1470])

tive was developed by the US Food and Drug Administration to address these challenges [31]. The initial application of the program demonstrated some success but also highlighted the need for additional steps to improve the efficiency of early device testing and approval. The futuristic theme for an ideal device development process features efficient EFS start-up, centralized institutional review board approval, smooth transition to pivotal trials, and increasing utilization of pragmatic trial designs [31, 32]. Furthermore, ascertainment of safety and efficacy in real-world cohorts, an essential part of ensuring the long-term success of novel devices, has been achieved by constructing dedicated post-market and device-specific registries. However, these can be hampered by cost, short-term follow-up, and limited generalizability. Recently, innovative solutions have emerged to bridge this gap such as using claim-based data to provide a timely assessment of device performance and to extend the follow-up of patients enrolled in randomized trials and national procedural registries (e.g., TVT registry) [33–36]. With further improvement in billing code validation, events adjudication, and increasing partnership between various stakeholders, it is likely that future evaluation of devices will routinely take a hybrid approach that incorporates both randomized and observational data.

Stroke Prevention and Treatment

Stroke is a leading cause of death and long-term disability, with over 800,000 strokes occurring annually in the United States. Hence, concerted efforts across multiple disciplines have aimed to reduce the burden of this morbid condition. Interventional cardiologists have had their share of these efforts, which have been crowned with notable successes. Today, two stroke prevention therapies with excellent safety and efficacy profiles are performed routinely and with increasing frequency in most cath labs: LAAO (pioneered by David Holmes et al. at the Mayo Clinic) and patent foramen ovale (PFO) closure [37, 38]. The future of these interventions appears to be bright; more standard and niche devices will become available, minimalist approaches will become dominant, and long-term data will become abundant [5, 39, 40]. Opportunities of innovations in these areas will likely be incremental such as adding pressure sensors to closure devices, mitigating long-term safety issues (e.g., reducing device thrombus with novel device coating), and improving device profiles to allow combined and ad hoc procedures. However, the area with the greatest potential for growth and advancements is the area of mechanical thrombectomy for the treatment of ischemic stroke with large vessel occlusion. Unfortunately, ICs have been effectively excluded from acute stroke care to date. Nonetheless, the increasing recognition of the unmet clinical needs in acute stroke care along with the growing collaboration between neurologists and ICs will likely change this theme in the future [41]. The benefits of such collaboration are enormous and include not only improving patient outcomes but also driving innovations in stroke management, increasing cross-discipline learning, extending the geographical reach of stroke interventions, and addressing unresolved issues such as the issue of postprocedural strokes in the cath lab [42].

Interventional Heart Failure

The art of performing precise and credible hemodynamic studies has been gradually lost in most cath labs worldwide due to advances in echocardiography, reimbursement, and other logistical issues. However, the Earl Wood Cath Lab has maintained its leading position in exercise physiology, transseptal heart catheterization, and hemodynamic assessment of intricate cardiomyopathies. This branch of the cath lab practice continues to flourish under the leadership of renowned hemodynamic HF experts (Dr. Borlaug, Dr. Nishimura) and the addition of new hemodynamic specialists (Dr. Reddy and Dr. Miranda). In addition, SHD interventionalists are increasingly incorporating invasive hemodynamics not only to diagnose valvular disease but also to guide its treatment. Several investigations are ongoing at Mayo Clinic to assess the optimal techniques, utility, and prognostic value of intraprocedural hemodynamics during SHD interventions (Fig. 18.5). The results of these studies may change the way we perform transcatheter valvular interventions. Furthermore, the

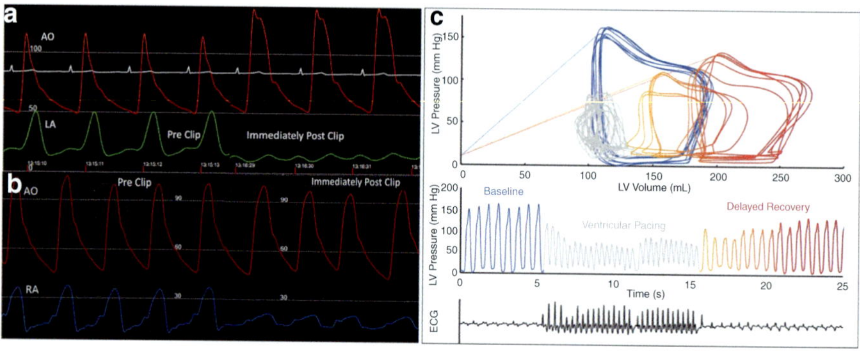

Fig. 18.5 Hemodynamic-guided transcatheter valve interventions. (**a**) Transcatheter mitral edge-to-edge repair. (**b**) Transcatheter tricuspid edge-to-edge repair. (**c**) Pressure volume loop monitoring during transcatheter aortic valve replacement. (Reprinted with permission; creative commons license [Sarraf et al. J Am Coll Cardiol Case Rep. 2021, 3 (1) 77–81])

role of the cath lab in managing HF will grow much further beyond its diagnostic capabilities, driven by the rapid growth in the HF population and in novel transcatheter therapeutics.

The prevalence of HF in the United States is expected to increase by 46% from 2012 to 2030, resulting in >8 million adults with HF [43]. These rising trends have been coupled with a growing interest in interventional HF therapies beyond coronary revascularization. Interventional HF therapies encompass a wide spectrum of preventive strategies and treatment strategies. Myocardial salvage in patients presenting with STEMI has recently gained momentum for its potential utility in mitigating subsequent HF after anterior wall STEMI [44]. The Door-To-Unload in STEMI Pilot Trial documented the safety and feasibility of mechanically unloading the LV with a microaxial blood pump prior to primary PCI to decrease infarct size and prevent future HF [45]. This concept is now being studied in a pivotal trial (DTU-STEMI) and, if proven efficacious, would change the landscape of interventional therapies specifically aiming to prevent HF. Transcatheter therapies for MV and TR are expected to become a cornerstone in the management of refractory HF. Another encouraging venue in interventional HF is related to iatrogenic shunt creation to decompress the left atrium in patients with advanced HF [46]. The primary shunt location that has been evaluated to date is in the intra-atrial septum, although a first-in-human report of levoatrial-to-coronary sinus shunting also has shown promising initial results [47]. Albeit long-term clinical and cost-effectiveness data remain needed, early trials on iatrogenic atrial shunts demonstrated improved functional status and hemodynamics in patients with preserved or reduced systolic function [46].

The largest unmet clinical need in HF continues to be among patients with preserved ejection fraction (HFpEF), in whom an effective therapy has not been established yet. In this realm, the opportunities for innovation are enormous. Creative concepts and transcatheter tools for the treatment of HFpEF already have started to emerge. The concept of "percutaneous pericardial resection" is being explored as a potential therapy for HFpEF patients using minimally invasive techniques. One device, invented at Mayo Clinic, is a scissors-like device that allows resection of the anterior pericardium to mitigate the increase in LV end-diastolic pressure during volume loading in HFpEF patients [48] (Fig. 18.6). Another intriguing concept that is being investigated is the use of transcatheter tools to improve lymphatic drainage which is known to be severely impaired in patients with HFpEF [49]. A different approach for unloading is by performing intermittent balloon occlusion of the superior vena cava, which reduces cardiac filling pressures in

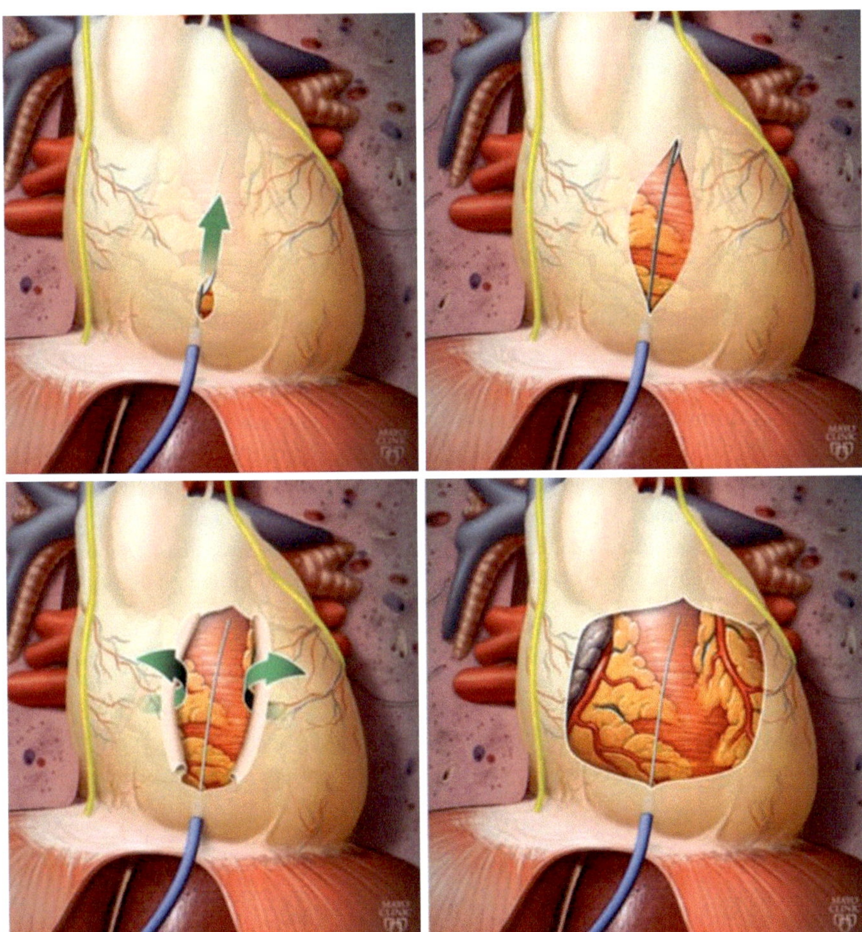

Fig. 18.6 Percutaneous pericardial resection tool for refractory heart failure

patients with decompensated HF [50]. Data from these investigations will contribute considerably to the potential evolution of interventional HF as a standalone subspecialty with substantial clinical impact and opportunities for growth.

Interventions on the Pulmonary Circulation

Venous thromboembolism (VTE) affects >900,000 patients in the United States every year. Yet the management of the acute and chronic sequalae of VTE remains primordial. Anticoagulation continues to be the only mainstream option in patients with large thrombus burden despite its modest efficacy. Nonetheless, the future of interventional management of VTE seems to be promising with several novel approaches being developed or refined to address submassive PE, deep venous thrombosis, and chronic thromboembolic pulmonary hypertension (CTEPH) (Fig. 18.7).

Creative solutions for flow restoration in acute submassive PE have demonstrated excellent safety and promising efficacy results [51]. Although randomized trials and comparative effectiveness data remain sparse, large opportunities for growth in this field exist. The current armamentarium for acute PE care includes safer and more effective methods of catheter-directed thrombolysis, ultrasound-facilitated lysis, and thrombolytic-free thrombus removal technologies [51, 52]. Mayo Clinic Cath Lab staff (Mohamad Alkhouli and Sam Asirvatham) have pioneered the first cryobased dedicated tool for vascular thrombus removal. This invention is based on the concept that cryo-enabled tools can act as "magnets" that allow grabbing and removal of thrombus and possibly other undesired materials (Fig.18.7). Initial animal studies yielded favorable results, and advanced prototype designs are underway. Pending further development and additional investigation, this method can potentially be a game changer not only in PE care but in addressing large thrombus burden in other vascular beds. Interventional cardiologists have also been a driving force in the establishment and refinements of balloon pulmonary angioplasty for

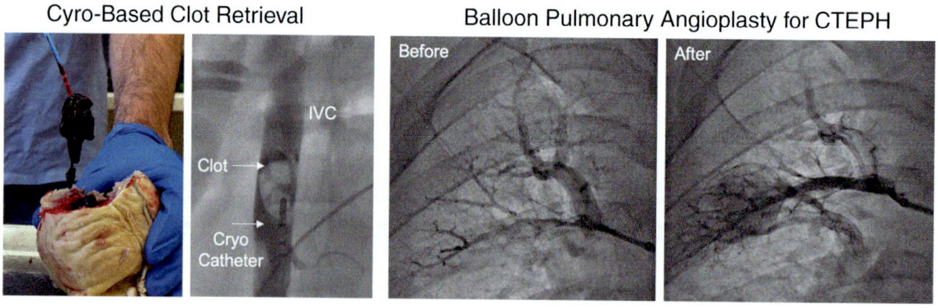

Fig. 18.7 Future of pulmonary vascular interventions. Left, Cryo-based clot retrieval system in benchtop and proof-of-concept early animal studies. Right, Balloon pulmonary angioplasty for chronic thromboembolic pulmonary hypertension

CTEPH [53]. Mayo Clinic has been on the vanguard of CTEPH management. Dr. Sandhu, Frantz, and others have built an extremely successful balloon pulmonary angioplasty program that became a national magnet for CTEPH patients [54]. Multidisciplinary collaboration such as the PERT (Pulmonary Embolism Response Team) and CTEPH team will be essential to optimize the overall care for patients with PE and to advance pulmonary vascular interventions.

Training and Education in Interventional Cardiology

The recent waves of transformational technologies in SHD interventions have brought forth new opportunities and challenges for IC training [14]. Duration and structure of training programs, the concept of ultraspecialization, and the future interactions between cardiology, cardiac surgeons, and other specialists are issues that are becoming increasingly relevant to everyday practice. In addition, the impact of the COVID-19 pandemic and the upswing in the role of social media (SoMe) in medical education demand serious consideration to reimagine future educational programs in IC [55].

The following changes are expected to take place in IC training and education in the near future:

1. Training future ICs will gradually evolve into a two-tiered approach. Level-1 training will focus on PCI and perhaps straightforward TAVRs. Operators seeking level-2 training will then choose between additional training in complex SHD interventions, vascular interventions, and high-risk PCIs (CHIP). Yet interest in ultraspecialization will likely be impacted by the practical issues of market need, reimbursement, and geographic limitations. Accreditation will likely remain limited to level-1 training for the foreseeable future but will eventually follow the evolution of other fields with certification exams emerging for tier-2 super-subspecialized training.

2. Smart training concepts will be incorporated into routine IC fellowship curricula. These include integrating mental skills training, virtual and augmented reality instruments, as well as robotics [56]. Training schemes will also depart from focusing on teaching "procedures" to teaching "skills," a concept known as "the building block," which was proposed and popularized by Charanjit Rihal et al. at Mayo Clinic [57]. In addition, the rapid and ongoing expansion of the interventional toolbox (new imaging modalities [OCT, ICE], new intricate therapies for valve dysfunction and PE, etc) will pose certain challenges for training of ICs who are already in practice. Newer strategies for training and retrofitting of current practitioners will become increasingly needed.

3. The dividing line between surgical and transcatheter interventions will become less discernible. Interest in training in transcatheter interventions will continue to rise among surgical trainees, and new platforms for training future "hybrid" surgeons will emerge. This will also pose new challenges to professional societ-

ies which will bear the burden of developing a creative vision for the heart team 2.0 [14].

4. The COVID-19 pandemic forced the cardiovascular community to find innovative solutions to the prolonged travel restrictions that accompanied the virus outbreak. This led to the widespread proliferation and improvement of "virtual" education. Considering the numerous advantages of virtual meetings, including their extraordinary global reach and affordability, this mode of learning will continue to grow and mature. In addition, efficient methods of live case transmission and virtual proctoring will allow unparalleled access to experts and will help advance patient care worldwide.

5. Social media has allowed a staggering democratization of medical education that has not been achieved with any other methods previously [58]. It is apparent that SoMe will become even more influential in the future not only in didactic, webinar-like, and case-based education but also fellowship recruitment and academic promotion. Yet certain pitfalls of SoMe will be increasingly realized and will require innovative strategies to remediate. For example, considering the ease of unvetted information sharing on SoMe, there is a risk of limiting the scope of intellectual discourse as is encouraged in live meetings, journal clubs, and peer review.

6. New strategies of learning will emerge. The flood of information in cardiovascular medicine is staggering: from the myriad number of journals, publications, guidelines, and consensus documents to SoMe, which is increasingly relied upon for information served up in either bites or bits. How will future practitioners and trainees be able to manage the deluge? One possibility will be the venue of frequent compendium topics carefully selected and reviewed and made readily available. This approach is gaining a growing popularity among both practitioners and professional societies alike and hence is expected to continue to grow in the future.

7. Yet another issue relates to how the mantle of teachers and leaders will be passed. Will there be places for mentors in our busy practices? The practice of see one, do one, and then teach one will never suffice. Instead, we will need learned discourse and exposure to experts' thoughts, as well as a groundswell of curiosity to address unmet clinical needs, the time to think and imagine and solve problems.

Advances in cath lab innovation, research, and practice can be at least partially credited for the substantial reduction in cardiovascular mortality in the last half century. However, major challenges persist, and key questions remain open. Evaluation of the history of interventional cardiology is essential to inform future leaders in the field along their journey to address these remaining obstacles.

References

1. Darmoch F, Alraies MC, Al-Khadra Y, Moussa Pacha H, Pinto DS, Osborn EA. Intravascular ultrasound imaging-guided versus coronary angiography-guided percutaneous coronary intervention: a systematic review and meta-analysis. J Am Heart Assoc. 2020;9:e013678.

2. Smilowitz NR, Mohananey D, Razzouk L, Weisz G, Slater JN. Impact and trends of intravascular imaging in diagnostic coronary angiography and percutaneous coronary intervention in inpatients in the United States. catheter Cardiovasc Interv. 2018;92:E410–5.

3. Sharma SP, Rijal J, Dahal K. Optical coherence tomography guidance in percutaneous coronary intervention: a meta-analysis of randomized controlled trials. Cardiovasc Interv Ther. 2019;34:113–21.

4. Ali ZA, Karimi Galougahi K, Maehara A, et al. Intracoronary optical coherence tomography 2018: current status and future directions. JACC Cardiovasc Interv. 2017;10:2473–87.

5. Alkhouli M, Chaker Z, Alqahtani F, Raslan S, Raybuck B. Outcomes of routine intracardiac echocardiography to guide left atrial appendage occlusion. JACC Clin Electrophysiol. 2020;6:393–400.

6. Alqahtani F, Bhirud A, Aljohani S, et al. Intracardiac versus transesophageal echocardiography to guide transcatheter closure of interatrial communications: Nationwide trend and comparative analysis. J Interv Cardiol. 2017;30:234–41.

7. Alkhouli M, Eleid MF, Michellena H, Pislaru SV. Complementary roles of intracardiac and transoesophageal echocardiography in transcatheter tricuspid interventions. EuroIntervention. 2020;15:1514–5.

8. Alkhouli M, Alqahtani F, Kalra A, et al. Trends in characteristics and outcomes of patients undergoing coronary revascularization in the United States, 2003-2016. JAMA Netw Open. 2020;e1921326:3.

9. Alkhouli M, Osman M, Elsisy MFA, Kawsara A, Berzingi CO. Mechanical circulatory support in patients with cardiogenic shock. Curr Treat Options Cardiovasc Med. 2020;22:4.

10. Alkhouli M, Al Mustafa A, Chaker Z, Alqahtani F, Aljohani S, Holmes DR. Mechanical circulatory support in patients with severe aortic stenosis and left ventricular dysfunction undergoing percutaneous coronary intervention. J Card Surg. 2017;32:245–9.

11. Brilakis ES, Banerjee S, Karmpaliotis D, et al. Procedural outcomes of chronic total occlusion percutaneous coronary intervention: a report from the NCDR (National Cardiovascular Data Registry). JACC Cardiovasc Interv. 2015;8:245–53.

12. Alkhouli M. Coronary calcifications in patients undergoing PCI: the forgotten enemy back in the spotlight. JACC Cardiovasc Interv. 2020;13:1429–31.

13. Ali ZA, Nef H, Escaned J, et al. Safety and effectiveness of coronary intravascular lithotripsy for treatment of severely calcified coronary stenoses: the disrupt CAD II study. Circ Cardiovasc Interv. 2019;12:e008434.

14. Holmes DR Jr, Alkhouli M. Past, present, and future of interventional cardiology. J Am Coll Cardiol. 2020;75:2738–43.

15. Partovi S, Sin D, Gill A. Less of a good thing - the paradox of reduced multidisciplinary team decision-making. Vasa. 2019;48:203–4.

16. Lopez-Jimenez F, Attia Z, Arruda-Olson AM, et al. Artificial intelligence in cardiology: present and future. Mayo Clin Proc. 2020;95:1015–39.

17. Attia ZI, Noseworthy PA, Lopez-Jimenez F, et al. An artificial intelligence-enabled ECG algorithm for the identification of patients with atrial fibrillation during sinus rhythm: a retrospective analysis of outcome prediction. Lancet. 2019;394:861–7.

18. Sardar P, Abbott JD, Kundu A, Aronow HD, Granada JF, Giri J. Impact of artificial intelligence on interventional cardiology: from decision-making aid to advanced interventional procedure assistance. JACC Cardiovasc Interv. 2019;12:1293–303.

19. Yang S, Koo BK, Hoshino M, et al. CT angiographic and plaque predictors of functionally significant coronary disease and outcome using machine learning. JACC Cardiovasc Imaging. 2020;

20. Howard JP, Cook CM, van de Hoef TP, et al. Artificial intelligence for aortic pressure waveform analysis during coronary angiography: machine learning for patient safety. JACC Cardiovasc Interv. 2019;12:2093–101.

21. Cho H, Lee JG, Kang SJ, et al. Angiography-based machine learning for predicting fractional flow reserve in intermediate coronary artery lesions. J Am Heart Assoc. 2019;8:e011685.

22. Alkhouli M, Rihal CS. The odyssey of risk framing in cardiovascular medicine: a patient-Centered perspective. Mayo Clin Proc. 2020;95:1315–7.

23. Alkhouli M, Friedman PA. Ischemic stroke risk in patients with nonvalvular atrial fibrillation: JACC review topic of the week. J Am Coll Cardiol. 2019;74:3050–65.
24. Alkhouli M, Sengupta PP. 3-dimensional-printed models for TAVR planning: why guess when you can see? JACC Cardiovasc Imaging. 2017;10:732–4.
25. Pereira NL, Farkouh ME, So D, et al. Effect of genotype-guided Oral P2Y12 inhibitor selection vs conventional clopidogrel therapy on ischemic outcomes after percutaneous coronary intervention: the TAILOR-PCI randomized clinical trial. JAMA. 2020;324:761–71.
26. Lander MM, Aldweib N, Abraham WT. Wireless hemodynamic monitoring in patients with heart failure. Curr Heart Fail Rep. 2021;18:12–22.
27. Shavelle DM, Desai AS, Abraham WT, et al. Lower rates of heart failure and all-cause hospitalizations during pulmonary artery pressure-guided therapy for ambulatory heart failure: one-year outcomes from the CardioMEMS post-approval study. Circ Heart Fail. 2020;13:e006863.
28. Holmes DR Jr, Krucoff MW, Mullin C, et al. Implanted monitor alerting to reduce treatment delay in patients with acute coronary syndrome events. J Am Coll Cardiol. 2019;74:2047–55.
29. Reddy VY, Neuzil P, de Potter T, et al. Permanent percutaneous carotid artery filter to prevent stroke in atrial fibrillation patients: the CAPTURE trial. J Am Coll Cardiol. 2019;74:829–39.
30. Khan JM, Rogers T, Greenbaum AB, et al. Transcatheter electrosurgery: JACC state-of-the-art review. J Am Coll Cardiol. 2020;75:1455–70.
31. Holmes DR Jr, Farb AA, Chip Hance R, et al. Early feasibility studies for cardiovascular devices in the United States: JACC state-of-the-art review. J Am Coll Cardiol. 2020;76:2786–94.
32. Sepehrvand N, Alemayehu W, Das D, et al. Trends in the explanatory or pragmatic nature of cardiovascular clinical trials over 2 decades. JAMA Cardiol. 2019;4:1122–8.
33. Butala NM, Strom JB, Faridi KF, et al. Validation of administrative claims to ascertain outcomes in pivotal trials of transcatheter aortic valve replacement. JACC Cardiovasc Interv. 2020;13:1777–85.
34. Strom JB, Faridi KF, Butala NM, et al. Use of administrative claims to assess outcomes and treatment effect in randomized clinical trials for transcatheter aortic valve replacement: findings from the EXTEND study. Circulation. 2020;142:203–13.
35. Alkhouli M, Alqahtani F, Harris AH, Hohmann SF, Rihal CS. Early experience with cerebral embolic protection during transcatheter aortic valve replacement in the United States. JAMA Intern Med. 2020;180:783–4.
36. Alkhouli M, Holmes DR Jr, Carroll JD, et al. Racial disparities in the utilization and outcomes of TAVR: TVT registry report. JACC Cardiovasc Interv. 2019;12:936–48.
37. Holmes DR Jr, Alkhouli M, Reddy V. Left atrial appendage occlusion for the unmet clinical needs of stroke prevention in nonvalvular atrial fibrillation. Mayo Clin Proc. 2019;94:864–74.
38. Alkhouli M, Sievert H, Holmes DR. Patent foramen ovale closure for secondary stroke prevention. Eur Heart J. 2019;40:2339–50.
39. Alkhouli M. Moving the needle forward for more relevant evidence on left atrial appendage occlusion. JACC Cardiovasc Interv. 2021;14:79–82.
40. Alkhouli M, Holmes DR. Remaining challenges with transcatheter left atrial appendage closure. Mayo Clin Proc. 2020;95:2244–8.
41. Alkhouli M, Graff-Radford J, Holmes DR. The heart-brain team-towards optimal team-based coordinated care. JAMA Cardiol. 2018;3:187–8.
42. Alkhouli M, Alqahtani F, Hopkins LN, et al. Clinical outcomes of on-site versus off-site endovascular stroke interventions. JACC Cardiovasc Interv. 2020;13:2159–66.
43. Rosamond WD, Johnson A. Trends in heart failure incidence in the community: a gathering storm. Circulation. 2017;135:1224–6.
44. Alkhouli M. Left ventricular unloading in ST-elevation myocardial infarction without cardiogenic shock. Artif Organs. 2020;44:773–8.
45. Kapur NK, Alkhouli MA, DeMartini TJ, et al. Unloading the left ventricle before reperfusion in patients with anterior ST-segment-elevation myocardial infarction. Circulation. 2019;139:337–46.
46. Emani S, Burkhoff D, Lilly SM. Interatrial shunt devices for the treatment of heart failure. Trends Cardiovasc Med. 2020;

47. Simard T, Labinaz M, Zahr F, et al. Percutaneous atriotomy for levoatrial-to-coronary sinus shunting in symptomatic heart failure: first-in-human experience. JACC Cardiovasc Interv. 2020;13:1236–47.
48. Borlaug BA, Carter RE, Melenovsky V, et al. Percutaneous pericardial resection: a novel potential treatment for heart failure with preserved ejection fraction. Circ Heart Fail. 2017;10:e003612.
49. Rossitto G, Mary S, McAllister C, et al. Reduced lymphatic reserve in heart failure with preserved ejection fraction. J Am Coll Cardiol. 2020;76:2817–29.
50. Kapur NK, Reyelt L, Crowley P, et al. Intermittent occlusion of the superior vena cava reduces cardiac filling pressures in preclinical models of heart failure. J Cardiovasc Transl Res. 2020;13:151–7.
51. Tice C, Seigerman M, Fiorilli P, et al. Management of acute pulmonary embolism. Curr Cardiovasc Risk Rep. 2020;14:24.
52. Sista AK, Bhatheja R, Rali P, et al. First-in-human study to assess the safety and feasibility of the Bashir endovascular catheter for the treatment of acute intermediate-risk pulmonary embolism. Circ Cardiovasc Interv. 2020; CIRCINTERVENTIONS120009611
53. Papamatheakis DG, Poch DS, Fernandes TM, Kerr KM, Kim NH, Fedullo PF. Chronic thromboembolic pulmonary hypertension: JACC focus seminar. J Am Coll Cardiol. 2020;76:2155–69.
54. Anand V, Frantz RP, DuBrock H, et al. Balloon pulmonary angioplasty for chronic thromboembolic pulmonary hypertension: initial single-center experience. Mayo Clin Proc Innov Qual Outcomes. 2019;3:311–8.
55. Alkhouli M, Coylewright M, Holmes DR. Will the COVID-19 epidemic reshape cardiology? Eur Heart J Qual Care Clin Outcomes. 2020;
56. Spoon DB, Vickers KS, Alkhouli M. Mental skills training in cardiology. J Am Coll Cardiol. 2020;76:1905–9.
57. Raphael CE, Alkhouli M, Maor E, et al. Building blocks of structural intervention: a novel modular paradigm for procedural training. Circ Cardiovasc Interv. 2017;10:e005686.
58. Parwani P, Choi AD, Lopez-Mattei J, et al. Understanding social media: opportunities for cardiovascular medicine. J Am Coll Cardiol. 2019;73:1089–93.

Index

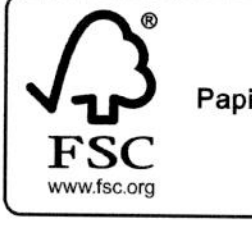